Obesity

For a catalogue of publications available from ACP–ASIM, contact:

Customer Service Center
American College of Physicians–American Society of Internal Medicine
190 N. Independence Mall West
Philadelphia, PA 19106-1572
215-351-2600
800-523-1546, ext. 2600

Visit our Web site at www.acponline.org

Obesity

Barry Gumbiner, MD
Editor

Associate Director
Clinical Research, Endocrinology and Metabolism
Merck Research Laboratories
Rahway, New Jersey

Former Medical Director
Indiana University Center for Weight Management
Associate Professor of Medicine
Indianapolis University School of Medicine
Indianapolis, Indiana

A|C|P

American College of Physicians
Philadelphia, Pennsylvania

Clinical Consultant: David R. Goldmann, MD
Manager, Book Publishing: David Myers
Production Supervisor: Allan S. Kleinberg
Acquisitions Editor: Mary K. Ruff
Developmental Editor: Victoria Hoenigke
Editorial Assistant: Alicia Dillihay
Interior Design: Kate Nichols
Cover Design: Elizabeth Swartz
Indexer: Nelle Garrecht

Copyright © 2001 American College of Physicians–American Society of Internal Medicine

Printed in the United States of America
Composition by Fulcrum Data Services, Inc.
Printing/binding by Versa Press

American College of Physicians (ACP) became an imprint of the American College of Physicians–American Society of Internal Medicine in July 1998.

Library of Congress Cataloging-in-Publication Data

Gumbiner, Barry.
    Obesity/Barry Gumbiner.
        p.   cm.
    Includes bibliographical references and index.
    ISBN 0-930513-12-7 (alk. paper)
        1. Obesity—Handbooks, manuals, etc.   I. Title.

RC628.G85 2001
616.3′98—dc21   00-069962

The authors and publisher have exerted every effort to ensure that drug selection and dosage set forth in this book are in accordance with current recommendations and practice at the time of publication. In view of ongoing research, occasional changes in government regulations, and the constant flow of information relating to drug therapy and drug reactions, the reader is urged to check the package insert for each drug for any change in indications and dosage and for added warnings and precautions. This care is particularly important when the recommended agent is a new or infrequently used drug.

01 02 03 04 05 / 9 8 7 6 5 4 3 2 1

Contributors

Robert I. Berkowitz, MD
Associate Professor of Psychiatry
Department of Psychiatry
Weight and Eating Disorders Program
University of Pennsylvania School
of Medicine
Philadelphia, Pennsylvania

Jorge Calles-Escandon, MD
Associate Professor of Medicine
Department of Medicine
Endocrine Unit
University of Vermont College of
Medicine
Burlington, Vermont

Graham A. Colditz, MD, DrPH
Professor of Medicine
Department of Medicine
Channing Laboratory
Brigham and Women's Hospital
Harvard Medical School
Boston, Massachusetts

Robert V. Considine, PhD
Assistant Professor of Medicine
Department of Medicine
Division of Endocrinology and
Metabolism
Indiana University School of Medicine
Indianapolis, Indiana

Jamie Dananberg, MD
Director
Endocrine Discovery and
Clinical Investigation
Lilly Research Laboratories
Eli Lilly & Company
Indianapolis, Indiana

Lou-Ann Galibert, MD
Assistant Professor of Surgery
Department of Surgery
New York Medical College
White Plains, New York

John C. Guare, PhD
Associate Professor of Psychology
Department of Psychology
Indiana University Purdue University -
Indianapolis
Indianapolis, Indiana

Mehmood A. Khan, MD, FACE
Senior Associate Consultant
Mayo Clinic
Rochester, Minnesota

John Kral, MD, PhD
Professor of Surgery
Department of Surgery
SUNY Health Science Center at
Brooklyn
Brooklyn, New York

Leonard I. Mastbaum, MD, FACE
Clinical Associate Professor
of Medicine
Indiana University School of Medicine
Ft. Wayne, Indiana

John V. St. Peter, PharmD, BCPS
Department of Medicine
Division of Endocrinology
Hennepin County Medical Center
University of Minnesota College of
Pharmacy
Minneapolis, Minnesota

David B. Sarwer, PhD
Assistant Professor of Psychology in
Psychiatry and Surgery
Department of Psychiatry
Weight and Eating Disorders Program
University of Pennsylvania School of
Medicine
Philadelphia, Pennsylvania

Angela Schulze, BS
Department of Psychology
Indiana University Purdue University -
Indianapolis
Indianapolis, Indiana

Helmut O. Steinberg, MD
Assistant Professor of Medicine
Department of Medicine
Division of Endocrinology and
    Metabolism
Indiana University School of Medicine
Indianapolis, Indiana

Patricia A. Stewart, PhD, RD
Postdoctoral Fellow
Department of Community and
    Preventive Medicine
University of Rochester Medical Center
University of Rochester School of
    Medicine and Dentistry
Rochester, New York

Celia Topping, MNS, RD, CDE
Nutrition/Weight Management Center
University of Rochester Medical Center
University of Rochester School of
    Medicine and Dentistry
Rochester, New York

Lloyd B. Williams, MS
Department of Medicine
Division of Endocrinology and
    Metabolism
Indiana University School of Medicine
Indianapolis, Indiana

Nellie Wixom, RD
Program Director
Nutrition/Weight Management Center
University of Rochester Medical Center
University of Rochester School of
    Medicine and Dentistry
Rochester, New York

Leslie G. Womble, MD
Assistant Professor of Psychology in
    Psychiatry
Department of Psychiatry
Weight and Eating Disorders Program
University of Pennsylvania School of
    Medicine
Philadelphia, Pennsylvania

Contents

Clinical Vignettes

Introduction

■ ■ ■

Objectives of a Clinical Text on Obesity

Barry Gumbiner, MD

O besity will be the major chronic health problem of this century (1). Obesity has reached epidemic proportions in some nations (2), and as the Information Age and the global economy bring homogeneity to lifestyles its incidence is rapidly increasing in developing nations and traditional cultures (3). Although the underlying causes of this epidemic are debated, the social and economic ramifications of this problem can no longer be ignored. Unfortunately, despite the vast medical literature on the topic, progress in understanding obesity has not kept pace with the magnitude of the problem. Nevertheless, new basic and clinical research has advanced the field dramatically. Therefore the objectives of this text are to pragmatically translate the current state of knowledge in obesity into clinical practice and to provide a framework for treatment in the primary care setting.

Standards of Practice

Despite the well-documented health ramifications of obesity, only recently have definitive reports been issued by recognized institutions: the 1997 World Health Organization publication "Obesity: Preventing and Managing the Global Epidemic—Report of a WHO Consultation on Obesity" (3), and the 1998 National Institutes of Health (NIH) publication "Clinical Guidelines on the Identification, Evaluation, and Treatment of Overweight and

Obesity in Adults: The Evidence Report" (4). The NIH report is a major breakthrough in the field that finally establishes standards for clinical practice. Therefore it serves as the foundation for this text and is often referred to in generic terms when citing summaries of evidence and recommendations for treatment.

Objectives

What is particularly, perhaps uniquely, challenging about obesity is that everyone, professionals and nonprofessionals alike, has an opinion about the causes and remedies for the condition. Regrettably, these often are actually just opinions based on selective (or no) evidence for their derivation. Moreover, implicit in developing such opinions are the influences of personal experience, philosophical outlooks, and sometimes, unfortunately, bias and prejudice (2, 5-7). Even objectivity can suffer in our most respected medical journals (8). Ultimately, this detracts from effective and safe treatment for obesity. The strength of the NIH report is that it is evidenced-based and uses whenever possible randomized controlled trials, almost all of which are 4 months or greater in duration, to derive consensus recommendations. When evidence was limited by too few randomized controlled trials, reasoned, albeit usually conservative, consensus recommendations were established. Thus, to achieve the goals of *Obesity*, the NIH report is used as an authoritative framework for proposing how to implement treatment in a systematic fashion and, equally important, how to facilitate communication with the patient to counter the myths and misinformation so prevalent in this field.

Because the field is rapidly evolving, it is unavoidable that some of the information presented herein may become outdated. However, the main objective remains clear: to provide an understanding of the major issues so that, as new findings emerge, they can be placed into context. This difficult task was assigned to authors not necessarily known for their academic credentials but rather for their "hands-on" experience, the type of experience many widely recognized authorities in the field no longer have on a daily basis. Thus the approach of the writing (and editing) is pragmatic. In doing so, it is expected that the reader will identify some inconsistencies between authors. These inconsistencies are both a reflection of the rapid evolution of this field and valid differences in perspective. Rather than attempting to achieve a forced consensus, the editor intends to allow readers to arrive at their own conclusions.

Obesity has been written to provide the physician with breadth, not depth, of knowledge. Probably the most important role of the primary care physician is to coordinate all treatment activities to ensure overall effectiveness and safety. In the current state of health care delivery, it is unrealistic to directly provide all the elements of the treatment (7). For the physician to fulfill this role requires a familiarity not only with accepted treatment modalities but with those that are questionable or frankly dangerous and contraindicated (9-12). Moreover, it requires an understanding of the myths related to obesity, many of which are derived from nonclinical sources (7, 13). Thus even those chapters that may seem not directly applicable to patient care, such as those reviewing epidemiology (Chapter 1), etiology (Chapter 2), and pathophysiology (Chapter 3), contain clinically relevant information, the kind that answers the questions which savvy patients ask their doctors (e.g., "cocktail party" questions), whether they be about insulin resistance, "carbs", weight cycling, willpower, or a plethora of other popular topics and fads. This information provides a platform from which the physician can communicate effectively as well as make reasoned recommendations tailored to the needs of the individual patient.

Ultimately, what patients and practitioners have in common is that obesity is an overwhelming condition fraught with frustration. Both parties often have unrealistic expectations for fixing the problem quickly, completely, and permanently. As will become evident from this text, more can be accomplished when these misconceptions are recognized and addressed frankly.

The scope of this text is limited to adults. Childhood obesity is discussed minimally; a separate text is needed to address its unique social and developmental issues. Regrettably, less progress has been made in understanding and treating childhood obesity, and as an individual and public health issue it has different needs to be addressed. Nevertheless, it is clear that if long-lasting progress is to be made, adequate resources must be devoted to childhood obesity.

Definitions and Terminology

Although many terms are described, and even defined, within the text, the following provides a common reference point for all chapters, particularly those that use these terms without elaboration. These definitions are based primarily on those set forth in the NIH report, with clarifications by the editor:

1. *Obesity*—As defined in the NIH report, obesity is "the condition of having an abnormally high proportion of fat...a complex multifactorial chronic disease that develops from an interaction of genotype and the environment". Of note is that this definition neither quantifies parameters nor mentions weight or body habitus. Thus the usual standards used by practitioners and the public at large to describe obesity do not apply.

(This important concept is emphasized in Chapter 5.) Based on the combined biological and epidemiologic evidence in which the medical consequences of excess adiposity begin to be experienced, men with greater than 25% body fat and women with greater than 30% body fat are considered to be obese.

2. *Body Mass Index (BMI)*—BMI is now the accepted measure of body habitus that normalizes adiposity for height. The calculation is

$$BMI = Body\ Weight\ (in\ kilograms)/Height\ (in\ meters)^2$$
$$BMI = [Body\ Weight\ (in\ pounds)/Height\ (in\ inches)^2] \times 703$$

The categories are

Classification	BMI (kg/m^2)
Underweight	<18.5
Normal	18.5–24.9
Overweight	25.0–29.9
Obesity	30.0–39.9
Extreme obesity	≥40.00

Details about BMI are provided throughout the text.

3. *Regional Fat Distribution*—Just as important as the amount of fat tissue is the anatomical locations of fat depots. A major distinction between the predominance of upper versus lower body distribution is made throughout the text. A variety of terms are used in a synonymous manner, including *central, abdominal, visceral, gynoid, upper segment, upper body* versus *peripheral, android, lower segment,* and *lower body.* Indirect measures of fat distribution are waist-to-hip ratio and waist circumference alone. Waist circumference is the newly established NIH standard (men, >102 cm; women, >88 cm), but waist-to-hip ratio remains prevalent in the medical literature.

4. *"Long-term"*—"Long-term" is used in a variety of contexts but most often with reference to treatment outcomes. In medical terms, however, the gold standard for a determining the efficacy and safety of any treatment intervention is favorable health outcomes. Unfortunately, there is a paucity of prospective interventional data from randomized controlled clinical trials over a sufficient period of time demonstrating either favorable or deleterious health outcomes (i.e., morbidity and mortality) with weight loss. Thus other surrogate measures of health outcomes have been substituted until such data are available. Taking type 2 diabetes as an example, surrogate biomarkers, such as HbA1c, and disease burden, such as diabetic complications, are used for this purpose. Morbidity and

mortality outcomes should be forthcoming when some of the studies discussed in the text, such as the NIH SHOW trial (Study of Health Outcomes of Weight-loss) (14-17) and the SOS study (Swedish Obesity Subjects) (18), are completed. Until then, surrogate biomarkers (such as in the example above) and weight *per se* will be used as the marker of success, irrespective of health outcomes. In the surgery literature, 5-year outcomes of sustained loss of "excess" weight are the current standard. Although valid, this method mathematically distorts the percent weight loss (i.e., the percent weight loss is always higher than that reported for nonsurgical interventions because it is a figure that excludes baseline weight).

For interventions in general, per the NIH report, the weight loss goal is 10% of initial weight, and weight maintenance is defined as sustained weight loss within 3 kg (approximately 6.6 lb) and a waist circumference within 10 cm (4 in.) of baseline for 2 years. Until more health outcome and cost-effectiveness data are available, these will continue to be used as standards even with their inherent constraints and limitations.

Commentary

It is obvious that obesity is a complex, heterogeneous metabolic condition. In the clinical setting it is one of the most frustrating medical conditions to treat. Regrettably, it is sometimes treated with ignorance, prejudice, and disdain (2, 5, 6). Often forgotten is that body fat and adipose tissue are necessary for optimal health (19). Thus the current epidemic could be viewed as a maladaptation to an evolutionary process focused on protecting against the inadequate and unreliable energy sources that until recently were the major challenge to survival (20). To assign blame and identify lifestyle and willpower as the culprits will appear to the patient as a superficial and dismissive assessment. The sooner the chronic disease model applied to other metabolic disorders, such as diabetes and hypertension, is accepted as the paradigm needed to treat obesity, the more effectively physicians will be able to help their patients. This means

- Accepting the preponderance of evidence that obesity is a chronic disorder with serious consequences, including death (1, 21-25).
- Realistic goals for success need to be designed and accepted by the practitioner before expecting the patient to accept them.
- Combining multiple treatment strategies and resources that reflect the multitude of metabolic and environmental etiologies and influences, and doing so responsibly and professionally (24, 26, 27).
- Relying on the fundamentals of evidence-based principles of treatment yet remaining open-minded to new treatment modalities.

- Addressing deficiencies in knowledge and counseling efforts because, rightly or wrongly, the patient views the physician as a definitive authority and, more often than commonly perceived, attempts by the physician to address this issue are taken seriously by the patient (28-30).
- As with smoking cessation, lapse and relapse should be expected and anticipated and viewed only as setbacks rather than failure.
- Being sensitive to the psychological burden of the disease when talking with patients who already know they need to lose weight (5, 6).
- Defining success beyond quantifiable parameters and focusing on favorable behavior and quality-of-life outcomes that are meaningful to the patient on a daily basis rather than abstract consequences that are years away (31).

Though patients ultimately must be ready to address this medical condition, physicians can do a better job in counseling, educating, and intervening with a dispassionate and objective approach free of judgement and prejudice (28-30). It is never too late to begin treatment and have a favorable impact on health (32). Each chapter of *Obesity* can in some way enlighten the practitioner on these issues and in doing so help him or her serve the best interests of the patient.

■ ■ ▓

REFERENCES

1. **Pi-Sunyer FX, Laferrere B, Arrone LJ, Bray GA.** Therapeutic controversy: obesity - a modern-day epidemic. J Clin Endocrinol Metab. 1999;84:3-11.
2. **Mokdad AH, Serdula MK, Dietz WH, et al.** The spread of the obesity epidemic in the United States, 1991-1998. JAMA. 1999;282:1519-22.
3. **World Health Organization.** Obesity: Preventing and Managing the Global Epidemic. Report of a WHO Consultation on Obesity; 1997.
4. **NHLBI Obesity Education Expert Panel.** Clinical Guidelines on the Identification, Evaluation, and Treatment of Overweight and Obesity in Adults: The Evidence Report. Bethesda, MD: National Institute of Health/National Heart, Lung, and Blood Institute. NIH Publication 98-4083; 1998.
5. **Crandall CS, Schiffhauer KL.** Anti-fat prejudice: beliefs, values and American culture. Obes Res. 1998;6:458-60.
6. **Falkner NH, French SA, Jeffery RW, et al.** Mistreatment due to weight: prevalence and sources of perceived mistreatment in women and men. Obes Res. 1999;7:572-6.
7. **Frank A.** Conflicts in the care of overweight patients: inconsistent rules and insufficient money. Obes Res. 1997;5:268-70.
8. **Kassirer JP, Angell M.** Losing weight: an ill-fated New Year's resolution. N Engl J Med. 1999; 338:52-4.
9. Portions, foods in a diet won't determine weight loss, study says. US Department of Agriculture; 20 October 2000. [Electronic Citation (CNN.com)]

9a. **Freedman MR, King J, Kennedy E.** Popular diets: a scientific review. Obes Res. 2001;9(suppl 1):1S-40S.

10. **Angell M, Kassirer JP.** Alternative medicine: the risks of untested and unregulated remedies. N Engl J Med. 1998;339:839-41.

11. FDA warns of diet drug: government cautions users of Triax, calling it a dangerous hormonal drug. US Food and Drug Administration; 11 November 1999. [Electronic Citation (Associated Press/CNN.com)]

12. **Dugan IJ.** Parish the thought: how Bible-based diet angered true believers. Wall Street Journal. 30 October 2000.

13. **O'Neill M.** A growing movement fights diets instead of fat. New York Times. 12 April 1992.

14. **Yanovski SZ, Bain RP, Williamson DF.** Report of a National Institutes of Health/Center for Disease Control and Prevention workshop on the feasibility of conducting a randomized clinical trial to estimate the long-term health effects of intentional weight loss in obese persons. Am J Clin Nutr. 1999;69:366-72.

15. **Blackburn GL.** Benefits of weight loss in the treatment of obesity. Am J Clin Nutr. 1999;69:347-9.

16. SHOW: Studies of Health Outcomes of Weight-loss. National Institutes of Diabetes and Digestive and Kidney Diseases. [Electronic Citation (http://show.phs.wfubmc.edu/)]

17. **National Institutes of Diabetes and Digestive and Kidney Diseases.** Study of Health Outcomes of Weight-loss (SHOW) Trial. 2000. [Electronic Citation (www.niddk.nih.gov/patient/SHOW/showhmpg.htm)]

18. **Sjostrom L, Larsson B, Backman L, et al.** Swedish Obese Subjects (SOS): Recruitment for an intervention study and a selected description of the obese state. Int J Obes. 1992;16:465-79.

19. **Norgan NG.** The beneficial effects of body fat and adipose tissue in humans. Int J Obes. 1997;21:738-46.

20. **Neel JV.** Diabetes mellitus: a "thrifty" genotype rendered detrimental by "progress"? Am J Hum Genet. 1962;14:353-62.

21. **Must A, Spadano J, Coakley EH, et al.** The disease burden associated with overweight and obesity. JAMA. 1999;282:1523-9.

22. **National Task Force on the Prevention and Treatment of Obesity.** Overweight, obesity and health risk. Arch Intern Med. 2000;160:898-904.

23. **Allison DB, Fontaine KR, Manson JE, et al.** Annual deaths attributable to obesity in the United States. JAMA. 1999;282:1530-8.

24. **Bray GA.** To treat or not to treat: that is the question. Obes Res. 1997;5:634-5.

25. **Hubbard VS.** Defining overweight and obesity: what are the issues? Am J Clin Nutr. 2000;72:1067-8.

26. **Frank A.** Futility and avoidance: medical professionals in the treatment of obesity. JAMA. 1993;269:2132-3.

27. **Kushner R.** The treatment of obesity. Arch Intern Med. 1997;157:602-4.

28. **Galuska DA, Will JC, Serdula MK, Ford ES.** Are health care professionals advising obese patients to lose weight? JAMA. 1999;282:1576-8.

29. **Wee CC, McCarthy EP, Davis RB, Phillips RS.** Physician counseling about exercise. JAMA. 1999;282:1583-8.

30. **Fontanarosa PB.** Patients, physicians, and weight control. JAMA. 1999;282:1581-2.

31. **Fine JT, Colditz GA, Coakley MA, et al.** A prospective study of weight change and health-related quality of life in women. JAMA. 1999;282:2136-42.

32. **Sherman SE, D'Agostino RB, Silbershatz H, Kannel WB.** Comparison of past versus recent physical activity in the prevention of premature death and coronary artery disease. Am Heart J. 1999;138:900-7.

1

■ ■ ■

Epidemiology of Obesity

Graham A. Colditz, MD, DrPH

This chapter reviews the trends in obesity for adults and children in the United States over the past decades, international trends when data support such presentations, and the trends in lifestyle factors that may account for the increasing prevalence of obesity in the population. The health consequences of obesity are briefly reviewed as is the economic impact of obesity and lack of physical activity. Finally, the relation between obesity and mortality is discussed because this continues to be an area of disagreement among scientists and the lay public.

Trends

Obesity is a serious public health problem in the United States. The prevalence of obesity has been increasing sharply among children and adults over the past three decades. The age-adjusted prevalence of obesity increased by approximately 30% between 1980 and 1994 (1). According to the Third National Health and Nutrition Examination Survey (NHANES III), 32% of adults in the United States are overweight (approximately 60 million) and an additional 22.5% are obese (2, 3). The percentage of the adult population over 20 years of age that exceeds healthy weight ranges (i.e., the prevalence of BMI [body-mass index] > 25.0) breaks down to 59.4% of men and 50.7% of women, or overall 54.9% of the adult population; 24.8% of women and 20% of men, or overall 22.5% of the adult population, are obese (BMI > 30). For African Americans and Hispanics the percentages are

1

much higher. About 67% of adult African American and Hispanic women are overweight or obese compared with 46% of white women.

Obesity is also a public health problem in other developed and affluent countries and is now spreading to less affluent countries such as Mexico, Brazil, and Cuba (4). Data from Russia and Asia show similar rapid changes. Altered diets and decreased physical activity have led to increases in adult obesity and associated chronic medical conditions (5).

Lifestyle Trends

Trends in lifestyle habits that relate to the increasing burden of obesity may be considered in terms of diet and activity (i.e., energy intake and energy output). The trend in fat intake, as a percentage of calories, has been downwards for more than seven decades (6). In fact, caloric intake as assessed by the NHANES survey has been stable. This suggests that the output of energy has decreased, because energy balance must have been positive in the population to support the increase in obesity. Although energy expenditure has not been monitored historically, several societal features clearly support a decrease in the level of physical activity. Less walking and bicycle riding over the latter part of this century, a smaller portion of the population employed in farm activities (and those who are now use mechanized labor aids), and the advent of mechanization in numerous other occupations have all contributed to a reduction in occupational energy expenditure. A consequence of this is the potential for a positive energy balance (i.e., where energy intake exceeds energy output).

Despite its benefits, many people do not engage in regular physical activity. The Behavioral Risk Factor Surveillance System (BRFSS) from the Center for Disease Control has noted that in 1995 approximately 28.8% of the adult population reported no leisure-time physical activity (7). In some states, up to 48% reported no leisure-time physical activity.

*   *   *

To estimate the proportion of disease that could be prevented by eliminating inactivity or obesity the population-attributable risk percent (PAR%) is calculated. This is the maximum proportion of disease attributable to the specific exposure (obesity or lack of physical activity). PAR% is based on the incidence of disease in the exposed (i.e., inactive) group compared with the nonexposed group, taking relative risks from analyses that control for confounders (e.g., age, smoking, dietary intake). The equation is

$$\text{PAR\%} = P(\text{RR} - 1)/1 + P(\text{RR} - 1)$$

where P is the prevalence of exposure in the population and RR is the relative risk for disease.

Comorbidities

Obesity and higher relative weights in adults are risk factors for cardiovascular disease (CVD) (8, 9), certain cancers (10-13), diabetes (14, 15), and mortality (16, 17). The health effects of obesity act through several different mechanisms. For example, with weight gain and increasing adiposity, glucose tolerance deteriorates, blood pressure rises, and the lipid profile becomes more atherogenic. These physiologic responses clearly predispose to the development of CVD and diabetes. Many randomized trials, as summarized in the NIH report, show that weight reduction is associated with a reversal in the physiologic effects of weight gain. Simply put, weight loss is associated with reduction in blood pressure, improved glucose tolerance, and improved lipid profile (17).

In addition to these more acute effects, weight gain and obesity are related to cancers through hormonal and nonhormonal mechanisms. For female reproductive cancers the direct relation between postmenopausal weight and circulating estrogen levels provides a clear mechanism for the increased risk of breast and endometrial cancers. Alteration in glucose metabolism may contribute to the risk of colon cancer (18).

Excessive weight exacerbates many other chronic diseases, such as hypertension (19), osteoarthritis (OA) (20, 21), gallstones (22), dyslipidemia, and musculoskeletal problems (17, 23). In addition to the physical health problems related to obesity, there are numerous psychological and psychosocial effects (24). Because psychological and psychosocial factors ultimately influence health and general well-being, the social impact of obesity is far-reaching.

Heart Disease

Young and middle-aged men and women who are overweight or obese are more likely than their leaner peers to develop heart disease. Rimm et al (25) followed 29,122 men from 40 to 75 years of age. They observed that for men less than 65 years of age, the risk of developing coronary heart disease (CHD) increased with increasing BMI. Overweight men were almost twice as likely as leaner men with BMI < 23 kg/m^2 to develop CHD (RR = 1.7; 95% confidence interval [CI], 1.1-2.7), whereas men with BMI of at least 33 kg/m^2 were more than three times more likely to develop CHD (RR = 3.4; 95% CI, 1.67-7.09) during the three years of follow-up.

Coronary heart disease is less common among women than men, particularly before menopause; nevertheless, associations between excessive weight and CHD have been observed in adult women. Harris et al (26) observed that among 1259 white women in NHANES I those who were overweight (in that study, defined as BMI > 29 kg/m^2) and had fairly stable weights had a threefold risk (OR [odds ratio] = 2.7; 95% CI, 1.7-4.4) of developing heart disease (26). In addition, independent of overall adiposity (as measured by BMI), women with a large waist circumference (in that study, defined as 96.5 cm or 38 inch) or waist-to-hip ratio (WHR ≥ 0.88) were approximately three times more likely than their peers to develop CHD over an 8-year period (27). Overweight women are also at increased risk of ischemic stroke. Among 116,759 women aged 30 to 55 years in the Nurses' Health Study, women with BMI > 29 kg/m^2 were approximately twice as likely as women with BMI < 21 kg/m^2 to have an ischemic stroke during 16 years of follow-up (9).

Not only are obese adults more likely to develop CHD, they are also more likely to die from it. During 12-years of follow-up of 48,287 Dutch men and women aged 30 to 54, Seidell et al (28) observed that men and women who were obese (BMI ≥ 30 kg/m^2) were three times more likely than their nonoverweight peers (BMI < 25 kg/m^2) to die from CHD. Moreover, they estimated that 20% to 30% of CHD mortality could be attributed to being overweight. Excessive weight earlier in life is also predictive of CHD mortality. Must et al (29) followed 508 adolescents who participated in the Harvard Growth Study of 1922 to 1935. The adolescents who were overweight were twice as likely as their lean peers (RR = 2.3; 95% CI, 1.4-4.1) to die from CHD during adulthood.

There are several mechanisms through which obesity and weight gain might increase the risk of CHD. Hyperlipidemia is one mechanism. BMI is correlated with triglyceride levels as well as HDL levels. Low HDL levels are more predictive than high total cholesterol of developing heart disease. Thus obesity increases the risk of heart disease in part by increasing total triglycerides and making the HDL/LDL ratio less favorable (30). Increased blood pressure and glucose intolerance leading to hypertension and type 2 diabetes mellitus are other mechanisms, as described in more detail below.

Hypertension

Approximately 25% of adult Americans have high blood pressure. From 1986 to 1996 the death rate from high blood pressure increased 6.8%. Although hypertension is a highly treatable condition, if left untreated its consequences are severe; hypertension is a strong predictor of more severe CVD. The combination of obesity and hypertension is associated with an increased risk of cardiac failure due to thickening of the ventricular wall and increased heart volume (31).

Both weight (32-34) and weight gain (35, 36) are positively associated with the development of hypertension. Among men and women there is a linear relation between body weight and blood pressure. Witteman et al (32) observed that overweight women with BMI between 26 and 28 kg/m^2

were approximately three times more likely than nonoverweight women with BMI < 23 kg/m² (RR = 2.8) to develop hypertension over a four-year period, and women with BMI ≥ 32 kg/m² were almost six times more likely to develop hypertension.

Blood pressure is very sensitive to weight change. A maintained weight loss of 10% to 15% can result in a sustained lowering of blood pressure and improvement in other CHD risk factors (37). As summarized in the NIH report, review of a number of studies suggests an approximately 2 mm Hg decline in both systolic and diastolic blood pressure for each kilogram (2.2 lb) of sustained weight loss. Thus, weight loss is recommended to patients with mildly elevated blood pressure or risk factors for developing CVD.

The risk of developing hypertension also decreases with weight loss (38, 38a). Huang et al (38) observed that among 82,473 women in the Nurses' Health Study those who lost at least 10 kg and were able to maintain the loss for at least two years were 45% less likely to develop hypertension (RR = 0.55; 95% CI, 0.40-0.74) than their peers who were weight stable, whereas women who gained 10 to 19.9 kg were twice as likely (RR = 2.18; 95% CI, 1.98-2.40) to develop hypertension. There are several mechanisms through which obesity causes hypertension (see Chapter 4).

Diabetes

The incidence of type 2 diabetes has risen steadily over the past 30 years. Diabetes is a prevalent and serious disease that affects approximately 14 million people in the United States. Individuals with diabetes are at substantially elevated risk for blindness, kidney disease, heart disease, stroke, and death. Diabetes is the seventh leading cause of death in the United States.

Type 2 diabetes is characterized by peripheral insulin resistance, impaired regulation of hepatic glucose production, and impaired β-cell function. Excessive weight increases the risk of type 2 diabetes through insulin resistance (39). Not only are overweight men and women at a substantially increased risk for developing type 2 diabetes (14, 15, 40, 41) but adults at the upper end of the normal BMI range are at an increased risk as reflected by the strong linear relation between BMI and risk. In addition, even after adjusting for weight, weight gain has been observed to be strongly associated with the risk of developing diabetes mellitus (14, 42). Colditz et al (14) observed that among 114,281 women aged 30 to 55 even modest weight gain (5-7.9 lb) since age 18 was associated with a 50% increase in risk of diabetes mellitus (RR = 1.5; 95% CI, 1.20-1.80). Moreover, similar results were observed in a parallel study among men (15).

Independent of weight, fat distribution has an important role in the development of type 2 diabetes. Carey et al (43) observed that women with a large waist circumference (in that study, defined as 92 cm or 36.2 inches) were more than five times as likely as their peers with small waists (67 cm or 26.2 inches) to develop type 2 diabetes, regardless of their overall adiposity (measured by BMI). Moreover, among 15,432 women Hartz et al (44) found that within each weight stratum (nonobese, moderately obese, and severely obese) the prevalence of diabetes increased with WHR. Among the nonobese women, the risk increased in a gradual linear fashion, whereas among the severely obese women the risk increased sharply from approximately 6% for those with a WHR < 0.72 to 16.5% among women with a WHR > 0.81. Similar associations have been seen in men. Ohlson et al (45) observed that BMI and WHR were both significant independent predictors of developing diabetes over a 13.5-year follow-up of 792 Swedish men. Approximately 15% of the men in the highest tertile of both WHR and BMI developed diabetes compared with only 0.5% of the men in the lowest tertile of both factors.

Cancers

Excessive weight is associated with the development of numerous types of cancer, including breast (among postmenopausal women), endometrial, gastric, and colon. Racial differences in the prevalence of excessive weight may partially explain the elevated rate of certain cancers among African Americans. The obesity-related increase risk of developing cancer is thought to be mediated through the effects on hormones and hormones metabolism. However, certain cancers, such as renal cell carcinoma, are related to obesity through other, not well understood mechanisms.

Among premenopausal women, those who are overweight are less likely to develop breast cancer (46). The decrease in risk may be due to a higher prevalence of menstrual irregularities and the associated low estrogen levels in overweight women. The relation is quite different in postmenopausal women, among whom o\besity is associated with an increased risk of developing breast cancer. Adipose tissue is the primary source of estrogen among postmenopausal women who do not use hormone replacement therapy. Therefore, it is not surprising that the obesity-related increase in risk is restricted to women who do not use hormone replacement therapy (10). Breast cancer is more common among postmenopausal than premenopausal women, which suggests that obesity promotes more breast cancers than it prevents. In addition, among women diagnosed with breast cancer, obesity is associated with a higher mortality rate (47). Nevertheless, the roles of excess adiposity, menopause, hormones, and cytokines in the risk for developing breast cancer is quite complex, and extrapolating epidemiologic studies to underlying mechanistic causes is problematic (48).

Overweight women are more likely than their leaner peers to develop endometrial cancer (49), which is the most common gynecologic cancer in the United States and the fourth most common cancer overall in women. The increase in risk is strongest in older women (50). Although data are limited, the results from primarily case control studies suggest that the risk of ovarian cancer increases with relative weight (51).

In addition to increasing the risk of developing hormone-related cancers, obesity is also associated with the development of other types of cancer, such as esophageal, stomach, and colon. Obesity has a known relationship with gastroesophageal reflux, which in turn is a risk factor for esophogeal adenocarcinoma (52). Obese adults are up to 16 times as likely as lean adults to develop this type of cancer (53). The increasing prevalence of obesity, coupled with the strength of the association between obesity and adenocarcinoma of the gastric cardia, may explain, in part, why the incidence of the tumor has been increasing dramatically in the United States (52). Colon cancer is the third most common cancer in the United States. Among the 13,420 men and women in the NHANES I follow-up study, the risk of colon cancer associated with excess weight was similar in men and women (54). Although other researchers have observed an increase in risk associated with weight only among men (55, 56), more recent data show an elevated risk in women (12).

Gallstones

Gallstones are a fairly common, often quite painful condition that is most common among overweight adults (see Chapter 4). Although gallstones do form in lean adults, the relationship between weight, weight change, and gallstone formation is very strong. Moreover, women are more likely than men to develop gallstones. Among 16,884 adults in NHANES III, the prevalence of gallbladder disease significantly increased with weight status (57). The relationship was stronger among women than men and stronger in those less than 55 years of age. Compared with women in the healthy weight range, overweight women were twice as likely to report gallbladder disease (OR = 1.94; 95% CI, 1.25-3.00), and women with BMI ≥ 40 kg/m^2 were more than five times as likely to report the diagnosis (OR = 5.20; 95% CI, 2.92-8.82).

The association between body weight and gallbladder disease also has been observed prospectively. Over an 8-year period, 2122 cases of symptomatic gallstones were diagnosed among the 90,302 women in the Nurses' Health Study (58). The risk of developing symptomatic gallstones that were not removed and the risk of having a cholecystectomy increased linearly with BMI. Women with BMI between 25 and 26 kg/m^2 were approximately 60% more likely than women with BMI < 24 kg/m^2 to have a cholecystectomy or to develop gallstones that were not removed (RR = 1.6; 95% CI,

1.36-1.88); women with BMI of 30 to 34.9 kg/m^2 were more than three times as likely to develop gallstones (RR = 3.52; 95% CI, 3.11-3.98).

Osteoarthritis

Approximately 16 million people in the United States have osteoarthritis. The hips, knees, and spine are the most common sites of OA. Although the condition has not been as well studied as other chronic diseases, such as CHD and cancer, it does appear that overweight adults are more than twice as likely as their leaner peers to develop OA in the hip (59). In addition, excessive weight is associated with the development and progression of OA of the knee (60, 61). It is presumed that excessive weight acts through biomechanical means to cause additional strain on the joints that leads to their degradation rather than through metabolic mechanisms.

Benign Prostatic Hyperplasia

Prostate enlargement is common among men. Benign prostatic hyperplasia (BPH) rarely causes symptoms among young men; however, more than 50% of men in their sixties and an estimated 90% in their seventies and eighties have some symptoms of BPH. Surgical treatment is very common. An estimated 350,000 prostatectomies are performed annually in the United States. Among 25,892 men in the Health Professionals Follow-up Study, independent of age, smoking, and BMI, men with a large waist circumference (in that study defined as ≥43 inches [109 cm] versus <35 inches [89 cm]) were more than twice as likely (OR = 2.38; 95% CI, 1.42-3.99) to develop BPH and have a prostatectomy (62). Centrally located adiposity may increase the risk of developing benign prostatic hyperplasia by increasing the estrogen-to-androgen ratio and sympathetic nervous activity.

Mental Health and Lifestyle Outcomes

Despite the rapid increase in the prevalence of overweight persons, societal acceptance of the condition is limited and there are considerable psychosocial consequences of being overweight in a Westernized society that values thinness and fitness. Obese women are less likely to be hired, more likely to have their performance rated negatively, and less likely to be promoted (63, 64). Moreover, among both normal and overweight women, weight gain is associated with poorer well-being (65). Among approximately 1000 adults in a weight gain prevention program, 22% of the women and 17% of the men reported that they had been mistreated because of their weight (66). The prevalence increased across quartiles of BMI from 5.7% for the leanest quartile to 42.5% for the heaviest participants. Gortmaker et al (67) followed a sample of 16- to 24-year olds over eight years. They observed that women who were overweight were approximately 20%, and overweight men 11%, less likely to marry. Sonne-Holm and Sorensen observed 3267 men in Copenhagen at each level of education attainment; the attained level of social class was significantly lower for obese men (68).

Obesity has an impact on many aspects of quality of life. The association between quality of life and body weight has been assessed in women in the Nurses' Health Study. In both cross-sectional (69) and prospective (24) analyses using Medical Outcomes Study SF-36, a well-validated standard instrument for measuring health-related quality of life, there was a linear association between increasing BMI and decreases in physical functioning and vitality. Moreover, weight change over a four-year period was associated with changes in quality of life. Women who gained more than 20 lb over the four years had significant decreases in physical functioning, whereas weight losses were associated with increases in functioning and vitality.

Economic Impact

Though mortality is commonly used as a measure of disease burden, it does not account for the morbidity associated with chronic conditions. Further, it omits any accounting of the impact of lifestyle on health-related quality of life. One can use an economic measure to summarize this broad range of health effects. Such a measure can account for both nonfatal and fatal conditions.

The direct costs of illness include the costs of diagnosis and treatment related to any disease (hospital stay, nursing home, medications, physician visits). The value of lost productivity is an indirect cost of illness. This includes wages lost by people unable to work because of disease and also the forgone wages due to premature mortality. These future earnings after death are translated into current monetary value using an inflation or discount factor, usually 3%. Note that these costs are not quantified in the current analysis.

In the United States, the direct cost of obesity has been estimated to be 70 billion dollars, or 7% of health care expenditures, compared with 2% in France (70) and Australia (71) and 4% in the Netherlands (72). The indirect costs of early retirement and increased risk of disability pensions are also considerable. Among adult women in Sweden, obese subjects were 1.5 to 1.9 times more likely to take sick leave, and 12% of obese women had disability pensions attributable to obesity (73). Overall, approximately 10% of sick leave and disability pensions for women may be related to obesity and obesity-related conditions.

Colditz estimated that the indirect costs (e.g., forgone earnings, premature mortality) attributable to obesity in the United States amounted to at least 48 billion dollars in 1995 (74). However, as Colditz noted, his estimate is at the lower end of health care cost because there are substantial additional costs incurred among those who are overweight (i.e., who have a BMI of 25-29.9 kg/m^2) but not obese (17, 75).

Gorsky et al simulated three hypothetical cohorts to estimate the costs of health care according to level of obesity over a 25-year period, discounting future costs at 3% per year (76). They estimate that 16 billion additional dollars will be spent over the next 25 years treating health outcomes associated with obesity among middle-aged women. Using an incidence-based approach to cost of illness, Thompson et al (77) estimated the excess costs of health services according to level of obesity. Using a conservative approach that does not include any future weight gain and starting with NHANES III population estimates for BMI, cholesterol, hypertension, and diabetes, they estimate the lifetime future costs per overweight person as comparable to those for a person who smokes.

The health care costs that have been estimated to date are an underestimation of the true costs because they do not consider the impact of reduced physical functioning (69, 78), the increased risk of infertility among young women (79), or the increased risk of asthma, all of which are directly associated with increasing adiposity. The costs associated with infertility, asthma treatment, and cataracts are substantial and should be included in future analyses of the costs of obesity.

Unfortunately, it is difficult to conduct studies that measure actual costs because collecting such data is highly complex. However, a recent study by Kaiser Permanente's Medical Care Program in the Northern California Region is uniquely organized to determine direct costs of health services (e.g., physician visits, hospital utilization, pharmacy, laboratory) for the medical care of obese patients (80). Compared with patients with BMI of 20.0 to 24.9, annual total costs are 25% higher for BMI of 30.0 to 34.9 and 44% higher for BMI > 35. Moreover, these higher costs were primarily the result of the association between BMI and the most common obesity-related illnesses: CHD, hypertension, and diabetes. This is the strongest direct evidence to date of the direct costs of obesity. Based on the above population estimates, if one assumes that indirect costs are comparable to direct costs, it is clear that for employers, in addition to the cost of providing health care insurance, the cost of lost productivity from employees in the obese range is quite substantial.

Controversies: Weight Guidelines and Treatment

Among the most debated and misunderstood issues in obesity is determining standards for weight and weight loss. This is in part due to overly simplistic approaches to studying this issue. When combined with the societal obsession with weight, it becomes an area of controversy. Thus, it is important to understand how these guidelines are established and their limitations in order to communicate with patients about their health status in relation to their weight and help correct their misconceptions surrounding this issue.

Weight Gain with Age

A major limitation of standard weight guidelines is that a person initially at the low end of the range can gain as much as 20 kg and still remain within the range. Yet, as noted earlier, even much smaller changes in weight are associated with significantly increased risks of many chronic diseases. Compared with men and women who maintained their weight within 2 kg of their weight at ages 18 to 20, those who gained 5 to 9.9 kg experienced 1.5- to two-fold risk of CHD, hypertension, and cholelithiasis, and two- to three-fold risk of type 2 diabetes. These risks were much greater with larger weight gains.

Weight changes since young adulthood are useful in assessing risks associated with body fat because they take into account individual differences in frame size and lean mass that are difficult to measure. At the completion of growth, about 18 years for women and 20 years for men, most individuals in our population are not overweight (81); excess body fat primarily accrues in the subsequent decades. Except for rare persons seriously engaged in muscle building, which would be evident in a clinical encounter, any substantial gains are largely fat. Also, change in weight provides a single, readily interpretable number that is known, at least approximately, to most persons. Lack of weight gain, particularly among men over 50, does not imply an absence of gain in fat. Above this age, muscle mass is to varying degrees redistributed to fat, much of it within the abdomen. This phenomenon may be manifested by an increasing waist circumference.

Considerations of Gender and Age

Other important considerations are whether weight guidelines should differ for men and women and whether weight guidelines should change with age. At identical levels of BMI, women will on average have more body fat (82). However, as the data described above indicate, morbidity appears to increase in a comparable fashion with increasing BMIs for men and women, and the same applies to mortality (83). Thus, although modest differences may exist in these relationships by gender, it can be argued that separate guidelines do not appear to be justified.

The relation between age and body weight is complex. In the large

American Cancer Society cohort, the relation between BMI and total or cardiovascular mortality was approximately linear for all age groups up to 75 years, although the magnitude of the relative risks declined with age (83). The declining relative risks with age do not necessarily mean that excess body fat becomes less important in older persons. Because mortality increases dramatically with age, the absolute excess risks of higher BMI increase rather than decrease with age. Also, as noted earlier, changes in body composition with age may make BMI a less valid indicator of body fatness with age, and it is possible that the reduced strength of association represents a lower validity of BMI as a measure of body fat. Among a cohort of men (84), BMI was a strong predictor of CHD among those under age 65 years but was minimally predictive among older men. Waist circumference predicted CHD only weakly among men under age 65 but was strongly predictive among older men, suggesting that body fat was important at all ages but that the optimal means of assessment may vary by age.

Definition of Healthy Weight

Traditionally, the criterion for setting weight guidelines has been the range of weights corresponding to minimal mortality rates. Mortality as an endpoint provides a simple, reliable, and consequential summary of health impacts. Despite its intuitive appeal, however, use of total mortality as an endpoint is fraught with methodological problems and is far from straightforward (16).

The most difficult problem with using total mortality as an outcome is reverse causation. Individuals frequently lose weight due to an illness that is ultimately fatal, creating the appearance of higher mortality among those with lower weights. For example, occult neoplasms that are likely to be diagnosed within a year or two cause weight loss. Weight loss can also result from undiagnosed conditions such as chronic lung or cardiac disease, alcoholism, and depression that may precede death by many years.

Several epidemiologic maneuvers can be used to minimize the impact of reverse causation. Individuals with diagnoses that might affect weight and those reporting previous weight loss, such as during the previous five years, can be excluded from an analysis. Also, deaths occurring during the first several years of follow-up in a prospective study can be excluded. Although important, neither of these procedures provides a perfect solution because of the variable period over which chronic conditions may influence weight loss. In addition, if the period for exclusion of deaths or the total follow-up is too long, many persons will have substantial changes in weight during follow-up that are not the result of underlying disease, and weight status will be misclassified. Thus, some compromise must be made. At least the first several years of follow-up should be excluded, and follow-up should probably not continue for longer than 10 or 15 years without some updating of weight status. In practice, it is useful to conduct different analyses that vary the censoring period and follow-up time to determine how sensitive the findings are to these decisions.

A second major concern, as in any epidemiologic study, is the possibility that confounding factors may distort the association between body weight and mortality. Smoking is of particular importance because smokers tend to weigh less and also have much higher mortality than nonsmokers. Again, this source of confounding will make leaner persons appear at higher risk because they include a higher proportion of smokers. Many large studies, including the Metropolitan Life insurance data that were used for years to set weight standards, did not include data on smoking and thus overstate desirable weights. Even if data on smoking are available, simple statistical adjustments for smoking are not entirely satisfactory because nuances such as depth of inhalation and genetic susceptibility cannot be accounted for and could influence the impact of smoking on both weight and mortality. The most satisfactory way to deal with smoking is to limit the analysis to those who have never smoked. Unfortunately, many studies have not been sufficiently large to have adequate statistical power (i.e., a study population size that is large enough to prove or disprove a hypothesis) among never smokers, in part because death rates are lower in this group. Other factors that can potentially confound the association between body weight and mortality include alcoholism, diet, and physical activity. Using statistical adjustments for physical activity may not be appropriate because activity is an important determinant of body weight.

A third problem that occurred in some earlier analyses of studies of weight and mortality is that the physiologic effects of excess fatness, such as hypertension, diabetes, and dyslipidemia, were "controlled" statistically, thus artificially removing the actual impact of being overweight. This is an important issue. Obesity-related illnesses were carefully accounted for in the Kaiser study (80), which concluded that they were the major determinant driving direct health care costs among obese patients.

The net effect of reverse causation and confounding by smoking is that lean persons are a mix of smokers, persons who have lost weight due to underlying disease, and individuals who have maintained a lean weight by consciously or unconsciously balancing physical activity and caloric intake. Thus, in analyses statistically adjusted only for age, the relation between body weight and mortality is typically U-shaped, with increased rates among both the leanest and heaviest persons. Also, in such analyses, the range of weights associated with lowest mortality tends to increase with age (85), which might be expected because the burden of chronic illness accumulates with age and enriches the low weight groups with persons at higher risk of death. Such observations, based on data biased by inadequate control for smoking and reverse causation, were the basis for the 1990 weight guidelines in which the range of healthy weights increased with age (from a BMI range of 19 to 25 kg/m² before age 35, to 21 to 27 kg/m² after age 35) (86). This increased range of healthy weights implied that a 10 to 15 lb weight gain at age 35 was acceptable and possibly interpreted as desirable. Moreover, these guidelines could be misconstrued to suggest that about 5% of middle-aged men and 17% of middle-aged women in the United States were at risk of poor health due to being underweight (81)!

Unfortunately, few studies have simultaneously made efforts to minimize reverse causation, to account for cigarette smoking, and to adjust statistically for the physiologic effects of excess body fat. In a review of the 25 major studies done up to 1986 (87), not one met these three criteria, and in a recent meta-analysis (88) only two studies among men (89, 90) provided data among never smokers and also attempted to account for reverse causation. One of these studies (89) included only 13 deaths, and in the other, which had sufficient numbers, mortality rates among nonsmokers increased linearly with greater weight (90). Among women in the Nurses' Health Study, the typical U-shaped relation between BMI and mortality became monotonically positive after accounting for reverse causation and limiting the analysis to never smokers (91). In the most powerful analysis to date, Stevens et al (83) examined mortality rates among never-smoking men and women in the American Cancer Society cohort over a ten-year period. After eliminating early mortality, mortality increased linearly with increasing body mass index from very lean to clearly obese at all ages up to 75 years, although the strength of association was weaker at older ages. Compared with persons with BMIs from 19 to 21 kg/m², total mortality rates were 10% to 35% higher at BMIs of 25 to 26.9 and 18% to 40% higher at BMIs of 27 to 28.9.

In addition to using total mortality as a criterion for weight guidelines, the incidence of diseases contributing importantly to morbidity should also be considered. Artifacts due to reverse causation are usually much less problematic in studies of disease incidence than in studies of death, which occurs at the end of the clinical process. Also, conditions such as CHD, stroke, diabetes, cancers, and OA contribute greatly to suffering even if they do not result in death. Furthermore, guidelines for weight should be based on more than statistical associations between weight and death. Information about the sequence of metabolic and physiologic effects of excess body fat that ultimately leads to specific diseases and finally to death is essential for interpreting these associations correctly. For example, any true causal increase in mortality among lean persons results from either an increased incidence of one or more common diseases among the lean or a higher case-fatality rate for those with these diseases. Lack of evidence for such causal biological relationships should have raised concern that the excess mortality in this group may have been due to artifacts.

Figure 1.1 shows the relationships between BMI and incidence of several common conditions caused by excess body fat—specifically CHD, type 2 diabetes, hypertension, and cholelithiasis— for men followed up to age 75 and for women up to age 72. Focusing on the range of BMI from 20 to 30 kg/m², the relationships are monotonic and approximately linear. For BMI of 26 kg/m² compared with BMI of less than 21, risks of myocardial infarction are increased by about two-fold in women and 1.5-fold in men; for both men and women, risk of diabetes is increased three-fold higher and risks of hypertension and cholelithiasis are two-fold higher. For the same comparison in BMI, risk of myocardial infarction is increased two-fold in women and 1.5-fold in men. For BMI of 29 and greater, these risks are greatly increased. Other important conditions increased by excess body fat include postmenopausal breast cancer (10, 92); cancers of the endometrium, colon, and kidney (92); stroke (93); OA (94); and infertility (80). Excess body fat appears to be beneficial for very few conditions. The incidence (but not mortality) of premenopausal breast cancer is slightly lower among heavier women (10), and hip fracture rates are inversely related to body weight (95); however, hip fractures contribute only slightly to overall total mortality rates.

Recommendations

Based on data such as these, the expert panel convened by the NIH concluded that treatment of obesity is indicated (17). This panel reviewed a substantial body of literature documenting the health consequences of obesity and the mechanisms through which excess weight causes disease and weight loss reduces risk of disease. These findings have been summarized in this chapter. The panel concluded that a variety of treatments are effective, including dietary therapy, altered physical activity patterns, behavior therapy, pharmacotherapy, surgery, and combinations of these. Ultimately, this led to three NIH-recommended general goals of weight loss and management:

1. At a minimum, prevent further weight gain.
2. Reduce body weight.
3. Maintain a lower body weight over the long term.

These approaches to assessment and treatment are discussed in greater detail in subsequent chapters.

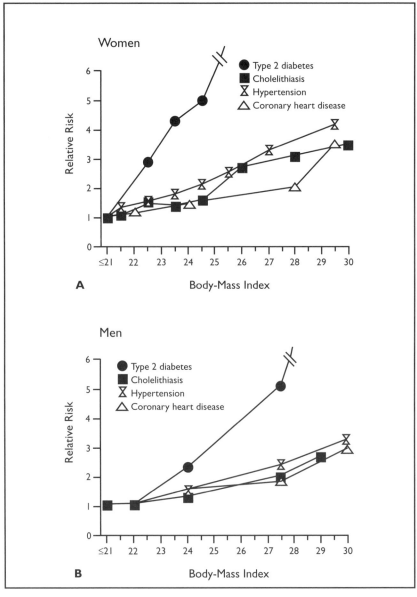

Figure 1.1   Relations between body-mass index up to 30 and the relative risk of type 2 diabetes, hypertension, coronary heart disease, and cholelithiasis. **A,** Relations for women in the Nurses' Health Study, initially 30 to 55 years of age, who were followed for up to 18 years. **B,** The same relations for men in the Health Professionals Follow-up Study, initially 40 to 65 years of age, who were followed for up to 10 years. (From Willett W, Dietz W, Colditz G. Guidelines for healthy weight. N Engl J Med. 1999; 341:427-34; with permission.)

■   ■   ■

Key Points

- The prevalence of obesity has increased dramatically over the past three decades; over 50% of Americans are overweight or obese.

- Obesity is a risk factor for cardiovascular disease, certain cancers, diabetes, hypertension, and overall mortality, and it exacerbates other chronic diseases such as osteoarthritis.

- Obesity has several psychosocial consequences, such as greater likelihood of remaining unmarried and negative evaluation of work performance, that contribute to a decreased quality of life.

- In the United States, direct and indirect costs attributed to obesity have been reported as at least 70 billion and 48 billion dollars, respectively.

- Determining standards for healthy weight has been fraught with limitations. Confounding factors and reverse causation distort the association between body weight and mortality, and the relation between older age and body weight is complex, making excess body weight as a predictor of disease more difficult to assess.

■   ■   ■

REFERENCES

1. **Kuczmarski RJ, Flegal KM, Campbell SM, Johnson CL.** Increasing prevalence of overweight among US adults. The National Health and Nutrition Examination Surveys, 1960 to 1991. JAMA. 1994;272:205-11.

2. **Flegal K, Carroll M, Kuczmarski R, Johnson C.** Overweight and obesity in the United States: prevalence and trends, 1960-1994. Int J Obes Relat Metab Disord. 1998;22:39-47.

3. **National Center for Health Statistics.** Monitoring Health Care in America; Quarterly Fact Sheet. June 1996.

4. **Popkin B.** The nutrition transition in low-income countries: an emerging crisis. Nutr Rev. 1994;52:285-98.

5. **Popkin B.** The nutrition transition and its health implications in lower-income countries. Public Health Nutr. 1998;1:5-21.

6. **Stephen AM, Wald NJ.** Trends in individual consumption of dietary fat in the United States, 1920-1984. Am J Clin Nutr. 1990;52:457-69.

7. State- and sex- specific prevalence of selected characteristics. Behavioral Risk Factor Surveillance System, 1994 and 1995. MMWR Morb Mortal Wkly Rep. 1997;46(SS-3):1-29.

8. **Manson JE, Colditz GA, Stampfer MJ, et al.** A prospective study of obesity and risk of coronary heart disease in women. N Engl J Med. 1990;322:882-9.

9. **Rexrode K, Hennekens C, Willett W, et al.** A prospective study of body mass index, weight change, and risk of stroke in women. JAMA. 1997;277:1539-45.

10. **Huang Z, Hankinson SE, Colditz GA, et al.** Dual effects of weight and weight gain on breast cancer risk. JAMA. 1997;278:1407-11.

11. **Giovannucci E, Ascherio A, Rimm EB, et al.** Physical activity, obesity, and risk for colon cancer and adenoma in men. Ann Intern Med. 1995;122:327-34.

12. **Martinez ME, Giovannucci E, Spiegelman D, et al.** Leisure-time physical activity, body size, and colon cancer in women. Nurses' Health Study Research Group. J Natl Cancer Inst. 1997;89:948-55.

13. **Grady D, Ernster V.** Endometrial cancer. In: Schotenfeld D, Fraumeni J (Editors). Cancer Epidemiology and Prevention. New York: Oxford University Press; 1996.

14. **Colditz GA, Willett WC, Rotnitzky A, Manson JE.** Weight gain as a risk factor for clinical diabetes in women. Ann Intern Med. 1995;122:481-6.

15. **Chan JM, Rimm EB, Colditz GA, et al.** Obesity, fat distribution, and weight gain as risk factors for clinical diabetes in men. Diabetes Care. 1994;17:961-9.

16. **Willett W, Dietz W, Colditz G.** Guidelines for healthy weight. N Engl J Med. 1999;341:427-34.

17. **NHLBI Obesity Initiative Expert Panel.** Clinical guidelines on the identification, evaluation, and treatment of overweight and obesity in adults: the evidence report. Obes Res. 1998;6(Suppl 2):51s-209s.

18. **Giovannucci E.** Insulin and colon cancer. Cancer Causes Control. 1995;6:164-79.

19. **Witteman JC, Willett WC, Stampfer MJ, et al.** Relation of moderate alcohol consumption and risk of systemic hypertension in women. Am J Cardiol. 1990;65:633-7.

20. **Davis M, Ettinger W, Neuhaus J, Hauck W.** Sex differences in osteoarthritis of the knee. Am J Epidemiol. 1988;127:1019-30.

21. **Carmen W, Sowers M, Hawthornes V, Weissfeld L.** Obesity as a risk factor for osteoarthritis of the hand and wrist: a prospective study. Am J Epidemiol. 1994;139:119-29.

22. **Maclure KM, Hayes KC, Colditz GA, et al.** Weight, diet and risk of symptomatic gallstones in middle-aged women. N Engl J Med. 1989;321:563-9.

23. **VanItallie TB.** Obesity: adverse effects on health and longevity. Am J Clin Nutr. 1979;32:2723-33.

24. **Fine J, Colditz G, Coakley E, et al.** A prospective study of weight change and health-related quality of life in women. JAMA. 1999;282:2136-42.

25. **Rimm EB, Stampfer MJ, Giovannucci E, et al.** Body size and fat distribution as predictors of coronary heart disease among middle-aged and older US men. Am J Epidemiol. 1995;141:1117-27.

26. **Harris TB, Ballard-Barbasch R, Madans J, et al.** Overweight, weight loss, and risk of coronary heart disease in older women. The NHANES-I Follow-up Study. Am J Epidemiol. 1993;137:1318-27.

27. **Rexrode K, Carey V, Hennekens C, et al.** Abdominal adiposity and coronary heart disease in women. JAMA. 1998;280:1843-8.

28. **Seidell J, Verschuren W, van Leer E, Kromhout D.** Overweight, underweight, and mortality: a prospective study of 48,287 men and women. Arch Intern Med. 1996;156:958-63.

29. **Must A, Jacques PF, Dallal GE, et al.** Long-term morbidity and mortality of over-weight adolescents: a follow-up of the Harvard Growth Study of 1922 to 1935. N Engl J Med. 1992;327:1350-5.

30. **Bray G.** Health hazards of obesity. Endocrinol Metab Clin North Am. 1996;25:907-19.

31. **Alpen M, Hashimi M.** Obesity and the heart. Am J Med Sci. 1993;306:117-23.

32. **Witteman JC, Willett WC, Stampfer MJ, et al.** A prospective study of nutritional factors and hypertension among US women. Circulation. 1989;80:1320-7.

33. **Ascherio A, Rimm EB, Giovannucci EL, et al.** A prospective study of nutritional factors and hypertension among US men. Circulation. 1992;86:1475-84.

34. **Folsom AR, Prineas RJ, Kaye SA, Soler JT.** Body fat distribution and self-re-ported prevalence of hypertension, heart attack, and other heart disease in older women. Int J Epidemiol. 1989;18:361-7.

35. **Yong L, Kuller L, Rutan G, Bunker C.** Longitudinal study of blood pressure: changes and determinants from adolescence to middle age. The Dormont High School follow-up study, 1957-1963 to 1989-1990. Am J Epidemiol. 1993;138:973-83.

36. **Field A, Byers T, Hunter D, et al.** Weight cycling, weight gain, and risk of hyper-tension in women. Am J Epidemiol 1999;150:573-9.

37. **Wing R, Jeffrey R.** Effect of modest weight loss on changes in cardiovascular risk factors: are there differences between men and women or between weight loss and maintenance? Obesity Res. In press.

38. **Huang Z, Willett W, Manson J, et al.** Body weight, weight change, and risk of hypertension in women. Ann Intern Med. 1998;128:81-8.

38a. **Mikhail N, Golub M, Tuck M.** Obesity and hypertension. Prog Cardiovasc Dis. 1999;42:39-58.

39. **Mahler R, Adler M.** Clinical Review 102. Type 2 diabetes mellitus: update on di-agnosis, pathophysiology, and treatment. J Clin Endo Metab. 1999;84:1165-71.

40. **Colditz GA, Willett WC, Stampfer MJ, et al.** Weight as a risk factor for clinical di-abetes in women. Am J Epidemiol. 1990;132:501-13.

41. **Lundgren H, Bengtsson C, Blohme G, et al.** Adiposity and adipose tissue distri-bution in relation to incidence of diabetes in women: results from a prospective population study in Gothenburg, Sweden. Int J Obes. 1988;13:413-23.

42. **Holbrook TL, Barrett-Connor E, Wingard DL.** The association of lifetime weight and weight control patterns with diabetes among men and women in an adult community. Int J Obes. 1989;13:723-9.

43. **Carey VJ, Walters EE, Colditz GA, et al.** Body fat distribution and risk of non-in-sulin-dependent diabetes mellitus in women. Am J Epidemiol. 1997;145:614-9.

44. **Hartz AJ, Rupley DC Jr, Kalkhoff RD, Rimm AA.** Relationship of obesity to dia-betes: influence of obesity level and body fat distribution. Prev Med. 1983;12:351-7.

45. **Ohlson LO, Larsson B, Svardsudd K, et al.** The influence of body fat distribution on the incidence of diabetes mellitus: 13.5 years of follow-up of the participants in the study of men born in 1913. Diabetes. 1985;34:1055-8.

46. **Hunter DJ, Willett WC.** Diet, body size, and breast cancer. Epidemiol Rev. 1993;15:110-32.

47. **Coates R, Clark W, Eley J, et al.** Race, nutritional status, and survival from breast cancer. J Natl Cancer Inst. 1990;82:1684-92.

48. **Stoll BA.** Adiposity as a risk determinant for postmenopausal breast cancer. Int J Obes. 2000;24:527-33.

49. **Shoff S, Newcomb P.** Diabetes, body size, and risk of endometrial cancer. Am J Epidemiol. 1998;148:234-40.

50. **Tornberg SA, Carstensen JM.** Relationship between Quetelet's index and cancer of breast and female genital tract in 47,000 women followed for 25 years. Br J Cancer. 1994;69:358-61.

51. **Farrow D, Weiss N, Lyon J, Daling J.** Association of obesity and ovarian cancer in a case-control study. Am J Epidemiol. 1989;129:1300-4.

52. **Vaughn T, Davis S, Fristal A, Thomas D.** Obesity, alcohol, and tobacco as risk factors for cancers of the esophagus and gastric cardia: adenocarcinoma versus squamous cell carcinoma. Cancer Epidemiol Biomarkers Prev. 1995;4:85-92.

53. **Lagergren J, Bergstrom R, Nyren O.** Association between body mass and adenocarcinoma of the esophagus and gastric cardia. Ann Intern Med. 1999;130:883-90.

54. **Ford E.** Body mass index and colon cancer in a national sample of US men and women. Am J Epidemiol. 1999;150:390-8.

55. **Le Marchand L, Wilkens L, Kolonel L, et al.** Associations of sedentary lifestyle, obesity, smoking, alcohol use, and diabetes with the risk of colorectal cancer. Cancer Res. 1997;57:4787-94.

56. **Lew EA, Garfinkel L.** Variations in mortality by weight among 750,000 men and women. J Chronic Dis. 1979;32:563-76.

57. **Must A, Spadano J, Coakley E, et al.** The disease burden associated with being overweight and obese. JAMA. 1999;282:1523-9.

58. **Stampfer M, Maclure K, Colditz G, et al.** Risk of symptomatic gallstones in women with severe obesity. Am J Clin Nutr. 1992;55:652-8.

59. **Cooper C, Inskip H, Croft P, et al.** Individual risk factors for hip osteoarthritis: obesity, hip injury, and physical activity. Am J Epidemiol. 1998;147:516-22.

60. **Cicuttini F, Baker J, Spector T.** The association of obesity with osteoarthritis of the hand and knee in women: a twin study. J Rheumatol. 1996;23:1221-6.

61. **Manninen P, Riihimaki H, Heliovaara M, Makela P.** Overweight, gender and knee osteoarthritis. Int J Obes Relat Metab Disord.1996;20:595-7.

62. **Giovannucci E, Rimm EB, Chute CG, et al.** Obesity and benign prostatic hyperplasia. Am J Epidemiol. 1994;140:989-1002.

63. **Larkin J, Pines H.** No fat person need apply. Soc Work Occup. 1979;6:312-27.

64. **Roe D, Eichwort K.** Relationship between obesity and associated health factors with unemployment among low income women. J Am Med Womens Assoc. 1976;31:193-204.

65. **Rumpel C, Ingram D, Harris T, Madans J.** The association between weight change and psychological well-being in women. Int J Obes. 1994;18:179-83.

66. **Falkner N, French S, Jeffery R, et al.** Mistreatment due to weight prevalence and sources of perceived mistreatment in women and men. Obes Res. 1999;7:572-6.

67. **Gortmaker S, Must A, Perrin J, et al.** Social and economic consequences of overweight in adolescence and young adulthood. N Engl J Med. 1993;329:1008-12.

68. **Sonne-Holm S, Sorensen T.** Prospective study of attainment of social class of severely obese subjects in relation to parental social class, intelligence, and education. Br Med J. 1986;292:586-9.

69. **Coakley E, Kawachi I, Manson J, et al.** Lower levels of physical functioning are associated with higher body weight among middle-aged and older women. Int J Obesity. 1998;22:958-65.

70. **Levy E, Levy P, Le Pen C, Basdevant A.** Economic cost of obesity: the French situation. Int J Obesity. 1995;19:788-92.

71. **Segal L, Carter R, Zimmet P.** The cost of obesity: the Australian perspective. PharmacoEconomics. 1994;5(suppl):45-52.

72. **Seidell J.** The impact of obesity on health status: some implications for health care costs. Int J Obesity. 1995;19(suppl):S13-S16.

73. **Narbro K, Jonsson E, Larsson B, et al.** Economic consequences of sick-leave and early retirement on obese Swedish women. Int J Obesity. 1996;20:895-903.

74. **Colditz G.** Economic costs of obesity and inactivity. Med Sci Sports Exerc. 1999;31:S663-7.

75. **U.S. Department of Agriculture, U.S. Department of Health and Human Services.** Nutrition and Your Health: Dietary Guidelines for Americans. Home and Garden Bulletin No. 232. Washington, DC: U.S. Government Printing Office; 1995.

76. **Gorsky R, Pamuk E, Williamson D, et al.** The 25-year health care costs of women who remain overweight after 40 years of age. Am J Prev Med. 1996;12:388-94.

77. **Thompson D, Edelsberg J, Colditz G, et al.** Lifetime health and economic consequences of obesity. Arch Intern Med. 1999;159:2177-83.

78. **Fontaine K, Cheskin L, Barofsky I.** Health-related quality of life in obese persons seeking treatment. J Fam Pract. 1996;43:265-70.

79. **Rich-Edwards JW, Goldman MB, Willett WC, et al.** Adolescent body mass index and ovulatory infertility. Am J Obstet Gynecol. 1994;171:171-7.

80. **Quesenberry CP, Caan B, Jacobson A.** Obesity, health services use, and health care costs among members of a health maintenance organization. Arch Intern Med. 1998;158:466-72.

81. **Kuczmarski RJ, Carroll MD, Flegal KM, Troiano RP.** Varying body mass index cutoff points to describe overweight prevalence among U.S. adults: NHANES III (1988 to 1994). Obes Res. 1997;5:542-8.

82. **Gallagher D, Visser M, Sepulveda D, et al.** How useful is body mass index for comparison of body fatness across age, sex, and ethnic groups? Am J Epidemiol. 1996;143:228-39.

83. **Stevens J, Jianwen C, Pamuk ER, et al.** The effect of age on the association between body-mass index and mortality. N Engl J Med. 1998;338:1-7.

84. **Rimm EB.** Height, obesity, and fat distribution as independent predictors of coronary heart disease. Am J Epidemiol. 1993;138 (abstract):601-2.

85. **Andres R, Elahi D, Tobin JD, et al.** Impact of age on weight goals. Ann Intern Med. 1985;103:1030-3.

86. **U.S. Department of Agriculture, U.S. Department of Health and Human Services.** Nutrition and Your Health: Dietary Guidelines for Americans; 3rd ed. Washington, DC: U.S. Government Printing Office; 1990.

87. **Manson JE, Stampfer MJ, Hennekens CH, Willett WC.** Body weight and longevity: a reassessment. JAMA. 1987;257:353-8.

88. **Troiano RP, Frongillo EA Jr., Sobal J, Levitsky DA.** The relationship between body weight and mortality: a quantitative analysis of combined information from existing studies. Int J Obesity Relat Metab Disord. 1996;20:63-75.

89. **Tuomilehto J, Salonen JT, Marti B, et al.** Body weight and risk of myocardial infarction and death in the adult population of Eastern Finland. Br Med J (Clin Res Ed). 1987;295:623-7.

90. **Garrison RJ, Castelli WP.** Weight and thirty-year mortality of men in the Framingham Study. Ann Intern Med. 1985;103:1006-9.

91. **Manson JE, Willett WC, Stampfer MJ, et al.** Body weight and mortality among women. N Engl J Med. 1995;333:677-85.

92. **World Cancer Research Fund, American Institute for Cancer Research.** Food, Nutrition and the Prevention of Cancer: A Global Perspective. Washington, DC: American Institute for Cancer Research; 1997.

93. **Walker SP, Rimm EB, Ascherio A, et al.** Body size and fat distribution as predictors of stroke among US men. Am J Epidemiol. 1996;144:1143-50.

94. **Felson DT.** Weight and osteoarthritis. Am J Clin Nutr. 1996;63 (suppl):430-2.

95. **Meyer HE, Tverdal A, Falch JA.** Body height, body mass index, and fatal hip fractures: 15 years' follow-up of 674,000 Norwegian women and men. Epidemiology. 1995;6:299-305.

2

■ ■ ■

Etiology of Obesity

Lloyd B. Williams, MS
Robert V. Considine, PhD

uch progress has been made in recent years in our understanding of the physiology of body weight maintenance. This chapter focuses on the concepts of energy balance, the signaling mechanisms by which the central nervous system monitors energy intake, and the genetic and environmental effects on body weight. Recent discoveries with potential impact on the treatment of obesity, such as leptin and the novel uncoupling proteins, are discussed in the context of energy balance.

Whole-Body Energy Balance

For the purpose of understanding the mechanisms regulating body weight, the following simple equation is often used:

$$\text{Energy stores} = \text{Energy intake} - \text{Energy expenditure}$$

Energy stores are primarily considered to be maintained in the adipose tissue as triglyceride because these stores are very large compared with the energy stored as glycogen (the complex carbohydrate storage form of sugar) or protein. As can be seen in the equation, when energy intake equals energy expenditure, energy stores (and therefore body weight) are at equilibrium and stable. If intake is persistently greater than expenditure, the excess energy will be stored in the body, primarily as triglyceride in the adipose tissue. Despite the increasing incidence of obesity, the fact that most adults maintain a fairly constant body weight, or only change body weight very slowly over the course of years, implies that the mechanisms that balance energy expenditure to energy intake are tightly regulated.

Energy expenditure is essentially calories burned (thermogenesis: generation of heat) and is quantified as metabolic rate (1). Over the course of a 24-hour day, total daily energy expenditure can be divided into three components: 1) resting metabolic rate (RMR), 2) thermic effect of food (TEF), and 3) physical activity. The sympathetic nervous system mediates much of the metabolic activity accounting for energy expenditure (2). RMR is the energy by a person at rest under conditions of thermal neutrality. The basal metabolic rate (BMR) is more precisely defined as the RMR measured soon after awakening in the morning, at least 12 hours after the last meal. From a clinical perspective, RMR and BMR are synonymous and are used interchangeably. RMR is measured under fasting conditions in the morning with the subject at rest in bed. Approximately 60% of the total daily energy expenditure can be accounted for by the RMR. TEF is the increase in RMR in response to food intake due to energy expended to digest, oxidize (burn), and store nutrients, which in humans accounts for about 10% of the total daily energy expenditure. Physical activity is the most variable component of the total daily energy expenditure and accounts for approximately 30% of energy expenditure in sedentary adults (1, 3).

Total daily energy expenditure can be quantitated by placing subjects in respiratory chambers that measure oxygen consumption and carbon dioxide production (the key variables in calculating metabolic rate) as well as monitor movement to account for the contribution of physical activity. Studies suggest that fat-free mass (FFM), fat mass, age, spontaneous physical activity, and gender are all significant determinants of total daily energy expenditure, accounting for 88% of the variance between subjects. Of these variables, FFM is the single most important determinant of total 24-hour energy expenditure (1). FFM is also the main determinant of the RMR, which is consistent with RMR accounting for 60% of the total daily energy expenditure. Unlike most animal models of obesity, which increase in fat mass only, human FFM increases in proportion to body weight. Consequently, RMR and total daily energy expenditure increase as body weight increases. Therefore, obese subjects have greater total daily energy expenditure than do lean individuals. Thus, if the commonly held belief that a "slow metabolism" is true, such a postulate must reconcile that the total energy expenditure and RMR are higher in obese individuals. The contribution of the three components to energy balance is illustrated in Figure 2.1.

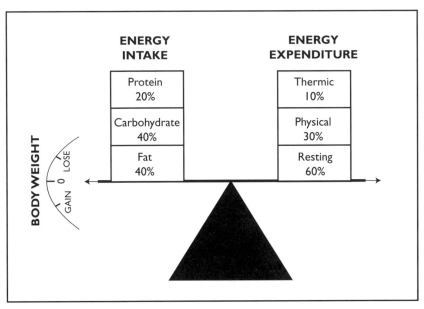

Figure 2.1   Energy balance in humans. The concept of energy balance can be simplified to a balance beam. When energy intake is equal to energy expenditure, body weight remains constant. An acute increase in energy intake is countered by a compensatory reduction in energy expenditure to return energy stores back to the original state. Chronic increases in energy intake are not offset by energy expenditure, and body weight increases to a new set point.

The Role of Energy Expenditure in the Development of Obesity

The three components of energy expenditure have been carefully examined in an attempt to detect defects, particularly deficiencies in energy expenditure, which could contribute to the development of obesity. As discussed above, the absolute (total) RMR is greater in obese subjects than in lean subjects. More importantly, on average, RMR is relatively comparable to lean individuals when normalized for differences in FFM. However, there is significant variability in the relation between RMR and FFM. Consequently, at any given body size some individuals have a high, some a low, and some a normal *relative* metabolic rate compared with the general population (1).

Several longitudinal studies have been carried out to determine if a relatively low RMR could contribute to, or predict the development of, obesity. In adult Pima Indians, a population with high rates of obesity and type 2 diabetes mellitus, a low relative RMR was associated with an approximately seven times greater risk of becoming obese within four years compared with subjects with the highest RMR (4). However, only 40% of the weight gain in this study could be accounted for by the low RMR, which suggests that weight gain is caused by additional factors. Other longitudinal studies in adult males (5), women who have lost weight (6), children (7), and infants (8) did not find that resting energy expenditure predicted weight gain. Furthermore, unlike the common misperception that weight loss causes a decline in metabolic rate that predisposes one to regain weight, carefully controlled studies indicate that sustained weight loss (postobese or reduced obese) does not result in a disproportionate reduction in metabolic rate in the overwhelming majority of people (9, 10). However, there may be a subpopulation that has a slightly lower RMR in the postobese state (11, 12), a finding consistent with the heterogeneity in RMR variability that may be predictive of the propensity towards obesity (4), but in general it is not a cause for relapse (12). Taken together these studies suggest that a relatively low RMR may be a risk factor for the development of obesity in specific populations or individuals but that its contribution to the development of obesity in the general population is small (3, 13, 14).

TEF as a potential defect causing obesity has been examined in a large number of studies, but a consensus has not been reached (1). However, the small differences in the TEF that have been reported for lean and obese subjects could, at best, only account for a minor increase in body weight (14, 15). Moreover, reduced TEF is a consequence of insulin resistance (16), a finding reinforced by studies demonstrating reduced TEF in nonobese patients with type 2 diabetes mellitus that can be accounted for by reduced rates of glucose uptake, the standard research measurement to quantify insulin resistance (17). Therefore, because most obese individuals are insulin resistant, insulin resistance is not likely to contribute significantly to the development of obesity and, in fact, is more likely a consequence rather than a cause of obesity.

Physical activity is the most variable component of the total daily energy expenditure. Studies of energy expenditure using the double-labeled water technique indicate that energy expended in physical activity is a predictor of weight gain (18) and that physical activity is reduced in obese subjects compared with lean (1, 14). Again, there are additional factors to consider such as possible racial differences in energy expenditure, the physical activity component, and regional differences in body composition that contribute to disproportionate rates of obesity among different subpopulations (19). Spontaneous physical activity (e.g., fidgeting), one component of the total physical activity, is itself a significant predictor of subsequent weight gain (20). As discussed below, spontaneous physical activity also appears to play an important role in preventing weight gain during periods of increased energy intake.

Even more subtle metabolic perturbations may occur, however, that contribute to the propensity for some individuals to gain weight. Recent studies suggest that, although total and resting expenditure may not account for weight gain, the nutrient partitioning to the metabolic pathways that contribute to these metabolic rates may have an influence. Specifically, there may be a reduction in fat oxidation in some individuals that may predispose them to obesity as well as recidivism (weight regain after weight loss) (21-27). In addition, subtle gender and ethnic/racial differences in metabolism may be important contributors to body weight regulation (28-30). Finally, a complex interaction between lifestyle habits (e.g., smoking, fat consumption) and energy expenditure may have a significant impact (31).

In summary, reduced total energy expenditure is a potential risk factor for the development of obesity. The sympathetic nervous system may modulate this risk and has until recently been the primary target of pharmacotherapeutic treatment strategy (2). Of the three components of daily energy expenditure, reduction in physical activity is the major significant predictor of weight gain, a finding reinforced by the observation that exercise is the strongest predictor of maintaining weight after successful obesity intervention. Certain subpopulations may also have lower RMR and other characteristics that increase risk for developing obesity. However, the degree to which altered energy expenditure can account for weight gain and obesity must be assessed within the context of the environment in which it occurs, an interaction that clearly facilitates developing the obese phenotype.

Changes in Energy Expenditure To Maintain Energy Stores

The stability of body weight in most adults over the course of years indicates that energy intake and energy expenditure are highly regulated and finely tuned. This would suggest, given the potentially large variation in food intake and energy expenditure on both a short- and long-term basis, that energy expenditure is altered to match energy intake such that energy stores (body weight) are maintained. Indeed a number of studies have demonstrated under defined experimental conditions that changes in body weight result in compensatory changes in energy expenditure that oppose the maintenance of the altered body weight, although it must be noted that historically most of these studies have been conducted in normal weight individuals and therefore may not accurately reflect the heterogeneity in metabolism that may contribute to body weight. In a study by Leibel et al (32) a 10% reduction in body weight was associated with a significant reduction in both resting and nonresting metabolic rate. A 10% increase in body weight resulted in a significant increase in energy expenditure, primarily nonresting energy expenditure. Both lean and obese subjects responded similarly to changes in body weight and there was no difference between males and females. These results demonstrate that mechanisms are in place which favor the maintenance of a stable body weight. These findings are important to consider in relation to weight loss programs because compensatory physiologic mechanisms that resist weight loss will be activated by caloric restriction.

Levine et al (33) examined the energetic response to overfeeding in humans to determine why some individuals gain weight more easily than others. These investigators identified a component of physical energy expenditure, termed *nonexercise activity thermogenesis* (NEAT), that is a major determinant of the amount of fat gain with overeating. NEAT is the energy expended in physical activities other than volitional exercise and includes daily living, activities, fidgeting, spontaneous muscle contraction, and maintenance of posture. In response to a 1000-kcal increase in energy intake, total daily energy expenditure increased and, on average, NEAT accounted for two-thirds of this increase. Furthermore, the greater the increase in NEAT, the less energy that was stored in the body as adipose tissue. These observations suggest that a reduced NEAT response to overfeeding could predispose some individuals to weight gain. The mechanisms leading to the activation of NEAT are currently under study but may involve sympathetic nervous system activity (34). The behavioral components accompanying NEAT also need to be elucidated.

Body Weight, Energy Metabolism, and Uncoupling Proteins

Mammals possess two types of adipose tissue: 1) white adipose tissue that functions to store energy in the form of lipid and 2) brown adipose tissue that is active in thermogenic energy expenditure. Adipocytes in brown adipose tissue contain, in addition to lipid droplets, numerous mitochondria that enable this tissue to have a very active metabolism. Brown fat is important in maintaining core body temperature in rodents exposed to cold temperatures, and activation of this tissue can account for ~40% of the twofold increase in RMR (35). Heat is generated in brown fat by the dissociation of ATP synthesis in the mitochondria from the oxidation of nutrients. Within the mitochondria the oxidation of substrates results in the generation of a proton gradient across the inner mitochondrial membrane. ATP synthase utilizes the energy released when these protons flow back across the inner membrane to synthesize ATP from ADP and P_i(36). Nutrient oxidation is dissociated from ATP synthesis by activation of uncoupling protein-1 (UCP-1), which allows the protons to flow across the inner mitochondrial membrane independent of ATP synthase. The energy produced by the flow of protons uncoupled from ATP synthesis is released as heat (37). In addition to cold, food intake can also increase the thermogenic activity of brown fat, and targeted ablation of the brown fat pad in mice results in the development of obesity. Energy expenditure by brown fat is therefore important in maintaining body weight stores in rodents (38).

Although humans are born with brown fat, there is very little of this tissue present in adults (39). For this reason the activation of UCP-1 is not believed to play a major role in energy expenditure in humans. However, several novel uncoupling proteins have recently been discovered that may be important regulators of metabolism in humans. Uncoupling protein-2 (UCP-2) is 55% homologous at the amino acid level to UCP-1 (40, 41). In contrast to UCP-1, which is expressed solely in brown adipose tissue, UCP-2 is expressed in most tissues examined. Interestingly, UCP-2 is present in several hypothalamic nuclei (paraventricular, arcuate, and suprachiasmatic) (42), which, as discussed below, are important in regulating energy intake and expenditure. UCP-3 is 57% identical to UCP-1, 73% identical to UCP-2, and is expressed primarily in skeletal muscle (43, 44). An additional message for a short UCP-3 is also present in skeletal muscle. Each of the novel uncoupling proteins can increase proton leak in yeast mitochondria in vitro, thus demonstrating that these proteins can function to uncouple nutrient oxidation from ATP synthesis (45).

The homology of UCP-2 and UCP-3 with UCP-1 suggests that these proteins could function in regulating thermogenesis in response to cold or food intake. Furthermore, UCP-2 and UCP-3 are present in human skeletal muscle, which plays an important role in energy expenditure in humans. Some studies suggest that UCP-2 and UCP-3 in brown fat may regulate thermogenic energy expenditure (37, 45), but a number of seemingly contradictory observations indicate their role has yet to be clearly understood. Some but not all studies indicate UCP-2 and UCP-3 are increased in skeletal muscle of obese individuals (46). The proteins also increase during fasting/starvation in both rodents and humans, despite this being a time during which whole-body energy expenditure is reduced. Carbohydrate intake and insulin do not acutely regulate UCP-2 gene expression (47). In contrast, a lipid infusion raising plasma triglyceride levels induces UCP-3 but not UCP-2 gene expression in human skeletal muscle that is counteracted by raising insulin levels with an intravenous infusion (48). In the aforementioned Pima Indians, UCP-3 gene expression is a determinant of total energy expenditure (49).

These findings argue against a general physiologic role for the novel uncoupling proteins in reactive thermogenesis in humans but demonstrate a complex differential cellular and tissue regulation of these proteins that requires further elucidation (37). Furthermore, UCP-2 and UCP-3 are important in regulating other metabolic processes (37, 45). UCP-2 may function to limit the production of reactive oxygen species by the mitochondrial electron transport chain. Reactive oxygen species can be produced when the amount of ADP available for phosphorylation is low, thus resulting in a high-proton electrochemical gradient. UCP-2 may dissipate this gradient to lessen the generation of reactive oxygen species. UCP-2 and UCP-3 are likely important in ATP synthesis in muscle. The ability to generate ATP is very much in excess of need when the muscle is at rest. During rest the uncoupling proteins may act to dissipate the proton gradient so that nutrient metabolism does not need to be reduced. In this way, when ATP is needed for contraction fuel metabolism does not need to rapidly increase to meet demand. Finally, uncoupling proteins may be involved in energy partitioning. Expression of UCP-2 and UCP-3 increases concomitantly with fat metabolism, which suggests a role for these proteins in fatty acid oxidation. Data also support a role for UCP-2 and UCP-3 in glucose metabolism in several tissues.

In summary, although a physiologically relevant role for the uncoupling proteins in energy expenditure in humans is not readily apparent, these novel proteins are important to mitochondrial function (Table 2.1). Pharmacologic manipulation of uncoupling protein activity to increase nutrient oxidation/energy expenditure may be a viable means of inducing weight loss in the future (see Chapter 11).

Central Mechanisms Regulate Energy Homeostasis

As stated above, energy intake and energy expenditure are tightly matched to maintain body weight fairly constant over many years. To achieve such a high degree of coordination the central nervous system regulates energy intake and expenditure (50, 51). Early lesion studies in rodents established that the ventromedial hypothalamus was a satiety center and that the lateral hypothalamus was a feeding center (52). Since those early studies, the role of specific nuclei within the hypothalamus in controlling energy balance has been better defined (53). The arcuate and ventromedial nuclei, which lie just above the median eminence at the base of the brain, process information about energy stores from hormonal signals such as insulin, leptin, and others, which gain access to these nuclei through the "leaky" blood brain barrier of the median eminence. The paraventricular nucleus integrates signals from the arcuate, ventromedial, and dorsomedial nuclei and transmits this information through the pituitary and autonomic neurons

Table 2.1   Uncoupling Proteins in Humans

	Location	Activity
UCP-1	Brown fat	Thermogenesis in newborns
UCP-2	Most tissues	ATP synthesis Energy partitioning
UCP-3	Skeletal muscle	ATP synthesis Energy partitioning

back to the body. The arcuate and lateral hypothalamic area also signal to the cortex to regulate behavioral responses to energy intake (54).

In addition to long-term regulation of energy balance, the brain receives short-term information about food intake from mechanosensitive and chemosensitive vagal afferent neurons that line the alimentary canal (55). These feeding-induced signals are transmitted via vagal afferent fibers to second-order neurons in the brainstem (nucleus of the solitary tract). Major outputs from the nucleus of the solitary tract project to medullary motor nuclei and to forebrain areas including the hypothalamic nuclei (arcuate, dorsomedial, and paraventricular), the lateral hypothalamus, and the insular cortex. Short- and long-term signals of energy intake and energy expenditure are therefore integrated in the hypothalamic nuclei. For a detailed discussion of the neurotransmitters involved in processing information from the alimentary canal the reader is referred to the paper by Berthoud et al (55) and the references therein.

Central Monoamines Regulate Energy Intake

The monoamines norepinephrine, epinephrine, dopamine, and serotonin were the first neurotransmitters to be studied for effects on feeding behavior. Neuronal pathways that utilize the neurotransmitters norepinephrine, epinephrine, and dopamine arise in the brainstem and innervate several nuclei in the hypothalamus as well as in the cerebral cortex, hippocampus, and thalamus (56). Serotonin-containing neurons are located in the paraventricular, ventromedial, and suprachiasmatic nuclei in the hypothalamus (57). Norepinephrine and epinephrine act in the paraventricular nucleus to stimulate food intake and are involved in the state of arousal to prepare for food intake (56, 58). Hypothalamic serotonin reduces overall food intake through a decrease in the size and duration of meal intake (57). Agents that prolong the synaptic availability of serotonin (re-uptake inhibitors) also reduce food intake and are effective as part of a weight reduction program (see Chapter 9).

Peptide Neurotransmitters Regulate Energy Intake and Expenditure

Rapid progress over the past five years has identified novel peptide neurotransmitters regulating energy stores. Defects in several of these peptides result in monogenetic syndromes of obesity in mice (50). These novel neuropeptides function in the long-term regulation of energy balance in two discrete hypothalamic areas: the arcuate nucleus and the lateral hypothalamus. However, evidence suggests that the arcuate nucleus and lateral hypothalamus do not function independently and that complex cross-talk exists between these two areas of the hypothalamus. Extrapolating these defects found in mice to etiologies of obesity in humans remains a major challenge in this field of research. However, rare syndromes (described later), as well as potential roles in the subpopulations of morbidly obese patients with unique phenotypes, are being discovered. Consequently, it is conceivable that in the near future many of these defects will be found to have a role in human etiologies of obesity.

α-Melanocyte stimulating hormone (α-MSH) is produced by cleavage of proopiomelanocortin (POMC) neurons in the arcuate nucleus. α-MSH binds to the melanocortin-4 receptor (MC-4) and decreases food intake. MC-4 receptors are highly expressed by neurons in the paraventricular and dorsomedial nuclei and in the lateral hypothalamic area (59). The binding of α-MSH to the MC-4 receptor is antagonized by another neuropeptide in the arcuate nucleus, the agouti-related peptide (AGRP) (60). This neuropeptide is a homolog of the agouti protein, which alters pigmentation of hair follicles by antagonizing the binding of α-MSH to the MC-1 receptor but whose ectopic and unregulated expression results in obesity in lethal yellow mice (50).

Aberrations in the genes regulating these neuropeptides are now being found in humans. Mutations in the POMC gene have been identified in a rare syndrome of obesity (61). The first mutations in the MC-4 receptor were reported in 1998 in women with long-standing obesity and a dominant inheritance pattern for the gene (62, 63). Since then, related defects have been described in a subpopulation of morbidly obese patients with a variety of inheritance patterns, which suggests a more common etiology for an obesity phenotype (64, 65).

Neuropeptide-Y (NPY) is found in many regions of the hypothalamus but is highly expressed in the arcuate nucleus (51). Expression of NPY in the arcuate is increased by energy deficits such as fasting, food restriction, and exercise. Intracerebroventricular injection (ICV) of NPY induces profound hyperphagia (51). NPY neurons project to the PVN, dorsomedial, and ventromedial nuclei of the hypothalamus to regulate food intake and energy expenditure. Four related receptors that bind NPY have been identified. Of these the Y1 and Y5 receptors appear the most relevant to the regulation of food intake by NPY (66).

One additional neuropeptide regulating food intake was originally discovered during a screen for genes induced by addictive drugs. CART (cocaine and amphetamine regulated transcript) containing neurons are found in the arcuate and paraventricular nuclei and in the lateral hypothalamus. CART in the arcuate nucleus is reduced in fasted or leptin-deficient animals, implicating this neuropeptide in the regulation of food intake in response to physiologic stimuli, and ICV injection of CART suppresses food intake (67).

In the lateral hypothalamus two neuropeptides that increase food intake have recently been found. Melanocyte-concentrating hormone (MCH) is present in the magnocellular neurons of the lateral hypothalamus (68). MCH neurons project to many sites including autonomic preganglionic neurons and the medial prefrontal cortex. The connection to the medial prefrontal cortex suggests that MCH may be involved in regulating the behavioral responses to feeding. Fasting increases expression of MCH, and ICV administration of the neuropeptide stimulates feeding (67). Orexin (69) or hypocretin (70) is found in neurons distinct from those expressing MCH but with overlapping projections to the autonomic preganglionic neurons and cerebral cortex. As observed for MCH, orexin expression is increased with fasting and ICV injection of orexin increases food intake. CART, which is an inhibitor of food intake, is also expressed in the lateral hypothalamus (67).

Table 2.2 summarizes the rapidly accumulating data on neuropeptides within the hypothalamus that regulate energy balance. The signalling pathways through which these neurotransmitters interact to regulate food intake under normal and pathophysiologic conditions are being investigated by many laboratories with the intent of identifying targets for future pharmacologic treatment of obesity in humans. Information on additional signaling molecules involved in energy homeostasis can be found in the recent review by Woods et al (51).

Leptin Signals Energy Stores to the Brain

To efficiently match energy intake and energy expenditure so that energy stores can be maintained constant, the hypothalamic centers regulating energy balance need to monitor the amount of energy stored in the adipose tissue. While adipose tissue has long been viewed simply as a passive repository for fuel storage, it is now recognized to be an extremely active endocrine organ that is critical not only to energy homeostasis but to reproduction and overall metabolism under both acute and chronic conditions (71). After decades of indirect research evidence indicating that there must be a signal generated by adipose tissue as part of an energy feedback loop

Table 2.2   Central Neuropeptides Regulating Food Intake

Neuropeptide	Hypothalamic Location	Receptor	Effect on Food Intake
NPY	Arcuate nucleus	Y1/Y5	Stimulate
α-MSH	Arcuate nucleus	MC-4	Inhibit
AGRP	Arcuate nucleus	MC-4	Stimulate
CART	Arcuate nucleus/Lateral hypothalamus	?	Inhibit
MCH	Lateral hypothalamus	?	Stimulate
Orexin	Lateral hypothalamus	Orexin receptor	Stimulate

with the CNS, the first adipose tissue hormone discovered that fulfills the role, leptin, was finally identified in the obese (*ob/ob*) mouse model and found to be present in humans (72). Leptin is the 146 amino acid peptide product of the *ob* gene, which is most highly expressed in adipose tissue (73) but is also detectable in other tissues including muscle (74) and placenta (75). Unlike polypeptide hormones such as insulin, which are stored in secretory vesicles and released upon the appropriate signal, leptin is not stored to any appreciable extent in the adipose tissue but is synthesized and released in a constitutive manner.

If *ob* gene defects are a significant etiology for obesity in humans, presumably there should be obese patients with low levels of leptin. Indeed, individual cases have been identified and these patients have been successfully treated with leptin replacement (76-78), but this is otherwise an extremely rare syndrome. Rather, the more common observation is that serum leptin concentrations are actually elevated in obese patients and highly correlated with the mass of adipose tissue in humans, which suggests there may be a resistance to leptin hormone action or a compensatory increase to protect against further weight gain (79). However, there is a large variance in leptin per fat mass in the population. One factor that accounts for the variance in leptin is gender. Leptin is significantly greater in women than in men with an equivalent amount of fat. Reproductive hormones, as well as body fat distribution, appear to contribute to the difference in leptin with gender (80). Leptin is also highly correlated with adiposity in children and newborns (81). Alterations in the amount of energy stored as adipose tissue change both *ob* gene expression and circulating leptin. The reduction in adipose tissue mass with weight loss results in a decrease in serum leptin. An increase in the adipose tissue mass significantly increases circulating leptin. However, serum leptin levels respond quickly (within 24 hours) to both quantitative and qualitative changes in energy intake and expenditure (82-85). These observations demonstrate that serum leptin is an adjustable signal to the CNS of the amount of energy stored in the adipose tissue (81).

In addition to providing information to the CNS of current energy stores, serum leptin signals caloric intake. Serum leptin falls dramatically during fasts of 24 hours or longer and will increase again within 4 to 5 hours of refeeding despite the fact that adipose tissue mass does not change over this time period (81). The fall in serum leptin with fasting provides a signal to the CNS that food intake has not recently occurred and, in part, initiates the complex response of the body to defend energy stores (86). The reduction in leptin with caloric restriction may have important implications with respect to success in dieting. The decrease in leptin that occurs with hypocaloric diets, independent of any reduction in adipose tissue, signals to the hypothalamus to increase food intake (discussed below) and decrease energy expenditure in an attempt to maintain energy stores constant. This normal physiologic response to caloric restriction is therefore counterproductive to the goal of a weight loss program and theoretically could contribute to difficulties in adherence to a treatment plan.

The receptor for leptin is a member of the class I cytokine receptor family (87). Binding of leptin to its receptor activates a receptor-associated janus kinase (JAK) that phosphorylates tyrosine residues within the receptor itself as well as STAT (signal transducer and activator of transcription) proteins. After phosphorylation STATs dimerize and translocate to the nucleus to initiate gene transcription. STAT-3 is the major STAT protein activated by the leptin receptor. Several leptin receptor isoforms have been identified including a short receptor (OB-Ra) with a truncated intracellular domain that is highly expressed in the choroid plexus membrane. The short leptin receptor does not appear to activate STAT proteins but may function in the transport of leptin across the blood-brain barrier.

The leptin receptor is detectable in several areas of the CNS but is highly expressed in the arcuate, paraventricular, ventromedial, and dorsomedial nuclei of the hypothalamus. Leptin may access the arcuate, ventromedial, and dorsomedial nuclei directly from the blood through the median eminence which lacks a blood-brain barrier. Alternatively, or in addition, leptin may be actively transported into the CSF through the choroid plexus. Leptin binding to its receptor in the arcuate nucleus reduces the expression of neuropeptides that stimulate food intake and increases expression of neuropeptides that reduce feeding. As such, leptin treatment suppresses NPY and induces the expression of POMC (88). α-MSH is the product of the POMC gene that inhibits food intake by binding to the MC-4 receptor. AGRP antagonizes the binding of α-MSH to the MC-4 receptor to increase food intake. Because AGRP mRNA is found in NPY expressing neurons in the arcuate, leptin likely reduces expression of AGRP as well as NPY to reduce food intake. Leptin also regulates the expression of CART in the arcuate nucleus as exogenous administration of the hormone reverses the reduction in CART induced by fasting (54).

Low levels of leptin receptors are also detectable in the lateral hypothalamic region. Leptin-deficient mice have elevated levels of MCH (stimulus for food intake) in the lateral hypothalamus that normalize with leptin administration, which suggests that MCH expression is leptin responsive. It is not yet clear whether leptin regulates neurons in the lateral hypothalamus by directly binding to receptors located in this region or if neural outputs from the arcuate nucleus to the lateral hypothalamus are responsible (54).

Whether leptin has a therapeutic role in controlling weight remains to be determined. The generally higher serum levels of leptin in obese individuals has led to the postulate that there is resistance to the hormone actions of leptin and that this is a compensatory response to obesity that protects against further weight gain (89). Moreover, leptin must cross the blood-brain barrier, which may be a significant obstacle. CSF concentrations in humans is half of what is present in the blood and reaches a maximal CSF concentration, which suggests the transport system is saturable (90). Nevertheless, leptin administration is being pursued as a pharmacotherapy for obesity. A report of an early clinical trial suggests that a subpopulation of obese patients responds favorably (91). Interestingly, in a very small study, a tight correlation between CSF and serum leptin levels was observed in response to exogenous administration of leptin (92).

Although the initial descriptions of leptin focused on its integral role in energy regulation, leptin has been implicated in many other metabolic processes including regulation of glucose homeostasis, stimulation of the development and differentiation of hematopoietic cells, and induction of cellular proliferation and action as an angiogenic factor. Yet its most pivotal role in metabolism may be in orchestrating the signals for the onset of puberty and in fetal/neonatal growth and development (93). Changes in body composition, fat mass, and nutrition all are important components, which suggests that leptin has a fundamental role in the regulation of reproductive function and integrating energy homeostasis with hypothalamic-pituitary-gonadal function. (For detailed discussion see Reference 94.)

Adiposity: From the Adipocyte to Whole-Body Composition

Overall body fatness and its medical ramifications ultimately stem from the number, volume, and differential metabolism of adipocytes. Seminal work in rodents (95), later confirmed and extended in research on humans (96-98), indicates that key periods in development result in the irreversible acquisition of fat cells and that this is in part related to adipocytes reaching a critical volume, after which additional cells are needed for fat storage. As would be expected, this primarily occurs very early in life, but it also continues during adulthood. Extrapolating these findings to adults indicates that, at one end of the spectrum, those who are overweight are afflicted primarily with hypertrophic obesity (i.e., increased cell volume due to lipid accumulation) (99, 100). At the other end of the spectrum, morbid obesity is associated with severe hyperplastic (increased adipoctye number) and hypertrophic obesity (99). Reducing hyperplasia does not appear possible, but hypertrophy is reversible (99, 100). These observations have particular implications for patients who believe that simply removing fat surgically (e.g., liposuction) will adequately address their problem with obesity. Similarly, those using more conventional approaches should understand that weight loss reduces adipocyte cell size but not cell number.

Adipose tissue in the body can be categorized into anatomically and metabolically distinguishable depots. The majority (~80%) of body fat is present as subcutaneous adipose tissue with the remainder distributed primarily to the visceral (omental), retroperitoneal, perirenal, muscular (intra- and inter-), and orbital depots. The distribution of subcutaneous fat is gender specific. Nonobese women have relatively more subcutaneous fat in the gluteofemoral area than do nonobese men, whereas nonobese men have subcutaneous fat more uniformly distributed. With weight gain and obesity, women generally accumulate subcutaneous fat in the lower part of the abdominal wall and the gluteofemoral region, whereas men accumulate fat in the subcutaneous abdominal region. The deposition of fat in the lower body in women is termed *gynoid, lower body,* or *pear-shaped* obesity, whereas the distribution of fat in men is to the upper body and referred to as *android, upper body,* or *apple-shaped* obesity.

Visceral adipose tissue mass is relatively similar in lean women and men; however, visceral adipose tissue is usually increased in obese men compared with obese women (101, 102). Some women tend to distribute excess fat in the upper body, similar to men. Likewise, although less commonly, some men distribute excess fat to the lower body.

Factors other than gender need to be considered as well. Race and ethnicity may affect body composition. For a given amount of fat, when gender and age are controlled, nonwhites have substantially lower BMIs than do whites (thus higher percent lean body mass) (103, 104). From a medical perspective, this suggests that the cutpoints for overweight and obesity (BMI 25 and 30 respectively) are too high for most nonwhite ethnic groups (i.e., medical complications of obesity occur at lower BMIs than observed in whites). Sex hormones, particularly menopause, can have significant effects on body composition and fat distribution, favoring increased adiposity and abdominal distribution of fat in conjunction with menopause (105). Finally, nongenetic influences also contribute to adiposity and fat distribution, smoking being of paramount importance (106). Thus, the determinants of body composition and fat distribution are quite complex.

Fat distribution has significant metabolic and medical implications. Regional differences in adipose tissue metabolism, specifically visceral fat, exist that are linked to the development of some of the most common and serious risk factors associated with coronary heart disease (i.e., type 2 diabetes mellitus, hyperlipidemia, and hypertension). Prospective studies suggest that fat distribution is a stronger predictor of cardiovascular risk and mortality than is overall adiposity (107-109). Typically, the visceral fat depot performs a major role in the rapid mobilization of lipid stores for energy when the physiologic need is present (110, 111). This depot has direct access to the liver via the portal circulation, and the liver can then function to process and distribute fat appropriately. To accomplish this, visceral fat is both more responsive to lipolytic hormones (i.e., the hormones that facilitate the catabolism of fat such as catecholamines) and less responsive to inhibition of lipolysis by insulin than is the abdominal subcutaneous fat. Moreover, peripheral subcutaneous depots (gluteofemoral) are the least responsive to lipolytic hormones. Intrinsic to the metabolisms of these fat depots is the differential gene expression regulating these functions (110, 111), which in conjunction with more global changes in metabolism and physiology, such as changes in body composition that accompany aging (112, 113), account for these observations. Although in the context of evolution these metabolic responses may have been critical to survival, they are maladaptive in the modern era. Several studies indicate that in obese individuals the increased rate of triglyceride and free fatty acids (a triglyceride breakdown product) release from the visceral fat depot has undesirable effects on liver function. Elevated release of free fatty acids into the portal vein leads to increased glucose production, decreased insulin breakdown, and increased triglyceride/VLDL synthesis by the liver, all of which are thought to contribute to the development of diabetes, dyslipidemia, and cardiovascular disease.

Recent studies suggest there are other fat depots associated with increased metabolic perturbations that are associated clinically with cardiovascular risk factors. These depots are associated with skeletal muscle, both intramuscular and subfascial, in addition to subcutaneous fat (114, 115). Whether these depots prove to be directly linked to the development of serious metabolic diseases associated with cardiovascular disease remains to be determined, but such research highlights the previously underappreciated heterogeniety in adipose tissue and underscores, along with new discoveries related to body weight regulation, that it is much more than a passive repository of energy stores.

Genes and the Environment

Obesity is a polygenic disease resulting from the actions of an unknown number of genes, several of which appear to account for a substantial amount (~40%) of the phenotypic variation and others that likely account for only a small portion of the variation (116). Thus, it is estimated that 60% of obesity is caused by environmental factors (e.g., lifestyle); the complex interaction between the environment and genetics results in the obese phenotype. This interaction between the environment and genetics is reflected in the variability of both developmental and familial influences on adiposity. Based on epidemiological studies, young obese children (<3 years old) have a low risk of becoming obese adults if their parents are not obese, but older children who are obese are more likely to become obese adults independent of their parents' body composition (117-119). This observation is consistent with the irreversible deposition of adipocytes that occurs during key periods of growth and development as children mature, even in older children at lower genetic risk, if preventative measures against excessive weight gain are not implemented. The landmark study by Stunkard et al used classical adoption methodology to provide strong evidence for the genetic influence on body composition, demonstrating that both leanness and obesity are highly heritable and most probably polygenic (120). Additional studies confirm body composition is a familial trait, with a wide range of heritability estimates for obesity, from a low of 25% in adoption studies to a high of 70% in studies of monozygotic twins (121). Regional fat distribution is similarly differentially affected by genetic and environmental influences, with genetics having a greater impact than overall body composition, and in which nongenetic influences have a significant determining role in adiposity (122, 123).

Two techniques for the identification of human obesity genes are candidate gene analysis and genome scanning. In candidate gene analysis, known genes, identified by their effects in animal models of obesity or by their role in physiologic processes of energy intake and expenditure, are evaluated for their relationship to the obese phenotype. In contrast, genome scanning makes no assumptions about the importance of a gene or chromosomal region to the development of obesity. Genome scanning is carried out through analysis of polymorphic regions equally spaced throughout the genome. The likelihood that a certain polymorphism is genetically transmitted with the obesity phenotype identifies a chromosomal region that may contain genes determining body weight. The linkage of a gene to a phenotype is quantitated by the LOD score (logarithm of the likelihood of linkage). An LOD score of 3 or greater is taken as evidence of strong linkage of a gene or chromosomal region to phenotype (116).

Analysis of candidate genes has identified associations between 26 genes and various phenotypes associated with obesity (124). Of these, UCP-2 is associated with sleeping and 24-hour metabolic rate and polymorphisms in the *ob* gene are associated with serum leptin levels. The number of single-gene mutations resulting in obesity in humans identified as of October 1999 is 25 cases with 12 mutations in 5 different genes. These include mutations in the *ob* gene (5 individuals), leptin receptor (3 individuals), POMC gene (2 subjects), and the MC-4 receptor gene (9 subjects). In addition, 20 Mendelian disorders have been mapped with obesity as one of their clinical manifestations. Besides gene candidates located in the CNS, peripheral sites may be involved. A mutation in the peroxisome-proliferator-activated receptor (PPAR) gamma-2 (the site at which thiazolidinediones act to improve insulin sensitivity and metabolic control in patients with type 2 diabetes) was found in four morbidly obese patients, which, when expressed *in vitro*, caused the differentiation of preadipoctyes to adipocytes with greater accumulation of triglyceride (125).

Over 200 genes, markers, and chromosomal regions have been linked or associated to obese phenotypes (124). Highly significant linkage has been found between chromosomal region 11q13, which includes the genes for UCP-2 and UCP-3, and RMR. Linkage to chromosomal region 7q31, which contains the *ob* gene, has been found in six studies; a significant linkage between the MC-4 receptor and obesity has also been reported. As noted above, mutations detected in the MC-4 receptor have led to the identification of subpopulations of morbidly obese patients with a potential genetic basis for their specific phenotype of obesity.

Utilizing five lines of evidence (single-gene mutations, Mendelian disorders, quantitative trait loci from crossbreeding experiments in animals, associaton studies, and linkage analyses), a human obesity gene map has been compiled and is updated each year (124). As of 1999, putative loci affecting obesity-related phenotypes in humans have been found on all but the Y chromosome. Although some of these loci will be proven false-positives and others shown more important than others, these findings illustrate the fact that excess body weight is the result of a complex interaction between many genes.

The rapid progress in molecular genetics could be interpreted to suggest that genes are the sole determinant of the likelihood of excess weight gain. However, the increase in the number of obese in the United States and other industrialized as well as developing nations has occurred much too rapidly to be explained solely by changes in gene expression. What has changed rapidly during the past 100 years is the environment, and it is this influence, acting in combination with certain genes, that is the major determinant of the propensity to gain excess weight. In 1962 Neal proposed the provocative thrifty gene hypothesis, which postulated that humans evolved a complex set of mechanisms to maximize survival during times of food deprivation by favoring the accumulation of fat stores during times in which food was abundant (126). Although this set of genes ensured survival during the early evolution of humans, the thrifty genotype has now become a liability in our current environment in which food is abundant and the energy expended to obtain nutrition much reduced. This environment thus places individuals in a chronic situation of positive energy balance that will ultimately lead to weight gain. While it is difficult to prove or refute this hypothesis, there is increasing epidemiologic and experimental evidence that the environment can have a significant impact on phenotypes. This has led to a field of investigation known as "metabolic imprinting" in which nutritional and other environment influences during the perinatal period have a significant impact on the development or prevention of chronic disease (127, 128).

Several environmental factors promote weight gain (129). The availability of inexpensive, energy-dense food, consumed in larger portions, results in excess nutrient consumption, a trend confirmed by three decades of USDA population surveys (130). Twin studies confirm that even when genetics are identical, environmental influences, such as smoking and family environment, can result in the discordant expression of the obese phenotype (131). Holiday consumption is particularly problematic. Although holiday weight gain actually averages only a pound or so, much lower than the popular belief of 5 to 10 lb, with less than 10% gaining over 5 lb (132), this weight gain tends to be permanent. High-fat diets contribute to excess intake because of the greater energy density of the food and because fat intake does not stimulate fat oxidation (1). As discussed above, low levels of physical activity are associated with an increased risk of weight gain. In the United States technology has largely reduced the requirement of strenuous physical activity for survival and many popular leisure time activities (e,g., television, computer games) also do not require physical exertion. The increase in sedentary activities among children is most troublesome, because this contributes to an earlier onset of positive energy balance, resulting in overweight/obesity at a younger age, and thus increasing the risk of cardiovascular disease and diabetes.

Summary

As more is learned about the genetics of body weight regulation, it is clear that although there is a significant genetic component in the etiology of obesity, the expression of the phenotype requires a genetic-environmental interaction (132, 133). This interaction is quite complex and not all who are genetically inclined to obesity manifest the phenotype, nor do those who make lifestyle choices that should result in manifestation of the phenotype become obese (31). Nevertheless, from a public health perspective, it is likely that the most effective means of addressing obesity is to focus on the environmental factors (increased caloric intake, reduced physical energy expenditure) that promote the development of the disease. Once obesity develops, metabolic forces are established that resist its reversibility.

■ ■ ■

Key Points

- Excess energy intake in combination with reduced physical activity is the most important determinant of weight gain.

- Energy intake and energy expenditure are coordinated within the central nervous system by nuclei in the hypothalamus.

- Leptin is a hormonal signal from the adipose tissue to the central nervous system of the amount of energy stored in the tissue.

- Obesity is a polygenic disorder resulting from the interaction of the environment with many different genes.

- Potential future targets for treatment of obesity include leptin, uncoupling proteins, and the novel peptide neurotransmitters regulating energy intake and energy expenditure within the hypothalamus.

■ ■ ■

REFERENCES

1. **Ravussin E, Swinburn BA.** Energy expenditure and obesity. Diabetes Rev. 1996;4:403-22.

2. **Snitker S, MacDonald I, Ravussin, E, Astrup, A.** The sympathetic nervous system and obesity: role in aetiology and treatment. Obesity Rev. 2000;1:5-15.

3. **Goran MI.** Genetic influences on human energy expenditure and substrate utilization. Behavior Genet. 1997;27:389-99.

4. **Ravussin E, Lillioja S, Knowler WC, et al.** Reduced rate of energy expenditure as a risk factor for body weight gain. N Engl J Med. 1988;318:467-72.

5. **Seidell JC, Muller DC, Sorkin JD, Andres R.** Fasting respiratory exchange ratio and RMR as predictors of weight gain: the Baltimore Longitudinal Study on Aging. Int J Obes. 1992;16:667-74.

6. **Weinsier RL, Nelson KM, Hensrud DD, et al.** Metabolic predictors of obesity: contribution of resting energy expenditure, TEF, and fuel utilization to four-year weight gain of post-obese and never-obese women. J Clin Invest. 1995;95:980-5.

7. **Goran MI, Shewchuk R, Gower BA, et al.** Longitudinal changes in fatness in white children: no effect of childhood energy expenditure. Am J Clin Nutr. 1998;67:309-16.

8. **Stunkard AJ, Berkowitz RI, Stallings VA, Schoeller DA.** Energy intake, not energy output, is a determinant of body size in infants. Am J Clin Nutr. 1999;69:524-30.

9. **Amatruda JM, Statt MC, Welle SL.** Total and resting energy expenditure in obese women reduced to ideal body weight. J Clin Invest. 1993;92:1236-42.

10. **Wyatt H, Grunwald GK, Seagle HM, et al.** Resting energy expenditure in reduced-obese subjects in the National Weight Control Registry. Am J Clin Nutr. 1999;69:1189-93.

11. **Astrup A, Gotzche PC, van de Werken K, et al.** Meta-analysis of resting metabolic rate in formerly obese subjects. Am J Clin Nutr. 1999;69:1117-22.

12. **Hill JO, Wyatt HR.** Relapse in obesity treatment: biology or behavior? Am J Clin Nutr. 1999;69:1064-5.

13. **Schoeller DA.** Recent advances from application of doubly labeled water to measurement of human energy expenditure. J Nutr. 1999;129:1765-8.

14. **Weinsier RL, Hunter GR, Heini AF, et al.** The etiology of obesity: relative contribution of metabolic factors, diet and physical activity. Am J Med. 1998;105:145-50.

15. **Tataranni PA, Larson DE, Snitker S, Ravussin E.** TEF in humans: methods and results from the use of a respiratory chamber. Am J Clin Nutr. 1995;61:1013-9.

16. **Ravussin E, Zawadzki JK.** Thermic effect of glucose in obese subjects with non-insulin-dependent diabetes mellitus. Diabetes. 1987;36:1441-7.

17. **Gumbiner B, Thorburn AW, Henry RR.** Reduced glucose-induced thermogenesis is present in noninsulin-dependent diabetes mellitus without obesity. J Clin Endocrinol Metab. 1991;72:801-7.

18. **Schoeller DA.** Balancing energy expenditure and body weight. Am J Clin Nutr. 1998;68(suppl):956S-961S.

19. **Hunter GR, Weinsier RL, Darnell BE, et al.** Racial differences in energy expenditure and aerobic fitness in premenopausal women. Am J Clin Nutr. 2000;71:500-6.

20. **Zurlo R, Ferraro R, Fontvieille AM, et al.** Spontaneous physical actvity and obesity: cross-sectional and longitudinal studies in Pima Indians. Am J Physiol. 1992:263:E296-E300.

21. **Ballor DL, Harvey-Berino JR, Ades PA, et al.** Decrease in fat oxidation following a meal in weight-reduced individuals: a possible mechanism for weight recidivism. Metabolism. 1996;45:174-8.

22. **Filozof CM, Murua C, Sanchez MP, et al.** Low plasma leptin concentration and low rates of fat oxidation in weight-stable post-obese subjects. Obes Res. 2000;8:205-10.

23. **Larson DE, Ferraro RT, Robertson DS, Ravussin E.** Energy metabolism in weight-stable postobese individuals. Am J Clin Nutr. 1995;62:735-9.

24. **Marra M, Scalfi L, Covino A, et al.** Fasting respiratory quotient as a predictor of weight changes in non-obese women. Int J Obes. 1998;22:601-3.

25. **Ranneries C, Bulow J, Buemann B, et al.** Fat metabolism in formerly obese women. Am J Physiol. 1998;274:E155-E161.

26. **Wyatt H, Grunwald GK, Seagle HM, et al.** Resting energy expenditure in reduced-obese subjects in the National Weight Control Registry. Am J Clin Nutr. 1999;69:1189-93.

27. **Zurlo F, Lillioja S, Puente AE-D, et al.** Low ratio of fat to carbohydrate oxidation as predictor of weight gain: study of 24-h RQ. Am J Physiol. 1990;259:E650-E657.

28. **Ferraro R, Lillioja S, Fontvieille AM, et al.** Lower sedentary metabolic rate in women compared with men. J Clin Invest. 1992;90:780-4.

29. **Weinsier RL, Hunter GR, Zuckerman PA, et al.** Energy expenditure and free-living physical activity in black and white women: comparison before and after weight loss. Am J Clin Nutr. 2000;71:1138-46.

30. **Gannon B, DiPietro L, Poehlman ET.** Do African Americans have lower energy expenditure than Caucasians? Int J Obes. 2000;24:13.

31. **Blundell JE, Cooling J.** Routes to obesity: phenotypes, food choices and activity. Br J Nutr. 2000;83:S33-S38.

32. **Leibel RL, Rosenbaum M, Hirsch J.** Changes in energy expenditure resulting from altered body weight. N Eng J Med. 1995;332:621-8.

33. **Levine JA, Eberhardt NL, Jensen MD.** Role of nonexercise activity thermogenesis in resistance to fat gain in humans. Science. 1999;283:212-4.

34. **Ravussin E, Danforth E Jr.** Beyond sloth: physical activity and weight gain. Science. 1999;283:184-5.

35. **Foster DO, Frydman ML.** Tissue distribution of cold-induced thermogenesis in conscious warm- or cold-acclimated rats reevaluated from changes in tissue blood flow: the dominant role of brown adipose tissue in the replacement of shivering by nonshivering thermogenesis. Can J Physiol Pharmacol. 1979;57:257-70.

36. **Mitchell P.** Keilin's respiratory chain concept and its chemisomotic consequences. Science. 1979;206:1148-59.

37. **Boss O, Hagen T, Lowell BB.** Uncoupling proteins 2 and 3: potential regulators of mitochondrial energy metabolism. Diabetes. 2000;49:143-56.

38. **Schrauwen P, Walder K, Ravussin E.** Human uncoupling proteins and obesity. Obesity Res. 1999;7:97-105.

39. **Lean ME, James Wp, Jennings G, Trayhurn P.** Brown adipose tissue uncoupling protein content in human infants, children and adults. Clin Sci. 1986;71:291-7.

40. **Fleury C, Neverova M, Collins S, et al.** Uncoupling protein-2: a novel gene linked to obesity and hyperinsulinemia. Nature Genet. 1997;15:269-72.

41. **Gimeno RE, Dembski M, Weng X, et al.** Cloning and characterization of an uncoupling protein homolog: a potential molecular mediator of human thermogenesis. Diabetes. 1997;46:900-6.

42. **Richard D, Rivest R, Huang Q, et al.** Distribution of the uncoupling protein-2 mRNA in the mouse brain. J Comp Neuro. 1998;397:549-60.

43. **Boss O, Samec S, Paoloni-Giacobino A, et al.** Uncoupling protein-3: a new member of the mitochondrial carrier family with tissue-specific expression. FEBS Lett. 1997;408:39-42.

44. **Vidal-Puig A, Solanes G, Grujic D, et al.** UCP3: an uncoupling protein homologue expressed preferentially and abundantly in skeletal muscle tissue and brown adipose tissue. Biochem Biophys Res Commun. 1997;235:79-82.

45. **Ricquier D, Bouilland F.** The uncoupling protein homologues: UCP1, UCP2, UCP3, StUCP and AtUCP. Biochem J. 2000;345:161-79.

46. **Gura T.** Uncoupling proteins provide new clue to obesity's causes. Science. 1998;280:1369-70.

47. **Pinkney JH, Boss O, Bray GA, et al.** Physiological relationships of uncoupling protein-2 gene expression in human adipose tissue *in vivo.* J Clin Endocrinol Metab. 2000;85:2312-7.

48. **Khalfallah Y, Fages S, Laville M, et al.** Regulation of uncoupling protein-2 and uncoupling protein-3 mRNA expression during lipid infusion in human skeletal muscle and subcutaneous adipose tissue. Diabetes. 2000;49:25-31.

49. **Schrauwen P, Xia J, Bogardus C, et al.** Skeletal muscle uncoupling protein-3 expression is a determinant of energy expenditure in Pima Indians. Diabetes. 1999;48:146-9.

50. **Flier JS, Maratos-Flier E.** Obesity and the hypothalamus: novel peptides for new pathways. Cell. 1998;92:437-40.

51. **Woods SC, Seeley RJ, Porte D Jr, Schwartz MW.** Signals that regulate food intake and energy homeostasis. Science. 1998;280:1378-83.

52. **Hetherington AW, Ranson SW.** Hypothalamic lesions and adiposity in the rat. Anat Rec. 1940;78:149-72.

53. **Levin BE, Routh VH.** Role of the brain in energy balance and obesity. Am J Physiol. 1996;271:R491-R500.

54. **Elmquist JK, Maratos-Flier E, Saper CB, Flier JS.** Unraveling the central nervous system pathways underlying responses to leptin. Nature Neuroscience. 1998;1:445-50.

55. **Berthoud H-R, Kelly L, Zheng H, Patterson LM.** Gut and brain interactions in the control of food intake and energy metabolism: neural pathways of postingestive satiety signals. In: Nutrition, Genetics and Obesity. Bray GA, Ryan DH, eds., Baton Rouge: Louisiana State Univ Pr; 1999:208-26.

56. **Angel I.** Central receptors and recognition sites mediating the effects of monoamines and anorectic drugs on feeding behavior. Clin Neuropharmacol. 1990;13:361-91.

57. **Leibowitz SF, Alexander JT.** Hypothalamic serotonin in control of eating behavior, meal size, and body weight. Biol Psychiatry. 1998;44:851-64.

58. **Hoebel BG, Hernandez L, Schwartz DH, et al.** Microdialysis studies of brain norepinephrine, serotonin, and dopamine release during ingestive behavior. Ann NY Acad Sci. 1989;575:171-91.

59. **Montjoy KG, Wong J.** Obesity, diabetes and functions for propiomelanocortin-derived peptides. Mol Cell Endocrinol. 1997;128:171-7.

60. **Ollman MM, Wilson BD, Yang YK, et al.** Antagonism of central melanocortin receptors *in vitro* and *in vivo* by agouti-related protein. Science. 1997;278:135-8.

61. **Krude H, et al.** Severe early-onset obesity, adrenal insufficiency and red hair pigmentation caused by POMC mutations in humans. Nat Genet. 1998;19:155-7.

62. **Yeo GS, Farooqi IS, Aminian DJ, et al.** A frameshift mutation in MC4R associated with dominantly inherited human obesity. Nat Genet. 1998;20:111-2.

63. **Vaisse C, Clement K, Guy-Grand B, Froguel P.** A frameshift mutation in human MC4R is associated with a dominant form of obesity. Nat Genet. 1998;20:113-4.

64. **Farooqi IS, Giles SH, Keogh JM, et al.** Dominant and recessive inheritance of morbid obesity associated with melanocortin-4 receptor deficiency. J Clin Invest. 2000;106:271-9.

65. **Vaisse C, Clement K, Durand E, et al.** Melanocortin-4 receptor mutations are frequent and heterogenous cause of morbid obesity. J Clin Invest. 2000;106:253-62.

66. **Walker MW.** NPY and feeding: finding a role for the Y5 receptor subtype. In: Nutrition, Genetics and Obesity. Bray GA, Ryan DH, eds., Baton Rouge: Louisiana State Univ Pr; 1999:287-305.

67. **Elmquist JK, Elias CR, Saper CB.** From lesions to leptin: hypothalamic control of food intake and body weight. Neuron, 1999;22:221-32.

68. **Nahon JL.** The melanin-concentrating hormone: from the peptide to the gene. Crit Rev Neurobiol. 1994;8:221-62.

69. **Sakurai T, Amemiya A, Ishii M, et al.** Orexins and orexin receptors: a family of hypothalamic neuropeptides and G protein-coupled receptors that regulate feeding behavior. Cell. 1998;92:573-5.

70. **de Lecea L, Kilduff TS, Peyron C, et al.** The hypocretins: hypothalamus-specific peptides with neuroexcitatory activity. Proc Nat Acad Sci USA. 1998;95:322-7.

71. **Mohamed-Ali V, Pinkney JH, Coppack SW.** Adipose tissue as an endocrine and paracrine organ. Int J Obes. 1998;22:1145-58.

72. **Zhang Y, Proenca R, Maffei M, et al.** Positional cloning of the mouse obese gene and its human homologue. Nature. 1994;372:425-32.

73. **Friedman JM.** Leptin, leptin receptors, and the control of body weight. Nutr Rev. 1998;56:S38-S46.

74. **Wang J, Liu R, Hawkins M, et al.** A nutrient-sensing pathway regulates leptin gene expression in muscle and fat. Nature. 1998;393:684-8.

75. **Holness MJ, Munns MJ, Sugden MC.** Current concepts concerning the role of leptin in reproductive function. Mol Cell Endocrinol. 1999;157:11-20

76. **Montague CT, Farooqi IS, Whitehead MA, et al.** Congenital leptin deficiency is associated with severe early-onset obesity in humans. Nature. 1997;387:903-8.

77. **Clement K, Vaisse C, Lahlou N, et al.** A mutation in the human leptin receptor gene causes obesity and pituitary dysfunction. Nature. 1998;392:398-401.

78. **Farooqi IS, Jebb SA, Langmack F, et al.** Effects of recombinant leptin therapy in a child with congenital leptin deficiency. N Engl J Med. 1999;341:879-84.

79. **Considine RV, Sinha MK, Heiman ML, et al.** Serum immunoreactive-leptin concentrations in normal weight and obese humans. N Eng J Med. 1996;334:292-5.

80. **Rosenbaum M, Leibel RL.** Role of gonadal steroids in the sexual dimorphisms in body composition and circulating concentrations of leptin. J Clin Endocrinol Metab. 1999;84:1784-9.

81. **Considine RV, Caro JF.** Leptin and the regulation of body weight. Int J Biochem Cell Biol. 1997;29:1255-72.

82. **Guven S, El-Bershawi A, Sonnenberg GE, et al.** Plasma leptin and insulin levels in weight-reduced obese women with normal body mass index: relationships with body composition and insulin. Diabetes. 1999;48:347-52.

83. **Havel PJ, Townsend R, Chaump L, Teff K.** High-fat meals reduce 24-h circulating leptin concentrations in women. Diabetes. 1999;48:334-41.

84. **Havel PJ.** Mechanisms regulating leptin production: implications for control of energy balance. Am J Clin Nutr. 1999;70:305-6.

85. **van Aggel-Leijssen DPC, van Bank MA, Tenenbaum R, et al.** Regulation of average 24 h human plasma leptin level: the influence of exercise and physiological changes in energy balance. Int J Obes. 1999;23:151-8.

86. **Flier JS.** What's in a name? In search of leptin's physiologic role. J Clin Endocrinol Metab. 1998;83:1407-13.

87. **Tartaglia LA.** The leptin receptor. J Biol Chem. 1997;272:6093-6.

88. **Elias CF, Aschkenasi C, Lee C, et al.** Leptin differentially regulates NPY and POMC neurons projecting to the lateral hypothalamic area. Neuron. 1999;23: 775-86.

89. **Arch JRS, Stock MJ, Trayhurn P.** Leptin resistance in obese humans: does it exist and what does it mean? Int J Obes. 1998;22:1159-63.

90. **Caro JF, Kolaczynski JM, Nyce MR, et al.** Decreased cerebrospinal-fluid/serum leptin ratio in obesity. Lancet. 1996;348:159-61.

91. **Heymsfield SB, Greenberg AS, Fujioka K, et al.** Recombinant leptin for weight loss in obese and lean adults: a randomized, controlled, dose-escalation trial. JAMA. 1999;282:1568-75.

92. **Fujioka K, Patane J, Lubina J, Lau D.** CSF leptin levels after exogenous administration of recombinant methionyl human leptin. JAMA. 1999;282:1517-8.

93. **Hileman SM, Pierroz DD, Flier JS.** Leptin, nutrition, and reproduction: timing is everything. J Clin Endocrinol Metab. 2000;85:804-7.

94. **Considine RV, Caro JF.** Pleotropic cellular effects of leptin. Curr Opin Endocrinol Diab. 1999;6:163-9.

95. **Knittle JL, Hirsh J.** Effects of early nutrition on development of rat epididymal fat pads: cellularity and metabolism. J Clin Invest. 1968;47:2091-7.

96. **Hager A, Sjostrom B, Arvidsson B, et al.** Body fat and adipose tissue cellularity in infants: a longitudinal study. Metabolism. 1977;26:607-15.

97. **Knittle JL, Timmers K, Ginsberg-Fellner F, et al.** The growth of adipose tissue in children and adolescents: cross-sectional and longitudinal studies of adipose cell number and size. J Clin Invest. 1979;63:239-45.

98. **Prins JB, O'Rahilly S.** Regulation of adipose cell number in man. Clin Sci. 1997;92:3-11.

99. **Leibel RL, Berry EM, Hirsch J.** Biochemistry and development of adipose tissue in man. In: Health and Obesity. Conn HL, DeFelice EA, Kuo P, eds. New York: Raven Press; 1983;21-48.

100. **Sjostrom L.** Fat cells and body weight. In: Obesity. Stunkard AJ, ed. Philadelphia: WB Saunders; 1980;72-100.

101. **Jensen MD, Kanaley JA, Reed JE, Sheedy PF.** Measurement of abdominal and visceral fat with computed tomagraphy and dual-energy x-ray absorptiometry. Am J Clin Nutr. 1995;61:274-8.

102. **Arner P.** Regional adiposity in man. J Endocrinol. 1997;155:191-2.

103. **Wagner DR, Heyward VH.** Measures of body composition in blacks and whites: a comparative review. Am J Clin Nutr. 2000;71:1392-1402.

104. **Deurenberg P, Yap M, van Staveren WA.** Body mass index and percent body fat: a meta-analysis among different ethnic groups. Int J Obes. 1998;22:1164-71.

105. **Tchernof A, Poehlman ET.** Effects of the menopause transition on body fatness and body fat distribution. Obes Res. 1998;6:246-54.

106. **Samaras K, Campbell LV.** The non-genetic determinants of central adiposity. Int J Obes. 1997;21:839-45.

107. **Larsson B, Svardsudd K, Welin L, et al.** Abdominal adipose tissue distribution, obesity, and risk of cardiovascular disease and death: 13-year follow-up of participants in the study of men born in 1913. BMJ. 1984;288:1401-4.

108. **Lapidus L, Bengtsson C, Larsson B, et al.** Distribution of adipose tissue and risk of cardiovascular disease and death: a 12-year follow-up of participants in the population study of women in Gothenberg, Sweden. BMJ. 1984;289: 1257-61.

109. **Peiris AN, Sothmann MS, Hoffman RG, et al.** Adiposity, fat distribution and cardiovascular risk. Ann Intern Med. 1989;110:867-72.

110. **Large V, Arner P.** Regulation of lipolysis in humans: pathophysiological modulation in obesity, diabetes and hyperlipidaemia. Diabetes Metab. 1998;24:409-18.

111. **Arner P.** Not all fat is alike. Lancet. 1998;351:1301-2.

112. **Imbeault P, Prud'homme D, Tremblay A, et al.** Adipose tissue metabolism in young and middle-aged men after control for total body fatness. J Clin Endocrinol Metab. 2000;85:2462.

113. **Mauriege P, Imbeault P, Prud'homme D, et al.** Subcutaneous adipose tissue metabolism at menopause: importance of body fatness and regional fat distribution. J Clin Endocrinol Metab. 2000;85:2446-2454.

114. **Goodpaster BH, Thaete FL, Kelley DE.** Thigh adipose tissue distribution is associated with insulin resistance in obesity and in type 2 diabetes mellitus. Am J Clin Nutr. 2000;71:885-92.

115. **Kelley DE, Mandarino IJ.** Fuel selection in human skeletal muscle in insulin resistance: a re-examination. Diabetes. 2000;49:677-83.

116. **Comuzzie AG, Allison DB.** The search for human obesity genes. Science. 1998;280:1374-7.

117. **Whitaker RC, Wright JA, Pepe MS, et al.** Predicting obesity in young adulthood from childhood and parental obesity. N Engl J Med. 1997;337:869-73.

118. **Bouchard C.** Obesity in adulthood: the importance of childhood and parental obesity. N Engl J Med. 1997;337:926-7.

119. **Power C, Lake JK, Cole TJ.** Measurement and long-term health risks of child and adolescent fatness. Int J Obes. 1997;21:507-26.

120. **Stunkard AJ, Sorensen TIA, Hanis C, et al.** An adoption study of human obesity. N Engl J Med. 1986;314:193-8.

121. **Bouchard C.** Can obesity be prevented? Nutr Rev. 1996;54:S125-S130.

122. **Bouchard C, Perusse L, Leblanc C, et al.** Inheritance of the amount and distribution of human body fat. Int J Obes. 1988;12:205-15.

123. **Rose KM, Newman B, Mayer-Davis EJ, Selby JV.** Genetic and behavioral determinants of waist-hip ratio and waist circumference in women twins. Obes Res. 1998;6:383-92.

124. **Chagnon YC, Perusse L, Weisnagel SJ, et al.** The human obesity gene map: the 1999 update. Obes Res. 2000;8:89-117.

125. **Ristow M, Muller-Wieland D, Pfeiffer A, et al.** Obesity associated with a mutation in a genetic regulator of adipocyte differentiation. N Engl J Med. 1998;339: 953-9.

126. **Neel JV.** Diabetes mellitus: a "thrifty" genotype rendered detrimental by "progress"? Am J Hum Genet. 1962;14:353-362.

127. **Waterland RA, Garza C.** Potential mechanisms of metabolic imprinting that lead to chronic disease. Am J Clin Nutr. 1999;69:179-97.

128. **Okosun IS, Liao Y, Rotimi CN, et al.** Impact of birth weight on ethnic variations in subcutaneous and central adiposity in American children aged 5-11: a study from the Third National Health and Nutrition Examination Survey. Int J Obes. 2000;24:479-84.

129. **Hill JO, Peters JC.** Environmental contributions to the obesity epidemic. Science. 1998;280:1371-4.

130. **Harnack LJ, Jeffrey RW, Boutelle KN.** Temporal trends in energy intake in the United States: an ecologic perspective. Am J Clin Nutr. 2000;71:1478-84.

131. **Hakala P, Rissanen A, Koskenvuo M, et al.** Environmental factors in the development of obesity in identical twins. Int J Obes. 1999;23:746-53.

132. **Yanovski JA, Yanovski SZ, Sovik KN, et al.** A prospective study of holiday weight gain. N Engl J Med. 2000;342:861-7.

133. **Barsh GS, Farooqi IS, O'Rahilly S.** Genetics of body-weight regulation. Nature. 2000;404:644-51.

KEY REFERENCES

Boss O, Hagen T, Lowell BB. Uncoupling proteins 2 and 3: potential regulators of mitochondrial energy metabolism. Diabetes. 2000;49:143-56.

Excellent review of the novel uncoupling proteins and their role in mitochondrial function and cellular metabolism.

Comuzzie AG, Allison DB. The search for human obesity genes. Science. 1998;280:1374-7.

Explanation of the methods used to study the genetic contribution to the development of obesity with examples of genes implicated in this process.

Elmquist JK, Elias CR, Saper CB. From lesions to leptin: hypothalamic control of food intake and body weight. Neuron. 1999;22:221-32.

Review of the novel peptide neurotransmitters and neural pathways within the hypothalamus regulating food intake and energy expenditure. Excellent discussion of the effect of leptin signalling by these neurotransmitters.

Hill JO, Peters JC. Environmental contributions to the obesity epidemic. Science. 1998;280:1371-4.

Discussion of the role of the environment in the development of obesity.

Ravussin E, Swinburn BA. Energy expenditure and obesity. Diabetes Rev. 1996;4: 403-22.

Discussion of the role of energy expenditure as a determinant of weight gain.

3

Pathophysiology of Obesity and Metabolic Response to Weight Loss

Helmut O. Steinberg, MD
Barry Gumbiner, MD

The onset of obesity in humans is associated with an increase in fat mass, but unlike animal models of obesity there is also an increase in lean body mass, albeit usually disproportionately less than fat mass under usual clinical conditions. With the onset of obesity, a number of metabolic changes occur. However, it is important to note that most studies that purport to determine the effect of weight gain are cross-sectional and/or epidemiological. Thus, these studies only reveal the prevalence of obesity-related metabolic derangements and associations between the parameters measured. Such observations cannot be extrapolated to cause and effect. Likewise, the use of overfeeding studies as a model of weight gain, and weight loss studies as a model for the metabolic reversal of the underlying pathophysiology that led to deleterious effects of weight gain, also must be viewed with the same limitations on the generalizations from their results.

Unfortunately, the few studies that have prospectively assessed the effects of weight gain or weight loss on metabolism and pathophysiology have usually been of limited duration (i.e., weeks or months, not years or decades). Even among longitudinal studies, there are limitations. Among the best long-term studies are those in unique ethnic groups, such as the Pima Indians, that may not be representative of the heterogeneous nature of the disease. Therefore, extrapolation of results of these studies to the overall etiology and pathophysiology of obesity must be viewed with caution.

Effect of Weight Gain on Insulin Action and Secretion

Insulin Resistance

Among the most profound metabolic derangements associated with obesity is insulin resistance. Insulin resistance is the impairment in its metabolic hormone actions on a number of key target tissues, including glucose uptake by skeletal muscle and fat tissue, and suppression of hepatic glucose production under fasting and postprandial conditions (1). This condition is mirrored by an opposite metabolic state in which tissues are responsive to insulin, the insulin-sensitive state.

Insulin (hormone) action and the degree of resistance or sensitivity to insulin can be measured in humans using a specialized research technique, the glucose clamp method, which determines the rate at which the body takes up glucose under controlled conditions (2). Under physiological conditions (e.g., mixed meals), it can be inferred that insulin resistance is present when there are high plasma insulin levels relative to the ambient glucose level; that is, there is decreased hormonal action of insulin so more insulin is required to maintain normal glucose homeostasis. Finally, while the focus of insulin resistance has been on the impact on glucose metabolism, recent research indicates other hormone actions of insulin are also impaired, fat metabolism being among the most important from a medical perspective (1, 3-6). (The interaction of insulin with glucose and fat metabolism is discussed below in more detail.)

Although most obese people are insulin resistant, some are relatively insulin sensitive. Moreover, insulin resistance can be observed even in lean subjects and is associated with the same metabolic perturbations, cardiovascular risk, and morbidity and mortality observed in obese individuals who are insulin resistant (7, 8). How weight gain may induce insulin resistance is not well understood but, because insulin resistance can occur in nonobese persons, it is not simply due to an overall increase in fat mass. Thus, studies trying to reproduce conditions leading to obesity do not always result in the onset of insulin resistance, despite weight gain. Overfeeding test subjects for two to six weeks, despite average weight gains of nearly 10 lb, did not induce insulin resistance as determined by the glucose clamp technique (9-11). Overfeeding subjects for 100 days, however, which caused average weight gains of 17 lb and an increase in body fat mass of 12 lb, resulted in a measurable decrease of insulin-mediated glucose uptake (12).

One reason why obesity is not a necessary requirement for insulin resistance is because it may occur in subjects with stable weight who over time replace muscle with fat tissue (7, 13, 14). Thus, body composition, independent of weight, is a significant determinant of insulin sensitivity. Just as important as absolute fat mass is fat distribution (i.e., abdominal versus peripheral fat). Predominance of abdominal and, most likely, visceral (intraabdominal) accumulation of fat represents the male pattern of obesity, whereas peripheral fat accumulation is the typical female pattern (15-18). More importantly, male-type obesity can also occur in women and is associated with insulin resistance, which in turn is associated with increased rates of cardiovascular morbidity and mortality. In contrast, female-type obesity, which occurs infrequently in men, is metabolically and medically intermediate between abdominal obesity and the nonobese state, thus having a lesser effect on cardiovascular risk. Mechanistically, this has been confirmed in studies demonstrating that females are more insulin sensitive even though they exhibit higher degrees of obesity (19). A predominance of abdominal fat distribution can occur in nonobese individuals; thus even the nonobese state can be associated with insulin resistance (7). This is of particular concern in nonwhites in whom overt obesity may not be present and can lead to serious health outcomes (e.g., type 2 diabetes) (20).

Insulin Secretion

Insulin levels are often increased in obesity (8). It is thought that fasting insulin levels are elevated to constrain hepatic glucose output, particularly in the fasting state, to maintain fasting plasma glucose levels in the normal range. The hyperinsulinemia is mainly due to increased rates of pancreatic insulin secretion, and less so to decreased metabolic clearance of the liver or, more specifically, to decreased insulin extraction by the liver (21). Most investigators believe hypersecretion of insulin and the resultant hyperinsulinemia are compensatory responses to insulin resistance, independent of obesity (because insulin resistance can occur in nonobese individuals). However, studies have yet to prove this or determine the underlying mechanisms by which obesity, and insulin resistance in general, causes fasting insulin levels to increase.

Some studies report that acute elevation of plasma free fatty acid (FFA) levels in normal subjects causes increased fasting plasma insulin levels. A direct effect of FFA to stimulate insulin secretion has also been demonstrated in the isolated perfused pancreas (22). Because FFAs are elevated in obese individuals (23), FFAs could be a metabolic link between insulin resistance and insulin secretion. However, it is unknown whether insulin secretion is elevated during prolonged FFA elevation in normal subjects under experimental or naturally occurring conditions.

Interestingly, in a longitudinal study of middle-aged whites, continuing weight gain was not associated with further increases in fasting plasma insulin levels, which indicates that the relationship between weight and basal insulin secretion is not linear (23a). In contrast to fasting plasma insulin levels, plasma insulin levels in response to glucose challenge were found to be strongly and positively associated with changes in weight. This positive relationship was only seen in subjects with normal glucose tolerance. In subjects with impaired glucose tolerance, there was a strongly negative relationship between increments in weight gain and changes in insulin levels. In other words, weight gain in subjects with impaired glucose tolerance leads to further impairment of insulin secretion. The implications are significant because these data suggest that this situation may eventually lead to diabetes.

Even more intriguing are longitudinal studies suggesting that the development of insulin resistance in association with weight gain may retard further weight gain. In a study of Pima Indians followed over ~3.5 years, it was found that those who were most insulin sensitive gained more weight than those who were insulin resistant (24). This is in contrast to the widely held belief that insulin resistance promotes obesity, a misconception extrapolated from cross-sectional studies. This is another example of the need for prospective studies to determine the natural history of a disease. This observation also strongly questions the contention of popular diet plans that ignore these data, claim hyperinsulinemia as the driving force for obesity rather than a consequence of insulin resistance, and extrapolate a narrow perspective on research into an entire therapy.

Obesity-Related Effects on Glucose and Fat Metabolism

Insulin regulates lipolysis (fat breakdown), hepatic glucose production, and skeletal muscle glucose uptake (17). Research has demonstrated that insulin has direct effects on the vascular system where it modulates skeletal muscle blood flow, cardiac output (25), and sympathetic nervous system activity (26). Thus, insulin has a central role in metabolism and a pivotal role in obesity-related illness.

Insulin regulates the release of FFA from adipose cells that serve as fuel between meals and under other conditions of energy restriction intake (17). FFA levels are elevated in obesity, particularly in people with abdominal obesity (15). The elevation of FFA could be due to impaired insulin action (insulin resistance) on adipose cells that constrain release of FFA; conversely, it could be due to increased stimuli that release FFA, as can be seen with epinephrine or norepinephrine, or decreased clearance (17). However, despite a plethora of studies, the mechanistic relationship between the etiology and pathophysiology of obesity and increased FFA levels is not well understood. Moreover, no data are available that directly assess the effect of short- or long-term weight gain on systemic circulating FFA levels.

FFA levels are not only increased in obesity under basal (fasting) conditions but fail to suppress normally in response to insulin. This failure to suppress FFA release is more severe in subjects with visceral obesity than in subjects with peripheral obesity (27). The failure to suppress FFA in response to insulin is also associated with higher diastolic blood pressure in obese hypertensive subjects (27).

Insulin is one of the most important regulators of hepatic glucose production, which under fasting conditions correlates with fasting plasma glucose levels (28). Hepatic glucose production, under fasting conditions, appears to be normal during prolonged periods of weight gain. Maintaining normal glucose production with weight gain is achieved by increasing insulin secretion, which suggests hepatic resistance to the hormone action of insulin. However, in those predisposed to type 2 diabetes, hepatic glucose production increases, which indicates increased resistance to insulin hormone action on the liver and/or progressive beta-cell failure to adequately compensate for excess glucose production by the liver (29, 30). The mechanism by which obesity induces the hepatic insulin resistance associated with type 2 diabetes is unknown. Increased circulating FFA levels may contribute to the hepatic resistance through a variety of metabolic influences, but other modulators, such as high glucagon levels, are also important. Obesity contributes to the development of these metabolic derangements and makes diabetes more metabolically resistant to treatment (30-33).

Insulin regulates glucose uptake into skeletal muscle (1, 28). Insulin-mediated glucose uptake decreases with significant weight gain (24, 30). However, as noted above, the decrease in insulin-mediated glucose uptake longitudinally with weight gain may be protective against further weight gain, thus suggesting that insulin resistance is an adaptive mechanism to attempt to maintain energy homeostasis. Although there are numerous studies describing the changes in molecular and cellular physiology associated with insulin resistance, the mechanism by which weight gain impairs insulin action at the level of the skeletal muscle is not understood. Elevated systemic circulating FFA levels may make a significant contribution to skeletal muscle insulin resistance (1, 2, 4, 17, 23, 28).

During euglycemic hyperinsulinemia, insulin increases skeletal muscle blood flow in a dose-dependent fashion in lean, insulin-sensitive subjects (34). This insulin effect on blood flow is impaired in obese insulin-resistant subjects, and obese subjects require much higher insulin concentrations to achieve equivalent blood flow responses (34). The normal increase in insulin-mediated elevation of skeletal muscle blood flow is associated with increased cardiac output and a small but significant drop in blood pressure, which indicates a profound decrease in skeletal muscle vasculature resistance (35). Obese subjects, however, do not exhibit this response (36). The effect of insulin to increase skeletal muscle blood flow is mediated via the release of endothelial nitric oxide (NO) (37, 38); this effect is impaired in obesity (36). Together, these data suggest that insulin exerts a well-orchestrated effect on the cardiovascular system, which is geared towards delivering substrate to the skeletal muscle, and that this hemodynamic effect is impaired by obesity.

No prospective studies have evaluated the effect of weight gain on endothelial function. However, it appears reasonable to speculate that weight gain with concomitant insulin resistance will result in defective endothelial function. Because FFAs are elevated in obesity and acute elevation of FFA has been associated with the induction of insulin resistance in normal subjects (4), FFAs have also been implicated in endothelial dysfunction in obesity (39). Other factors such as elevated endothelin levels or elevated sympathetic nervous system activity may also be involved in the development of endothelial dysfunction.

It is important to emphasize that the aforementioned metabolic and hemodynamic changes may have a profound impact on health, particularly on the development of cardiovascular disease. The clustering of metabolic changes in obesity/insulin resistance has been termed *Syndrome X, insulin resistance syndrome, metabolic syndrome*, and *dysmetabolic syndrome* (5). Subjects with the insulin resistance syndrome not only have impaired insulin action but frequently exhibit dyslipidemia characterized by higher triglyceride and lower HDL cholesterol levels. This is in fact a significant clinical sign of insulin resistance—the inability of insulin to suppress fat metabolism—as manifested by hypertriglyceridemia (1, 2, 4-6). Moreover, the LDL-cholesterol is smaller, denser, and more susceptible to oxidation, all characteristics associated with more atherogenic particles (1, 40). Subjects with the insulin resistance syndrome also have abnormalities in the clotting system with increased plasminogen inhibitor 1 (PAI1) and von Willebrand factor (6).

Simple regression analysis indicates a strong inverse relationship between these measures of obesity and endothelial function, which suggests that endothelial function worsens with each increment in obesity (36). Moreover, because waist circumference is the strongest predictor in males, fat distribution (peripheral versus central) may modulate the effect of fat accumulation on endothelial function. This could, in part, explain why patients with the male fat distribution pattern suffer from higher rates of cardiovascular disease.

Effect of Weight Gain on Other Hormones

Thyroid Hormone

The thyroid hormone is known to directly affect metabolism. However, a significant role of thyroid hormone in the development of obesity has yet to be established. In a study that measured basal metabolic rate to diagnose hypothyroidism, less than half of the 200 subjects were overweight and edema was a significant component of weight gain (41). Three weeks' overfeeding with a weight gain of 4.3 kg in a group of females resulted in a small decline in triiodothyronine (T3) levels (42). Similarly, no differences in thyroid hormone levels were found in a group of females who gained 5 kg over one year when compared with controls. Conversely, other studies showed an increase in T3 levels in response to short-term (14 to 25 days) overfeeding (43). In one other study, three weeks of overfeeding in a group of adult males also caused an increase in T3 levels (44). This was associated with higher-than-predicted calorie requirements to maintain the weight gain. However, the T3 levels were found to be normal after seven months of continued overfeeding. T4 and free T4 levels did not change in response overfeeding over a 100-day period (43). A recent study demonstrated that overfeeding in obese individuals has a similar effect on T3, indicating similar responses occur in obese and nonobese individuals independent of weight status (45). Taken together, these data suggest that the thyroid hormone is not a prime regulator of body mass, overfeeding-induced increments in T3 are probably an adaptive response, and these changes are likely to be insufficient or too short-lived to counteract weight gain.

Pituitary-Adrenal Axis

It has been shown by several studies that obesity is associated with elevated urinary cortisol secretion rates (46). However, after correcting for urinary creatinine excretion, differences between lean and obese subjects were not detectable (47). These data suggest that the higher cortisol excretion is a consequence of greater lean body mass and not due to dysregulation of the cortisol production. That cortisol is unlikely to play a major role in the development of obesity is underscored by a study in Pima Indians (48), who exhibit extremely high risk for development of obesity and diabetes. This study found no differences in fasting plasma ACTH levels and 24-hour urine free cortisol between age- and weight-matched Pima Indians and whites.

Recently, it has been reported that plasma aldosterone levels correlate strongly with visceral obesity as well as with blood pressure levels (49, 50). Together with observations that certain fatty acids stimulate aldosterone production in adrenal cells (51), these data suggest that increased obesity, especially with increased visceral fat mass, may modulate aldosterone production. The effect of weight gain on ACTH, cortisol, and aldosterone levels remains to be elucidated.

Sex Hormones

Overfeeding for three weeks, which resulted in a 4.3 kg weight gain, was associated with an increase in testosterone levels (42). However, testosterone levels fell after prolonged overfeeding as shown in the Quebec overfeeding study (52). This was accompanied by a proportional decrease in sex hormone binding protein which indicated that free testosterone levels, the bioactive form of the hormone, will remain relatively normal. Therefore, it is unlikely that typical cases of weight gain result in problems with the hypothalamic-pituitary-gonadal axis unless other problems, such as polycystic ovarian syndrome, are present.

Growth Hormone

Growth hormone (GH) secretion, both under native conditions and in response to secretagogues, is significantly impaired in obesity (53). However, insulin-like growth factor (IGF1) plasma levels—the mediator of GH action—and the related GH and IGF binding proteins are elevated in obesity. Although GH is important for normal growth, little is known about the effect of weight gain associated with obesity on GH secretion or levels. One study that assessed IGF1 levels, which are induced by GH secretion and provide a more integrated measurement of GH, demonstrated an increase in IGF levels after three weeks of overfeeding. However, the higher IGF1 levels may only represent a short-term response to the overfeeding because obesity is associated with decreased GH levels under basal and stimulated conditions (54, 55). The mechanism for the decrease in GH levels is not known. However, metabolic clearance of GH is increased in obesity, which may contribute to the lower plasma levels and is unrelated to regional body fat distribution unlike many of the abnormalities associated with obesity (56). The role of GH in the etiology and pathophysiology of obesity remains to be determined, but the foregoing studies may be interpreted as a compensatory or adaptive response to the obese state rather than as its cause (53).

Effect of Weight Loss on Insulin Action and Secretion

Obesity alters insulin secretion and action and a number of other hormonal systems that are associated with increased cardiovascular disease. The question arises as to whether weight loss will reverse or at least ameliorate these metabolic disturbances and, in turn, contribute to improved health outcomes.

Insulin Action

Data on the effect of weight loss on hepatic glucose production in simple obesity are scarce. One study reports that suppression of hepatic glucose production was not improved after ~20% weight loss (57). However, studies from obese type 2 diabetic subjects demonstrate quite clearly that this more severe condition of hepatic glucose output decreases with calorie restriction and weight loss, and that this effect occurs rapidly, within the first week of weight loss (58).

Weight loss induces an improvement in skeletal muscle glucose uptake in response to insulin. A ~35% increase from baseline was reported in a group of males after reducing an initial BMI from 37 to 31 (57). Even smaller reductions in weight improve insulin-mediated glucose uptake (59). In obese patients without diabetes, insulin sensitivity can normalize (60), but this does not occur in obese patients with diabetes, even with weight loss to levels of nonobese patients (61).

Some data suggest that the improvement in insulin action associated with weight loss is linked primarily to the reduction in visceral (intra-abdominal) adipose tissue. In rats, selective surgical removal of visceral fat with change in overall body fat resulted in improved hepatic insulin sensitivity and the associated derangements in key enzymes and gene expression of hepatic, as well as whole body, glucose metabolism (e.g., decreased hyperinsulinemia, PEPCK, glucose-6-phosphatase, leptin, and TNF mRNA, IGF binding protein-1) (62). Although comparable techniques are not available in humans, studies that precisely measure changes in total and regional body composition and fat distribution demonstrate that insulin action and related biomarkers correlate more strongly with intra-abdominal fat reduction than with whole-body decreases in adiposity (63, 64). Most (65) but not all (66) studies suggest, however, that there is not a selective decrease in abdominal obesity with weight loss, and no treatments yet exist that can focus only on this depot. More importantly, all data suggest that liposuction or surgical removal of subcutaneous fat (e.g., "tummy tuck") should have less significant medical benefits than a comprehensive weight management approach.

FFA levels decrease in response to weight loss (67). Furthermore, weight loss is associated with improved insulin-mediated suppression of FFA oxidation in skeletal muscle (68). Interestingly, FFA levels fall in insulin-resistant obese subjects in response to insulin sensitizing agents, such as thiazolidinedione (TZD) troglitazone, even though weight does not decrease and often increases (69). Therefore, these data suggest that decrease of fat mass, particularly visceral fat mass, may simply serve as a modality by which FFAs decrease and attenuate insulin resistance.

The effect of weight loss on the hemodynamic effects of insulin has not been evaluated.

Insulin Secretion

Given the important role of insulin in the pathophysiology of hyperglycemia, it is not surprising that most studies of the effect of weight loss on insulin secretion have been performed in obese type 2 diabetic subjects

(70-72). Weight loss of at least 10% resulted in decreased fasting insulin levels and improved insulin secretion to various stimuli (73). Ninety percent of the improvement can be accrued within three weeks of a very low calorie diet and occurs out of proportion to the degree of weight loss, which suggests caloric and/carbohydrate restriction rather than weight loss *per se* is the major determinant of the pancreatic response to weight loss (58, 74). The mechanism by which pancreas function improves is unknown, but it is probably related to less pancreatic stimulation due to decreased exposure to carbohydrates, improved insulin sensitivity during weight loss, and decreased FFA levels after achieving a new baseline, all of which reduce "stress" on pancreatic function.

Effect of Weight Loss on Other Hormones

Thyroid Hormone

Numerous studies have demonstrated that thyroid hormone levels change in response to acute weight loss. Total T3 and T4 levels decrease, reverse T3 increases, but free T4, the bioactive form of the hormone, and TSH levels remain unchanged (44, 75). After weight stabilization, T3 and T4 levels normalize. Only free T3 levels remain slightly lower compared with the basal levels. Similar to the response to weight gain, these changes are probably a compensatory or adaptive response to change in body weight.

Hypothalamic-Pituitary-Adrenal Axis

Because no significant effect of weight gain on cortisol or ACTH levels has been observed, it is not surprising that weight loss has no effect on either. Induction of nearly 50% weight loss in morbidly obese subjects did not cause any alterations in serum cortisol levels (76). Another study showed a decrease in 24-hour free cortisol levels during hypocaloric feeding, which returned to basal levels after weight stabilized (77). One study demonstrated a decrease in total plasma cortisol, and cortisol-binding globulin resulted in no change in bioactive-free hormone levels or in the response of corticotropin-releasing hormone, again suggesting that there is no significant dysregulation of the hypothalamic-pituitary-adrenal axis associated with obesity and that any changes that occur are adaptive rather than etiologic (78).

Sex Hormones

Weight loss attenuates obesity-induced abnormalities in sex hormones. In men, significant increases in testosterone, free testosterone, and dehydroepiandrosterone sulfate have been observed (77). The effect of weight loss on gonadotropins and sex-hormone binding globulin (SHBG) is less clear. Gonadotropins and SHBG values remained unaltered in one study (77) but increased in others (79, 80). In women, weight loss was associated with significant decreases in estradiol and total and free testosterone and an increase in FSH and SHBG.

Growth Hormone

A number of studies have demonstrated that weight loss normalizes the abnormalities in secretion of GH (53). Because of the anabolic effects of GH and IGF1, small clinical trials have been conducted to determine whether administering either during weight loss can attenuate the loss of lean body mass during weight loss. Although in the short-term this may occur, it appears tolerance develops and eventually lean body mass decreases to levels equal to those for subjects treated with weight-reducing diets alone (53).

Clinical Outcomes

The impact of weight gain, sustained obesity, and weight loss on clinical parameters and health outcomes is reviewed throughout the text and thus only an overview is provided here. Although many of these outcomes are related to the underlying pathophysiology of obesity described earlier, cause-and-effect relationships remain to be elucidated. There is a clear relationship between weight gain and the development of major metabolic diseases associated with obesity (i.e., type 2 diabetes, hypertension, hyperlipidema), all of which contribute to the major cause of mortality associated with obesity, cardiovascular disease (see Chapter 1). Weight loss improves all the major biomarkers associated with these co-morbidities (Table 3.1) (81, 82). However, results are highly variable and in part depend on the severity of the underlying co-morbidity, fat distribution, macronutrient composition of the diet, and genetic contributions to the disease. Thus, some individuals are below-average metabolic responders to

Table 3.1   Improvements in the Major Biomarkers Associated with Hypertension, Type 2 Diabetes, and Hyperlipidemia

Hypertension	−2.5 mm Hg systolic/kg
	−1.7 mm Hg diastolic/kg
Type 2 diabetes	$HbA1_c = 0.13\ (-kg) + 0.51$
Hyperlipidemia	−1.9 mg/dL cholesterol/kg
	−0.8 mg/dL LDL/kg
	−1.3 mg/dL triglycerides/kg

weight loss, may not achieve significant improvement in these parameters, and continue to require medication. In general, even with a poor metabolic response, it is believed that weight control helps slow the progression of the disease and makes individuals more responsive to medications for treatment of these problems.

Unfortunately, few reliable predictors of response are known and large-scale studies to identify or verify the determinants for responders have yet to be performed. Moreover, as noted throughout the text, whether these improvements in biomarkers can be extrapolated to better health outcomes is unknown. A recent study demonstrated normalization of the progression of carotid artery atherosclerosis, as measured by intima-media thickness during a four-year prospective trial, compared with the accelerated progression in obese control patients (83).

Summary

Obesity affects numerous metabolic and hormonal systems. Although the full extent to which obesity and weight gain influence the different hormonal and metabolic systems remains to be elucidated, it is believed that the greatest negative impact occurs at the level of the insulin-sensitive tissues. Weight loss attenuates many of these abnormalities. It is reasonable to speculate that successful weight loss will prevent or delay the onset of severe complications while awaiting definitive health outcome studies to prove that sustained weight loss decreases morbidity and mortality from obesity. It is hoped that the NIH multicenter weight loss trial now underway will provide more definitive answers on health outcomes (81).

■   ▩   ▩

Key Points

- One of the most significant metabolic conditions associated with obesity is insulin resistance, which causes not only derangements in glucose metabolism but impairment of other hormone actions such as fat metabolism.

- In contrast to the widely held belief that insulin resistance promotes obesity, some longitudinal studies have suggested that the insulin resistance that develops with weight gain may actually be protective of further weight gain. These findings highlight the need for further prospective studies.

- In persons with impaired glucose tolerance, weight gain results in further impairment of insulin secretion, which in turn may eventually lead to diabetes in those predisposed.

- Plasma free fatty acid levels are elevated in persons with obesity; however, the etiology of this association is not well understood.

- Endothelial function worsens with increasing obesity. Among other factors, elevated levels of free fatty acids have been implicated as a cause of endothelial dysfunction.

- Weight loss has been found to result in improved insulin action and secretion and decreased free fatty acid levels.

■   ▓   ▒

REFERENCES

1. **American Diabetes Association.** Consensus development conference on insulin resistance. Diabetes Care. 1998;21:310-4.

2. **DeFronzo RA, Tobin JD, Andres R.** Glucose clamp technique: a method for quantifying insulin secretion and resistance. Am J Physiol. 1979;237:E14-23.

3. **Roden M, Price TB, Perseghin G, et al.** Mechanism of free fatty acid-induced insulin resistance in humans. J Clin Invest. 1996;97:2859-65.

4. **Boden G.** Role of fatty acids in the pathogenesis of insulin resistance and NIDDM. Diabetes. 1997;46:3-10.

5. **Reaven GM.** Role of insulin resistance in human disease. Diabetes.1988;37:1595-607.

6. **Reaven GM.** Syndrome X: 6 years later. J Intern Med. 1994;236:13-22.

7. **Ruderman N, Chisholm D, Pi-Sunyer X, Schneider S.** The metabolically obese, normal-weight individual revisited. Diabetes. 1998; 47:699-713.

8. **Reaven GM, Moore J, Greenfield M.** Quantification of insulin secretion and in vivo insulin action in nonobese and moderately obese individuals with normal glucose tolerance. Diabetes. 1983;32:600-4.

9. **Ohannesian JP, Marco CC, Najm PS, et al.** Small weight gain is not associated with development of insulin resistance in healthy, physically active individuals. Horm Metab Res. 1999;31:323-5.

10. **Bouchard C, Tremblay A, Despres JP, et al.** Sensitivity to overfeeding: the Quebec experiment with identical twins. Prog Food Nutr Sci. 1988;12:45-72.

11. **Ogburn PL Jr, Kitzmiller JL, Hare JW, et al.** Pregnancy following renal transplantation in class T diabetes mellitus. JAMA. 1986;255:911-5.

12. **Oppert JM, Nadeau A, Tremblay A, et al.** Plasma glucose, insulin, and glucagon before and after long-term overfeeding in identical twins. Metabolism. 1995;44:96-105.

13. **Imbeault P, Prud'homme D, Tremblay A, et al.** Adipose tissue metabolism in young and middle-aged men after control for total body fatness. J Clin Endocrinol Metab. 2000;85:2455-62.

14. **Gallagher D, Ruts E, Visser M, et al.** Weight stability masks sarcopenia in elderly men and women. Am J Physiol Endocrinol Metab. 2000;279:E366-75.

15. **Arner P.** Regional adiposity in man. J Endocrinol. 1997;155:191-2.

16. **Peiris AN, Sothmann MS, Hoffman RG, et al.** Adiposity, fat distribution and cardiovascular risk. Ann Intern Med. 1989;110:867-72.

17. **Large V, Arner P.** Regulation of lipolysis in humans: pathophysiological modulation in obesity, diabetes and hyperlipidaemia. Diabetes Metab. 1998;24:409-18.

18. **Arner P.** Not all fat is alike. Lancet. 1998;351:1301-2.

19. **Yki-Jarvinen H.** Sex and insulin sensitivity. Metabolism. 1984;33:1011-5.

20. **Samaras K, Campbell LV.** Increasing incidence of type 2 diabetes in the third millennium: is abdominal fat the central issue? Diabetes Care. 2000;23:441-2.

21. **Polonsky KS, Given BD, Hirsch L, et al.** Quantitative study of insulin secretion and clearance in normal and obese subjects. J Clin Invest. 1988;81:435-41.

22. **Dobbins RL, Chester MW, Stevenson BE, et al.** A fatty acid dependent step is critically important for both glucose- and non-glucose-stimulated insulin secretion. J Clin Invest. 1998;101:2370-6.

23. **Boden G.** Fatty acids and insulin resistance. Diabetes Care. 1996;19:394-5.

23a. **Lemieux S, Prud'homme D, Nadeau A, et al.** Seven-year changes in body fat and visceral adipose tissue in women: association with indexes of plasma glucose-insulin homeostasis. Diabetes Care. 1996;19:983-91.

24. **Swinburn BA, Nyomba BL, Saad MF, et al.** Insulin resistance associated with lower rates of weight gain in Pima Indians. J Clin Invest. 1991;88:168-73.

25. **Baron AD, Brechtel-Hook G, Johnson A, et al.** Skeletal muscle blood flow: a possible link between insulin resistance and blood pressure. Hypertension. 1993;21:129-35.

26. **Scherrer U, Randin D, Tappy L, et al.** Body fat and sympathetic nerve activity in healthy subjects. Circulation. 1994;89:2634-40.

27. **Egan BM, Hennes MM, Stepniakowski KT, et al.** Obesity hypertension is related more to insulin's fatty acid than glucose action. Hypertension. 1996; 27:723-8.

28. **Olefsky JM, Molina JM.** Insulin resistance in man. In: Ellenberg and Rifkin's Diabetes Mellitus: Theory and Practice. Rifkin H, Porte D, eds. New York: Elsevier; 1990:121-54.

29. **Cahill GF Jr.** Beta-cell deficiency, insulin resistance, or both? N Engl J Med. 1988;318:1268-9.

30. **Weyer C, Bogardus C, Mott DM, Pratley RE.** The natural history of insulin secretroy dysfunction and insulin resistance in the pathogenesis of type 2 diabetes mellitus. J Clin Invest. 1999;104:787-94.

31. **Chung JW, Suh K, Joyce M, et al.** Contribution of obesity to defects of intracellular glucose metabolism in NIDDM. Diabetes Care. 1995;18:666-73.

32. **Perriello G, Misericordia P, Volpi E, et al.** Contribution of obesity to insulin resistance in noninsulin-dependent diabetes mellitus. J Clin Endocrinol Metab. 1995; 80:2464-9.

33. **Yki-Jarvinen H, Ryysy L, Kauppila M, et al.** Effect of obesity on the response to insulin therapy in noninsulin-dependent diabetes mellitus. J Clin Endocrinol Metab. 1997;82:4037-43.

34. **Laakso M, Edelman SV, Brechtel G, et al.** Decreased effect of insulin to stimulate skeletal muscle blood flow in obese men. J Clin Invest. 1990;85:1844-52.

35. **Baron AD, Brechtel G.** Insulin differentially regulates systemic and skeletal muscle vascular resistance. Am J Physiol. 1993;265:E61-7.

36. **Steinberg HO, Chaker H, Leaming R, et al.** Obesity/insulin resistance is associated with endothelial dysfunction: implications for the syndrome of insulin resistance. J Clin Invest. 1996;97:2601-10.

37. **Scherrer U, Randin D, Vollenweider L, et al.** Nitric oxide release accounts for insulin's vascular effects in humans. J Clin Invest. 1994;94:2511-5.

38. **Steinberg HO, Brechtel G, Johnson A, et al.** Insulin-mediated skeletal muscle vasodilation is nitric oxide dependent. J Clin Invest. 1994;94:1172-9.

39. **Steinberg HO, Paradisi G, Hook G, et al.** Free fatty acid elevation impairs insulin-mediated vasodilation and nitric oxide production. Diabetes. 2000;49:1231-8.

40. **Reaven GM, Chen Y-DI, Jeppesen J, et al.** Insulin resistance and hyperinsulinemia in individuals with small, dense, low density lipoprotein particles. J Clin Invest. 1993;92:141-6.

41. **Plummer WA.** Body weight in spontaneous myxedema. Trans Am Assoc Study Goiter. 1940;88-98.

42. **Forbes GB, Brown MR, Welle SL, Underwood LE.** Hormonal response to overfeeding. Am J Clin Nutr. 1989;49:608-11.

43. **Oppert JM, Dussault JH, Tremblay A, et al.** Thyroid hormones and thyrotropin variations during long term overfeeding in identical twins. J Clin Endocrinol Metab. 1994;79:547-53 [erratum in J Clin Endocrinol Metab. 1994;79:1810].

44. **Danforth E Jr, Horton ES, O'Connell M, et al.** Dietary-induced alterations in thyroid hormone metabolism during overnutrition. J Clin Invest. 1979;64:1336-47.

45. **Rosenbaum M, Hirsch J, Murphy E, Leibel RL.** Effects of changes in body weight on carbohydrate metabolism, catecholamine excretion, and thyroid function. Am J Clin Nutr. 2000;71:1421-32.

46. **Bjorntorp P.** Endocrine abnormalities of obesity. Metabolism. 1995;44(suppl 3):21-3.

47. **Strain GW, Zumoff B, Strain JJ, et al.** Cortisol production in obesity. Metabolism. 1980;29:980-5.

48. **Tataranni PA, Cizza G, Snitker S, et al.** Hypothalamic-pituitary-adrenal axis and sympathetic nervous system activities in Pima Indians and Caucasians. Metabolism. 1999;48:395-9.

49. **Goodfriend TL, Egan BM, Kelley DE.** Plasma aldosterone, plasma lipoproteins, obesity and insulin resistance in humans. Prostaglandins Leukot Essent Fatty Acids. 1999;60:401-5.

50. **Goodfriend TL, Kelley DE, Goodpaster BH, Winters SJ.** Visceral obesity and insulin resistance are associated with plasma aldosterone levels in women. Obes Res. 1999;7:355-62.

51. **Goodfriend TL, Egan BM, Kelley DE.** Aldosterone in obesity. Endocr Res. 1998;24:789-96.

52. **Pritchard J, Despres JP, Gagnon J, et al.** Plasma adrenal, gonadal, and conjugated steroids before and after long-term overfeeding in identical twins. J Clin Endocrinol Metab. 1998;83:3277-84.

53. **Scacchi M, Pincelli AI, Cavagini F.** Growth hormone in obesity. Int J Obes. 1999;23:260-71.

54. **Maccario M, Gauna C, Procopio M, et al.** Assessment of GH/IGF-I axis in obesity by evaluation of IGF-I levels and the GH response to GHRH+arginine test. J Endocrinol Invest. 1999;22:424-9.

55. **Kanaley JA, Weatherup-Dentes MM, Jaynes EB, Hartman ML.** Obesity attenuates the growth hormone response to exercise. J Clin Endocrinol Metab. 1999;84:3156-61.

56. **Langendonk JG, Meinders AE, Burggraaf J, et al.** Influence of obesity and body fat distribution on growth hormone kinetics in humans. Am J Physiol. 1999;277:E824-9.

57. **Webber J, Donaldson M, Allison SP.** The effects of weight loss in obese subjects on thermogenic, metabloic, and haemodynamic responses to the glucose clamp. Int J Obes Relat Metab Disord. 1994;18:725-30.

58. **Kelley DE, Wing R, Buonocore C, et al.** Relative effects of calorie restriction and weight loss in noninsulin-dependent diabetes mellitus. J Clin Endocrinol Metab. 1993;77:1287-93.

59. **Ross R, Dagnone D, Jones PJ, et al.** Reduction in obesity and related comorbid conditions after diet-induced weight loss or exercise-induced weight loss in men: a randomized, controlled trial. Ann Intern Med. 2000;133:92-103.

60. **Welle S, Statt M, Barnard R, Amatruda J.** Differential effect of insulin on whole-body proteolysis and glucose metabolism in normal-weight, obese, and reduced-obese women. Metabolism. 1994;43:441-5.

61. **Kelley D.** Effects of weight loss on glucose homeostasis in NIDDM. Diabetes Reviews. 1995; 3:366-77.

62. **Barzilai N, She L, Liu B-Q, et al.** Surgical removal of visceral fat reverses hepatic insulin resistance. Diabetes. 1999;48:94-8.

63. **Goodpaster BH, Kelley DE, Wing RR, et al.** Effects of weight loss on regional fat distribution and insulin sensitivity in obesity. Diabetes. 1999;48:847.

64. **Kopelman PG.** The effects of weight loss treatments on upper and lower body fat. Int J Obes. 1998;22:619-25.

65. **Purnell JQ, Kahn SE, Albers JJ, et al.** Effect of weight loss with reduction of intra-abdominal fat on lipid metabolism in older men. J Clin Endocrinol Metab. 2000;85:977-82.

66. **Smith SR, Zachwieja JJ.** Visceral adipose tissue: a critical review of intervention strategies. Int J Obes. 1999;23:329-35.

67. **Tappy L, Felber JP, Jequier E.** Energy and substrate metabolism in obesity and postobese state. Diabetes Care. 1991;14:1180-8.

68. **Kelley DE, Goodpaster B, Wing RR, Simoneau JA.** Skeletal muscle fatty acid metabolism in association with insulin resistance, obesity, and weight loss. Am J Physiol. 1999;277:E1130-41.

69. **Maggs DG, Buchanan TA, Burant CF, et al.** Metabolic effects of troglitazone monotherapy in Type 2 diabetes mellitus: a randomized, double-blind, placebo-controlled trial. Ann Intern Med. 1998;128:176-85.

70. **Gumbiner B, Polonsky KS, Beltz WF, et al.** Effects of weight loss and reduced hyperglycemia on the kinetics of insulin secretion in obese non-insulin dependent diabetes mellitus. J Clin Endocrinol Metab. 1990;70:1594-602.

71. **Gumbiner B, Van Cauter E, Beltz WF, et al.** Abnormalities of insulin pulsatility and glucose oscillations during meals in obese noninsulin-dependent diabetic patients: effects of weight reduction. J Clin Endocrinol Metab. 1996;81:2061-8.

72. **Henry RR, Brechtel G, Griver K.** Secretion and hepatic extraction of insulin after weight loss in obese noninsulin-dependent diabetes mellitus. J Clin Endocrinol Metab. 1988;66:979-86.

73. **Numata K, Tanaka K, Saito M, et al.** Very low calorie diet-induced weight loss reverses exaggerated insulin secretion in response to glucose, arginine and glucagon in obesity. Int J Obes Relat Metab Disord. 1993;17:103-8.

74. **Wing RR, Blair EH, Bononi P, et al.** Caloric restriction per se is a significant factor in improvements in glycemic control and insulin sensitivity during weight loss in obese NIDDM patients. Diabetes Care. 1994;17:30-6.

75. **Fisler JS, Drenick EJ.** Starvation and semistarvation diets in the management of obesity. Annu Rev Nutr. 1987;7:465-84.

76. **Yashkov YI, Vinnitsky LI, Poroykova MV, Vorobyova NT.** Some hormonal changes before and after vertical banded gastroplasty for severe obesity. Obes Surg. 2000;10:48-53.

77. **Pasquali R, Casimirri F, Melchionda N, et al.** Weight loss and sex steroid metabolism in massively obese man. J Endocrinol Invest. 1988;11:205-10.

78. **Yanovski JA, Yanovski SZ, Gold PW, Chrousos GP.** Differences in corticotropin-releasing-hormone stimulated adrenocorticotropin and cortisol before and after weight loss. J Clin Endocrinol Metab. 1997;82:1874-8.

79. **Strain GW, Zumoff B, Miller LK, et al.** Effect of massive weight loss on hypothalamic-pituitary-gonadal function in obese men. J Clin Endocrinol Metab. 1988;66:1019-23.

80. **Bastounis EA, Karayiannakis AJ, Syrigos K, et al.** Sex hormone changes in morbidly obese patients after vertical banded gastroplasty. Eur Surg Res. 1998;30:43-7.

81. **NHLBI Obesity Education Expert Panel.** Chapter 3: Examination of randomized controlled trial evidence. In: Clinical Guidelines on the Identification, Evaluation, and Treatment of Overweight and Obesity in Adults: The Evidence Report. NIH Publication 98-4083. Bethesda, MD: National Institute of Health/National Heart, Lung, and Blood Institute; 1988:29-55.

82. **Wing RR, Koeske R, Epstein LH, et al.** Long-term effects of modest weight loss in Type 2 diabetic patients. Arch Intern Med. 1987;147:1749-53.

83. **Karason K, Wikstrand J, Sjostrom L, Wendelhag I.** Weight loss and progression of early atherosclerosis in the carotid artery: a four-year controlled study of obese subjects. Int J Obes. 1999;23:948-56.

4

Medical Complications of Intentional Weight Loss

Barry Gumbiner, MD

The basic premise in the treatment of obesity is that intentional weight loss is both an effective and safe intervention and therefore should be recommended for most obese patients (1). Although debated by academics, the current public health perspective and standards of practice are that satisfactory data exist to support this supposition. Nevertheless, the metabolic and physiologic changes that occur in conjunction with weight loss can be associated with medical complications. These complications can occur independently of the therapeutic modality by which weight loss is achieved. Moreover, the patients at highest risk for complications are more likely to be those who benefit the most from treatment, the most obese who typically are afflicted with serious obesity-related illnesses.

Much of what is known about medical complications associated with intentional weight loss is from studies of patients treated with very low calorie diet plans or protein-sparing modified fasts, in which caloric intake is ≤800 cal/d (2). Although these are not the standard approaches to treating the typical obese patient in the primary care setting, it is reasonable to extrapolate from these experiences and related research because, in general, the overall medical risk from intentional weight loss is related to the rate of weight loss induced by caloric restriction. Thus, even without utilizing plans like very low calorie diets, treatment can unintentionally put patients at risk for complications by unknowingly creating a rigorous treatment plan that may seem reasonable in absolute level of caloric intake but inadvertently prescribes an excessive caloric deficit. Moreover, even when a plan is properly designed, patients can unintentionally put themselves at greater risk with overzealous behavior that further increases their caloric deficit, a situation patients often do not communicate to their health care team. Fortunately, medical complications from intentional weight loss are usually predictable, preventable, treatable, and, barring a catastrophic event, reversible. Thus, with proper planning, monitoring, and patient education, the overwhelming majority of patients can undertake weight loss treatment safely.

Acute Complications

Soon after initiating a weight-reducing meal plan, a number of physiologic and metabolic changes occur within the first 7 to 14 days that can result in significant medical problems (Table 4.1).

Sample Case—*Mr and Mrs Jones both weigh 275 lb (125 kg). However, Mr Jones is 6'2" (1.88 m), BMI = 35.3 kg/m², whereas Mrs Jones is 5'2" (1.57 m), BMI = 50.3 kg/m². Their physician prescribes a 1500 cal/d weight-reducing diet for both of them and asks a registered dietitian to assist in implementing the plan. Based on their resting metabolic rate (the energy expended during rest under conditions of thermal neutrality), activity level, and lifestyle (3-5), the dietitian estimates that Mr Jones consumes 3000 cal/d to maintain his current weight whereas Mrs Jones consumes only 2000 cal/d. After one week of treatment, Mr Jones has enthusiastically adhered to his new meal plan and reports no complaints. His weight has declined from 275 lb (125 kg) to 265 lb (120.5 kg). His physical exam reveals a supine heart rate and blood pressure of 85 and 120/80, respectively, and a standing heart rate and blood pressure of 100 and 105/70, respectively. In contrast, Mrs Jones states she is "constipated" and "does not quite feel like [herself]". Her weight has declined by 7 lb (3.2 kg). Her physical exam reveals a supine heart rate and blood pressure of 80 and 135/80, respectively, and a standing heart rate and blood pressure 85 and 130/80, respectively. A patient interview reveals she has been too enthusiastic in her attempt to lose weight, eating less than prescribed. A review of her food records by the dietitian indicates that she has been consuming approximately 1300 cal/d.*

This case illustrates some of the acute complications associated with weight loss that stem from prescribing what many consider a standard

Table 4.1   Medical Complications of Weight Loss

Acute
  Diuresis
  Vasomotor instability, orthostatic hypotension
  Electrolyte imbalance
  Altered bowel habits
  General malaise, fatigue
Subacute
  Cholelithiasis
  Hepatic dysfunction
  Exacerbated obesity-related illnesses
    Cardiovascular disease
    Gout
    Venous insufficiency
  Minor discomforts
    Headache
    Cold intolerance
    Integumentary changes
    Dysmenorrhea

weight-reducing meal plan that is seemingly safe. Although both individuals are prescribed the same 1500 cal/d meal plan, Mr Jones' intake is reduced by ~50% compared with the much more modest ~25% reduction prescribed for Mrs Jones. Both have significant weight loss (–3.6% for Mr Jones and –2.5% for Mrs Jones). However, her behavior has resulted in an additional caloric deficit, reducing her intake by ~35%, significantly more than planned by her health care team. This can result in a number of side effects and complications, some of which Mrs Jones suffers from, and which are of particular concern in patients suffering from obesity-related illnesses.

Fluid and Electrolyte Imbalance

Regardless of the intervention, a normal consequence of weight reduction is diuresis. In the idealized 70 kg (nonobese) male, over 70% of fat-free mass is composed of water (6). In response to the standard caloric deficits recommended by the NIH ($^1/_2$ to 2 lb/wk), 25% of the total weight lost will be fat-free mass (6). Thus, it is clear that water loss will be significant and, because fat-free mass loss occurs to some degree during active weight loss, it will be an ongoing concern throughout treatment. However, the most significant diuresis occurs within the first one to two weeks of dieting, particularly if severe caloric restriction is imposed. Depending on the macronutrient composition (i.e., carbohydrate vs. protein vs. fat), up to 70% of weight lost per 1000-cal deficit during the first three days of treatment can be due to water loss, a very significant amount in most patients (6, 7). Therefore, even in otherwise healthy individuals, unsafe and unmonitored approaches can be quite dangerous, and the most celebrated cases even make headlines in the tabloids (8). There are a number of underlying mechanisms accounting for this phenomenon (Table 4.2).

Glycogen Depletion

Glycogen, the major storage form of carbohydrate in humans, is an essential short-term energy reserve that is critical to moment-to-moment carbohydrate homeostasis. Under conditions of fasting, starvation, acute exercise, and caloric restriction, it is the first energy store called upon to meet metabolic fuel needs. Glycogen is a highly hydrated compound, and with its breakdown the associated water is freed and ultimately cleared through the kidney. The water loss can be quite substantial. In the postabsorptive (fasting) state of the typical, nonobese 70-kg man, the ~70 g of glycogen stored in the liver and ~250 g of glycogen stored in the muscle (9, 10) are associated with water equivalent to 2.5 to 4 times glycogen's dry weight (7, 9).

Obese people have larger livers that could result in more glycogen storage, although most of the increase in hepatic size is probably due to excess fat. However, obese individuals also have higher lean body mass, including more skeletal muscle, which results in even higher glycogen storage and associated water. Moreover, glycogen stores are highly variable, in part due to the impact of small changes in nutritional conditions (9, 11). In response to carbohydrate deprivation, 75% to 90% of the liver glycogen stores can be depleted within 24 hours (11). This can result in a significant contribution to the acute diuresis associated with initiation of weight loss therapy. Water derived from skeletal muscle glycogen breakdown should also contribute to acute diuresis even though the glucose from skeletal muscle glycogen is not available for systemic use. (Skeletal muscle lacks the enzyme glucose-6-phosphatase needed for the final reaction to generate glucose from glycogen.) Skeletal muscle glycogen stores can decline by as much as 50% after one week of severe caloric restriction (12), although the stores may be

---

Table 4.2   Mechanisms of Weight-Loss Associated Diuresis

•Glycogen depletion	•Decreased sodium intake
•Protein depletion	•Hormonal shifts
•Ketosis	•Medications, OTC products
•Altered renal physiology	

restored after two weeks of weight loss (13). Thus, although the glucose generated from muscle glycogen is not available for general fuel utilization, the kidney will eventually clear the water generated by skeletal muscle glycogenolysis (glycogen breakdown).

Protein Loss
Protein loss associated weight reduction also contributes to water loss, because protein is also hydrated, and to a degree similar to glycogen (7). However, the contribution of protein loss to water and overall weight loss is more subacute and of concern over the entire duration of treatment. Its impact on fluid and electrolyte balance during the first 7 to 14 days is more modest and in part related to its contribution to ketosis.

Ketosis
The role of ketoacids generated under various physiologic and pathologic conditions has been studied for nearly a century (14). It has long been recognized that high fat diets are ketogenic. In response to a significant caloric and/or carbohydrate deficit, fat becomes the primary source of fuel (15). Ketoacids (acetoacetate, beta-hydroxybutyrate, acetone) are breakdown products generated by fat oxidation. As these negatively charged molecules are cleared by the kidney, neutralizing cations, such as sodium, potassium, and magnesium, are excreted in conjunction with water (16, 17). To a certain degree, diet macronutrient composition can affect ketogenesis; 50 to 150 g/d of carbohydrate intake, even in the face of a caloric restriction, can substantially suppress ketosis (18). However, it may be the relative proportions of carbohydrate to fat and/or protein that may be modulating ketogenesis (14) and the urinary output of ketoacids as well as other anions (19), because caloric restriction is not necessary to generate significant ketosis (20). Thus, low-carbohydrate high-protein/fat weight loss plans can create a metabolic milieu that is unsafe. Fortunately, metabolic adaptation to acidosis precludes long-term diuresis due to ketosis (21).

Changes in Renal Physiology
Obesity is associated with a resetting of the mechanisms controlling natriuresis. This may be one of the causes for the propensity of obese individuals to develop hypertension (22, 23). In fact, weight gain rather than obesity *per se* is more closely associated with resetting of renal pressure natriuresis. Why this occurs is unknown, but as a consequence tubular reabsorption of sodium increases, in part due to higher renal plasma flow and increased GFR. Thus, these complex changes in renal physiology promote fluid retention, which is reversed with weight loss. Paradoxically, the decrease in intravascular volume that is necessarily associated with natriuresis/diuresis and should therefore occur with weight loss does not result in a

compensatory increase in blood pressure that otherwise occurs under most other physiologic conditions. This may be due to the absence of the increase in catecholamines that normally occurs with volume depletion (24, 25). Interestingly, when the focus of therapy for hypertension is salt restriction rather than weight loss, catecholamine levels increase about 20% to 30%, usually with a concomitant modest and probably unintended decrease in body weight (−0.4 to −3.0 kg) (26). Therefore, weight loss and natriuresis probably have unique and independent modulatory affects on blood pressure, and the balance and focus of these therapeutic interventions and subsequent metabolic adaptations will determine changes in blood pressure (25, 27-29).

Sodium Restriction
The USDA's Continuing Survey of Food Intakes of Individuals (1994-96), the most recent government survey available, indicates that the average *ad lib* sodium intake by the typical American is 3271 mg/d (30), which exceeds the recommended intake of 2400 mg/d by over 35%. Indeed, the average intake may be as high as 4000 mg/d (31). With weight loss, whether inadvertent or by meal plan design, this high level of sodium intake is decreased with caloric restriction. This contributes to the acute diuresis early in the course of weight loss. In addition, patients often change behaviors beyond what is prescribed in their treatment plan without communicating this to their health care professionals and may further decrease salt intake. Thus, the overall decrease in salt/sodium intake associated with weight reduction can be significantly underestimated. It should be noted, however, that sodium/salt intake is a highly controversial topic, and its role in health and disease continues to be actively debated (31-35).

Hormonal Shifts
In the more theoretical realm, changes in insulin and glucagon levels may contribute to alterations in fluid and electrolyte balance. The effects of insulin on renal function are under-appreciated (36), yet it is well known that insulin therapy in diabetes is associated with water retention that may be a consequence of insulin effects on sodium metabolism. In obese patients with normal glucose tolerance, as the insulin resistance of obesity is ameliorated (see Chapter 3) the compensatory pancreatic hypersecretion of insulin, as well as the decreased insulin clearance associated with obesity, is reversed, thus decreasing hyperinsulinemia (37-43). The same response occurs in patients with type 2 diabetes mellitus with the exception of insulin secretion; the relative impairment in insulin secretion is partially reversed by weight loss and insulin secretion increases. Nevertheless, the balance of metabolic changes also results in lower plasma insulin levels in weight-reduced patients with type 2 diabetes (41–44).

The role hyperinsulinemia may have in sodium regulation is still being debated. Some reviews of this topic suggest insulin resistance as a more likely culprit, with hyperinsulinemia simply serving as a marker of this condition (22, 23, 28, 36, 45). Moreover, even the role of insulin resistance in sodium metabolism is not universally accepted.

In contradistinction to insulin, glucagon can promote sodium excretion (46-48). Although plasma glucagon levels in obese individuals are quite variable, they are probably higher than those in nonobese individuals (49-51), particularly when measured with an accurate assay (50). The hyperglucagonemia of obesity is modulated by the interaction of glucose tolerance, insulin sensitivity, and body fat distribution (49-56). However, although plasma glucagon levels often fall with weight loss (49, 55, 57-60), levels can also increase in response to severe short-term caloric restriction, as one would expect when the metabolic conditions are more closely aligned with a near-starvation state (46). Metabolically what is crucial is the relation between glucagon and insulin levels. The glucagon:insulin ratio is well known to be critical in the regulation of carbohydrate and fat metabolism under most physiologic and pathophysiologic conditions (61, 62), including weight loss. The ratio is modulated by macronutrient composition and ketosis (59, 60, 62, 63).

Medication and Other Agents

A number of medications and other agents can have dehydrating effects that add to or potentiate the foregoing effects. Not only are prescribed diuretics of concern but so are over-the-counter products (e.g., over 70 herbal diuretic supplements (64)). Laxatives are another over-the-counter agent of concern; these are found not only in many products marketed for constipation but also in herbs promoted for a variety of uses (over 50 herbal "laxative" supplements and 14 listed as "bowel evacuant" (64)). Another common category of agents is the xanthines. This category includes not only prescription medications such as theophylline but, even more commonly, the nonprescription agent caffeine, found both in well-recognized food products (e.g., coffee, tea, cola) and in less well known over-the-counter agents used for other purposes (e.g., many analgesics). Xanthine's diuretic potency can be significant, with prescription agents like theophylline being more potent than nonprescription agents (65). However, given that some patients consume high quantities, caffeine can result in significant diuresis. The effects of caffeine are variable, but there are reports indicating 30% increases in urine volume; some acute circumstances increase urine output by greater than 1 L (66-68).

Summary and Medical Consequences

As a result of diuresis, some patients can develop orthostatic hypotension and/or become electrolyte depleted during the initiation of therapy. In addition to the aforementioned mechanisms, altered sympathetic nervous system activity can induce symptoms similar to those associated with volume depletion and can contribute to vasomotor instability without frank volume depletion. Typically, plasma norepinephrine levels increase twofold when moving from the supine to the standing position, a compensatory response to help maintain blood pressure (17). Catecholamine levels observed under resting supine conditions may decrease by half during the initial phase of weight loss therapy, and their increase in response to standing may be blunted (17). This is particularly true of protein-enriched diet. Interestingly, this response is counter to what is normally observed in sodium-depleted individuals studied under eucaloric conditions (69), and sodium intake can modulate the response of the sympathetic nervous system to weight loss (29). Thus a variety of mechanisms collude to place patients undergoing weight loss therapy at risk for complications related to fluid and electrolyte imbalances.

Altered Bowel Habits

Changes in bowel habits are a common side effect of intentional weight loss. Change in diet composition is the primary mechanism that accounts for this complication. Bowel habits can alter not only due to changes in fiber intake but also in response to the type of protein consumed (70). By the design of the dietitian's meal plan, changes in diet composition are expected. In addition, changes in diet composition can also occur by the instigation of the patient without the knowledge of the supervising health care professionals.

Constipation

Variation in individual bowel habits makes constipation difficult to define, but any decrease in the frequency of bowel movements, obstipation, or other related complaints may be what the patient indicates as constipation (70). This can occur at any time during weight loss. When constipation occurs early in treatment, it is usually due to inadequate hydration. Not only is fluid lost from diuresis but there is a decrease in overall food intake with its natural water content as well as a concomitant decline in water generated from metabolism. In addition, fiber intake is highly variable in the US population. Most patients do not consume adequate amounts of fiber, and this may be further reduced with caloric restriction, even with meal plans designed to incorporate fiber.

Although precise individualized recommendations for water intake can be calculated, generally patients need to consume at least 2 L/d over and above their meal plan (71), and the largest patients even more. Patients also need instruction on the types of fluids to consume. As noted above, for example, caffeinated drinks can induce mild diuresis and thus counterbalance fluid intake (65). A calorie-free fiber supplement is also recommended for most patients to prevent constipation (72), and in some cases prophylactic use of a stool softener can be used. Of particular concern, however, is the use of laxatives because they are a medication of abuse with some patients and thus should be used with caution. Should the patient be particularly uncomfortable, then mild laxatives (e.g., magnesium hydroxide) can be used short term.

Impaction
Should impaction occur, this should not be attributed to the meal plan. A medical evaluation is warranted under these circumstances.

Diarrhea
Some individuals may complain of diarrhea, which can occur at any time during weight loss, though it is more common early in treatment; it is typically short-lived (71). Diarrhea is usually attributable to changes in diet composition and often occurs in individuals who are not accustomed to a diet higher in fiber. It can also occur with protein formulas or amino acid supplements that irritate the bowel (70). However, true diarrhea does not actually occur. Rather, upon further inquiry, unformed stools with an increase in frequency compared with previous habits may be reported rather than true watery stools and significant frequency and urgency. It is imperative to ascertain whether there are other risk factors for diarrhea (e.g., recent travel to a foreign country) before concluding it has been caused by changes in diet. If it is determined that there are no other causes, short-term reduction in fiber intake followed by slow titration in conjunction with over-the-counter medications to control bowel movements will usually resolve the problem.

Related Issues

In addition to the acute metabolic and physiologic changes associated with weight loss described above, the Jones' scenario highlights related issues:

- The diuresis during the initial period of weight loss can be quite substantial and is one reason that diets both do and do not work. Any structured meal plan, whether designed by a health care professional or promulgated by the latest bestseller, will initially result in significant weight loss due to diuresis. This response misleads individuals into thinking their weight loss will last long term.

- An issue not often perceived as a problem is the patient's zealousness to lose weight by not consuming all the calories prescribed. Thus the patient may not be consuming all the nutrients of a balanced diet, particularly protein.

- General malaise with or without any other untoward signs or symptoms is quite common. Although there may be no overt signs of fluid and electrolyte imbalance, carbohydrate restriction *per se*, which necessarily occurs with most weight-reducing meal plans, can be associated with sympathetic nervous system instability leading to the nonspecific symptoms noted above (17). In addition, ketosis can be associated with nausea and fatigue, with or without weight loss (20). Consequently, carbohydrate and salt intake may need to be adjusted until individuals adapt to their new physiologic and metabolic milieu (70). The problem can be easily addressed by increasing salt intake. Instruct the patient to consume bouillon soup (CAUTION—*Not* the sodium-free brands!) or to salt food "to taste" until feeling better (73, 74). The symptoms should resolve within 24 hours, at which point added salt is no longer necessary. Adding back carbohydrates to the diet should be considered if increased salt intake does not resolve the problem (70).

Thus, rather than prescribe a "one size fits all" meal plan, it is better to advise an initial meal plan that is ~25% caloric deficit, a level that is generally safe for most patients. As the patient progresses, further reductions in intake can be initiated, with the caveat that the acute complications described above can occur coincident with additional major reductions in intake.

Obesity-Related Illnesses

The potential for acute complications can be further complicated by a number of obesity-related illnesses. Although these complications can occur at any time during weight reduction, they are more apt to occur early in the course of therapy. These complications are usually due to concomitant medications becoming more effective and/or mitigating pathophysiologic mechanisms improving rapidly at a rate disproportionate to weight loss. Therefore close monitoring and, in some cases, pre-emptive medication adjustments are warranted, particularly if caloric restriction will be quite severe (e.g., a very low calorie diet or a partial meal replacement plan substituting one to two meals with powder formula or nutrition bars).

Type 2 Diabetes Mellitus
Although weight loss is almost universally recommended for obese patients with type 2 diabetes, there are contraindications. It should not be embarked upon in the patient under poor metabolic control and showing signs and symptoms of a catabolic state. Typically these patients will report involuntary weight loss (e.g., "I have lost 20 lb in two months without dieting") and have very high fasting hyperglycemia (>270 mg/dL). Some of these individuals may be in a ketotic metabolic state and therefore at risk for worsening

ketosis with caloric restriction, resulting in its attendant effects on fluid and electrolyte balance described above. Moreover, although not widely appreciated, some patients with type 2 diabetes can develop diabetic ketoacidosis (DKA), and caloric restriction is a condition that will place them at higher risk for this complication. Finally, there are the occasional insulin-treated overweight/obese patients presumed to have type 2 diabetes who are actually afflicted with type 1 diabetes. Weight loss is important in such patients but treatment can be more complicated and difficult, and these patients would benefit from intervention by an endocrinologist and diabetes health care team. Thus, under all these circumstances, patients need to be under metabolic control in which they show no signs of ketosis or catabolism before embarking on weight reduction.

With the exception of those patients with poor metabolic control and signs of a catabolic state, most obese patients with type 2 diabetes are candidates for weight loss treatment. Unlike patients without diabetes they risk hypoglycemia as weight loss ensues. Typically this is more likely in those treated with antidiabetic medications, but under some conditions hypoglycemia can occur in those not being treated with pharmacotherapy. Weight loss partially reverses (75-77) all the major underlying pathophysiologic mechanisms contributing to hyperglycemia (78-81): decreased insulin-mediated glucose uptake (primarily by muscle and adipose tissue), excess hepatic glucose production, and relative impairment in pancreatic insulin secretion. The amelioration of hyperglycemia is often disproportionate to the amount of weight loss and can occur quite quickly if caloric restriction is severe. For example, during treatment with very low calorie diets, 90% of the improvement in hyperglycemia can occur within the first ten days (82, 83). More often, however, the decline is slower when conventional weight-reducing meal plans are used (84-87).

Even patients not being treated with medication occasionally develop hypoglycemia during weight loss therapy. This typically occurs when an individual has a particularly active day and goes for a long period without caloric intake (e.g., a busy shopping day) or an individual embarks on rigorous exercise without proper monitoring. A decrease of 50 mg/dL in blood glucose from a short bout (e.g., 45 min) of exercise is not unusual (88), despite a decrease in insulin levels that normally occurs during exercise (89). Exercise promotes insulin-mediated glucose uptake, primarily by increasing nonoxidative glucose metabolism and glycogen depletion followed by resynthesis (90, 91). At the cellular level, this is due in part to increasing the abnormally low levels of muscle glucose transporter (GLUT4) mRNA and protein, although not to levels comparable with those in patients without obesity or diabetes (92). Moreover, in patients on sulfonylureas who take their medication before exercise, the increase in insulin levels can be quite substantial, thus potentiating the effects of exercise on insulin action and increasing the likelihood of hypoglycemia (93). Thus, for all these reasons, basic diabetes education and monitoring, as recommended by the American Diabetes Association, should be reinforced with particular attention to high-risk scenarios (94). Moreover, it is often prudent to decrease doses of antidiabetic medication by 25% to 50% if initiating severe caloric restriction, to have all patients intensify home glucose monitoring, and to arrange close follow-up during the initial weeks of therapy.

Hypertension

Like type 2 diabetes, weight loss is almost universally recommended for obese patients with hypertension. The benefits of weight loss for prevention, as a primary treatment modality, or to facilitate pharmacotherapeutic management are well-documented (95-103). However, as is the situation with type 2 diabetes, this therapeutic approach should not be embarked upon in patients with severe, poorly controlled hypertension. Once controlled, the immediate risk for complications is from diuresis. Thus, discontinuation of diuretics should be considered upon initiation of weight loss therapy, especially if severe caloric restriction is used. Alternatively, very close follow-up and patient education may be effective in preventing a problem. This will reduce the risk of electrolyte abnormalities occurring within the first two weeks of treatment. Other medications may need reduction as well, but it is usually prudent to await further weight loss unless signs and/or symptoms warrant adjustments.

Peripheral Edema

Some patients are prone to peripheral edema, often due to venous stasis and related problems associated with obesity, and although edema can improve with weight loss, the response is highly variable. Thus a lower dose and/or less potent diuretic may need to be reintroduced later in therapy. Before doing so, further evaluation and restriction of sodium intake may alleviate the problem. Unfortunately, this is a daunting task due to the prevalence of salt incorporated in processed foods and in prepared food from outside sources (e.g., restaurants). Moreover, despite a number of studies demonstrating the efficacy of restricting salt intake, as noted previously, it is an issue that is under constant debate (31-35). In fact, some studies suggest severe salt restriction may actually be harmful to the individuals who are in greatest need of weight loss therapy (35). Nevertheless, from a public health and clinical perspective, there appears to be no harm in reducing salt intake as a component of the meal plan for weight control.

Subacute and Long-Term Complications

In addition to acute complications, there are other complications, subacute and long term, which usually occur weeks or even months after initiating treatment. However, it should be noted that the aforementioned acute side effects and complications can occur at any time during intentional weight loss. The most likely scenario is when there is a significant change in the meal plan and/or behavior (e.g., a patient who previously had adjustment problems has a breakthrough leading to a significant rapid weight loss). Thus monitoring of both acute complications (described above) and later-occurring complications is warranted.

Sample Case (continued)—*Mr Jones states he is doing well with his meal plan. Although he has struggled at times, his weight has decreased by 31 lb (14 kg) in 8 weeks. However, for the past week, he reports nausea, particularly with dinner, and one episode of abdominal pain that was relieved with multiple doses of antacids and acetaminophen. He does not report vomiting, changes in bowel habits, fever, or chills.*

This case illustrates the potential for a number of gastrointestinal complications that can occur well into the course of weight loss treatment.

Cholelithiasis

Obesity *per se* confers an increased risk for gallstone formation (see Chapter 1) (104, 105). There are three underlying mechanisms (105, 106):

1. Cholesterol supersaturation of the bile

2. A chemical milieu that promotes nucleation (i.e., a nidus for stone formation)

3. Decreased gallbladder motility resulting in a larger gallbladder volume and reduced ejection of bile

Although weight loss decreases the long-term risk of developing cholelithiasis, active weight loss promotes gallstone formation by potentiating the underlying mechanisms by which gallstones develop (105, 107). The risk is 15 to 25 times that of obese individuals not losing weight (105, 108) and occurs independently of the modality by which weight loss is achieved. This risk is in part related to the rapidity of weight loss, as attested to by the high rates of cholelithiasis with both surgically induced weight loss and very low calorie diet therapy (109), and in part to the duration of treatment (105, 108, 110). Usually gallstones will not develop until at least four weeks of weight loss but then can occur at anytime thereafter, even months later (108). Rates of weight loss greater than 1.5 kg/wk (~3 lb) put an individual at particularly high risk (110).

A number of interventions to prevent this problem have proven effective. Because the impairment in gallbladder contractility during weight loss is due in part to a reduction in intake of dietary stimuli, a minimum of 10 g of fat intake per day will significantly reduce the formation of gallstones during weight loss (111-113). It should be noted that most of the subjects in the studies assessing contractility also have higher protein intake than the control diet comparisons, but nevertheless it is thought that fat is the key dietary component for stimulating gallbladder contraction. Medications have also been shown highly effective (107, 109, 114-116). Ursodiol, a bile acid agent that reduces the cholesterol saturation of bile, results in the dissolution of gallstones or prevention of formation during weight loss. Aspirin and ibuprofen may be effective as well, but adequate large-scale efficacy and safety studies have yet to be conducted.

Despite the risk of cholelithiasis, it is not thought to be cost-effective to screen for gallstones before initiating weight loss intervention or to treat prophylactically with medication (106, 110, 117). It is problematic defining an endpoint to such treatment, particularly because these patients remain at risk, albeit less risk, after weight loss intervention because most are still obese. Moreover, one small study demonstrated that as many as half of the gallstones dissolve on their own (118). Most patients diagnosed for cholelithiasis will remain asymptomatic and not require intervention. What clearly can be recommended is for patients to consume a daily fat intake of at least 10 g/d to ensure gallbladder contraction; for this reason alone radical meal plans that are extremely low in fat intake are not advisable.

Pancreatitis

Pancreatitis can occur during weight loss as a complication of active gallbladder disease (e.g., choledocholithiasis). Furthermore, even without gallstones, the predisposition to biliary sludge during weight loss can lead to this problem (119). Some also believe it can occur if the patient has a lapse and "binges". This can happen when biliary sludge is suddenly excreted in higher quantities into the biliary tract in response to sudden increased gallbladder activity (70). This would be consistent with the rare reports of pancreatitis associated with refeeding syndrome in the treatment of anorexia and malnourished children (120-122).

Hepatic Dysfunction

Abnormal liver function tests are common in obese patients, particularly obese patients with type 2 diabetes and hyperlipidemia. This reflects the presence of steatosis, which is almost universally present in all obese patients (123). The inflammatory form of the disease, nonalcoholic steatohepatitis (NASH, "fatty liver"), is typically clinically silent but can have severe consequences. If left untreated, NASH can lead to cirrhosis and death (123, 124). The histopathology of NASH is similar to alcohol-related liver disease (125) and, although reports vary, in one report 60% of patients with liver test abnormalities not due to alcohol-induced, drug-induced, viral, genetic, or autoimmune disease had biopsy-proven inflammatory activity, including

30% with septal fibrosis and 11% with cirrhosis (126). The odds of having NASH increase by almost sixfold for a BMI > 28. Upper-body distribution of fat is more strongly correlated than obesity *per se*, and type 2 diabetes, independent of obesity, is also a risk factor (123). After accounting for all these confounders, it is unlikely that gender *per se* contributes to the risk of NASH.

A recent study implicates insulin resistance, the common link among these metabolic disturbances, as the most likely risk factor for steatosis in obesity (127). The normal suppression of fat oxidation by insulin is impaired, and it is postulated that this results in the accumulation of intracellular fatty acids. Abnormal cytokine production is another proposed mechanism (125). Of particular interest is the increased tumor necrosis factor α, which is increased in obesity and associated with insulin resistance (128). A more interesting mechanism recently hypothesized is oxidative stress and lipid peroxidation as the underlying insult (125), a condition also thought to promote cardiovascular disease (129).

It is common for individuals with steatosis to have mild elevations in plasma AST, ALT, and alkaline phosphatase concentrations but not bilirubin. Although sustained weight loss is the presumed treatment for steatosis and NASH, it does not universally resolve the problem (123, 124). In fact, one of the major complications that led to the discontinuation of the jejuno-ileal bypass procedure was the high rate of liver failure due to the rapid progression of NASH (125), a complication not associated with gastroplasty and gastric bypass (see Chapter 10).

During the normal course of weight loss there is an increase in liver enzymes due to mobilization of the liver's excess fat. Hepatocellular degeneration with focal necrosis accounts for an increase in liver biomarkers that peaks two to six weeks after treatment begins and then generally declines, with most individuals achieving normal values (111). However, despite the improvement in the vast majority of patients, steatosis can remain even after significant weight loss, and over 20% can develop or continue to have inflammatory lobular hepatitis, the long-term implications of which remain unknown (130, 131). Moreover, rapid weight loss on radical starvation-like treatment plans can cause increased morbidity from this problem when not adequately monitored; in fact, such treatments may be ineffective (123).

Whether it is cost-effective to more thoroughly evaluate hepatic dysfunction before or during treatment to confirm the presence of NASH is a challenging dilemma. Certainly if there are other historical features (e.g., hepatitis risk) or symptoms (e.g., biliary colic) that suggest a diagnosis other than NASH, a work-up should be pursued. As with other clinical circumstances, individuals with liver test abnormalities more than three times the upper limits of normal warrant further examination. Finally, if the predominant abnormalities are elevated plasma bilirubin and alkaline phosphatase concentrations, gallbladder disease should be considered. Nevertheless, there are no firm recommendations for patients who are asymptomatic with mild laboratory abnormalities, and a case-by-case assessment is prudent.

Obesity-Related Illnesses

Not only can acute complications occur in patients with type 2 diabetes and hypertension during weight loss therapy but diligent monitoring of these conditions is needed during the entire course of weight loss therapy. However, it is usually during periods of renewed rapid weight loss when problems will occur. Thus individualized follow-up schedules and, more importantly, patient education about when to contact the treatment team is the most reasonable approach.

In addition to diabetes and hypertension, there are other important obesity-related illnesses that may need special attention during the course of therapy and in which problems usually occur after the initial phase of treatment (Table 4.3).

Cardiac Disease

Obesity *per se* is associated with a number of ECG changes, most of which are not in the pathologic, and may not even be in the abnormal, range. These changes include increased heart rate and QRS voltage, slower conduction, leftward axis shift, and QT_c prolongation (132). In addition, obesity is associated with as much as a 30-fold increase in premature ventricular ectopy if the patient has left ventricular hypertrophy (133). QT_c prolongation is of particular concern and has been reported to occur in 28% of overweight individuals using older, more conservative standards to define overweight/obesity (132). This may be more common in the subgroup of individuals with upper-body obesity (134), which in turn may be a manifestation of the more common and severe metabolic perturbations associated with visceral obesity. This latter abnormality may explain the significantly higher rate of sudden death observed in a cohort of severely obese patients awaiting surgical intervention for obesity (i.e., before weight loss (135)).

Table 4.3 Comorbidities of Obesity to Monitor Attention During Weight Loss Therapy

•Type 2 diabetes mellitus	•Cardiac disease
•Hypertension	•Venous insufficiency
•Gout	

Historically, a particular area of concern is the issue of sudden death under conditions of severe caloric restriction. This concern stems from the initial experiences in the 1960s using the predecessors to the current very low calorie diets. There were a number of reports of sudden death in conjunction with these products (136-140), and an FDA review of 60 cases indicated a potential association with cardiac arrhythmia stemming from prolonged QT_c interval (141). Although cause-and-effect was never established (138, 141), obesity is probably associated with longer QT_c intervals than observed in nonobese individuals and ECG abnormalities are common at all stages of treatment with very low calorie diets (142). However, carefully conducted clinical trials noted that arrhythmias occurred in the absence of pretreatment QT_c abnormalities and, more importantly, arrhythmias were avoided if high-quality protein formulas properly fortified with minerals, electrolytes, trace elements, and vitamins were used (143, 144). Moreover, cardiac safety for the standard treatment approach with very low calorie diet followed by a conventional balanced deficit diet has been documented for a treatment duration as long as 45 weeks (145). Nevertheless, these diet plans should be carefully monitored by experienced health care professionals (2, 138). Caution is particularly warranted if a patient already has underlying risk (e.g., known cardiac disease, prolonged QT_c interval, arrhythmia).

A more recent concern is the relation between weight loss and valvular heart disease. The concern arises out of the association that occurred during long-term pharmacotherapy that led to the removal of fenfluramine and dexfenfluramine from the market (146) (see Chapter 9). However, due to the uncontrolled circumstances under which this problem was observed, the potential role of rapid weight loss *per se* as a contributor to the problem could not be determined. The baseline prevalence of valvular heart disease in obesity has previously only been extrapolated from larger studies designed for other purposes and cannot necessarily be considered an acceptable reference population (147, 148). However, because valvulopathy has never been observed with other weight loss treatment modalities, the possibility that rapid weight loss *per se* is the cause of valvulopathy is remote. Analyses of matched or placebo cohorts from the exposed populations (149-152), as well as a recent small prospective study of echocardiography designed specifically to address this question (153), indicate that it is highly unlikely that valvular heart disease develops as a consequence of weight loss *per se*.

If a comprehensive evaluation is performed before initiating therapy and an appropriate treatment plan is designed and implemented, cardiac complications are unlikely with weight loss. Only the presence of significant underlying cardiac disease may require special measures. If cardiac disease is unstable, weight loss should be postponed. For patients with recent events (typically within six months) in which patients are otherwise stable, a conservative and cautious approach is recommended. Otherwise, adherence to the principles outlined in Chapters 5 and 7 should be adequate.

Gout

Hyperuricemia occurs in obesity by a number of underlying mechanisms. Although decreased excretion/renal clearance of uric acid contributes to hyperuricemia in all obese patients, uric acid overproduction occurs in those with upper-body obesity (154). Additional increases in plasma uric acid levels are a normal physiologic response to weight loss independent of the treatment modality employed. It is a consequence of cellular breakdown that necessarily occurs under the catabolic conditions of therapy (70). In addition, there is competition at the renal tubular level between uric acid and ketoacids for reabsorption that favors uric acid, thus decreasing uric acid excretion (70, 155). Serum uric acid levels begin increasing soon after initiating therapy and peak as early as two weeks into therapy (156). Because uric acid elevation during weight loss is modulated in part by carbohydrate restriction and ketosis, minimal change in uric acid levels occurs when ketosis is suppressed (157).

Although one would expect gout to be common in dieters, this is not the case, perhaps because the initial decrease in uric acid excretion that occurs early in therapy improves over time (158). The patients who are at risk are those who have a documented history of gout or undiagnosed patients with a history of arthritis that may be consistent with gout but not necessarily proven by synovial fluid analysis. It is generally recommended that patients in these categories be treated prophylactically, usually with allopurinol. Some recommend that severe hyperuricemia (>10 mg/dL) be treated prophylactically as well (2, 159). However, as noted above, the underlying mechanisms causing the hyperuricemia of obesity may vary, and although decreased excretion/renal clearance of uric acid contributes to hyperuricemia in all obese patients, uric acid overproduction is a prominent feature in those with upper-body obesity (154). Therefore a blanket recommendation for allopurinol may need to be re-evaluated. Should a gout attack occur during weight loss, it should be evaluated and treated like any other case of gout. In addition, increasing carbohydrate intake is warranted to more effectively suppress ketogenesis and prevent future attacks.

Minor Side Effects

A variety of minor side effects are attributable to weight loss. Many of these conditions resolve without intervention; if not, increasing caloric intake usually reverses the condition.

Headache

Headache is a nonspecific complaint for which a cause often cannot be identified. The exception, based on anecdotal evidence, is caffeine withdrawal. Before treatment, many patients may be consuming large quantities of caffeinated beverages and upon initiation of a meal plan may drastically reduce their intake. This can result in severe headaches typical of caffeine withdrawal. Reinstitution of caffeine using noncaloric products should be considered followed by a deliberate weaning process if warranted or desired.

Cold Intolerance

The underlying cause of cold intolerance associated with weight loss is unknown. The adaptive decrease in T_3 levels resulting from decreased T_4 to T_3 conversion commonly occurs with weight loss (159) and is modulated by ketosis-induced carbohydrate restriction (157, 160). However, no studies have linked cold intolerance to declines in T_3 levels. Although T_3 replacement reverses the adaptive decline in resting metabolic rate (161), it also promotes protein loss and therefore has no place in the treatment of obesity (159). Like most of the minor side effects that occur with weight loss, cold intolerance may improve with increasing caloric intake, particularly carbohydrate.

Dry Skin, Rash, Brittle Nails, and Thinning Hair

One might expect that the onset of dry skin, rash, brittle nails, and thinning hair are related to nutritional deficiencies in the meal plan. Yet all reputable medically supervised programs use well-balanced meal plans that incorporate all the essential components for sound nutrition. Nevertheless, even in these programs, such side effects occasionally occur. After verifying that the meal plan is adequately fortified and being consumed appropriately, further evaluation by a dermatologist may be warranted.

Menstrual Irregularities

A variety of gynecologic conditions, many hormonally mediated, are associated with obesity (a review of which is beyond the scope of this chapter). Often manifested as menstrual irregularities, these problems usually improve with weight loss. However, some women develop menstrual irregularities in conjunction with weight loss therapy. Of particular importance is ruling out pregnancy. Since a medical and social history is sometimes misleading, and because significant caloric restriction is contraindicated during pregnancy, a pregnancy test is warranted. If ruled out, a general gynecologic evaluation should be considered.

Fatigue

Fatigue is a common nonspecific complaint, and there is no recommendation specific to weight loss therapy other than altering the nutrition and/or physical activity plan. If fatigue continues, a general medical evaluation is the usual course of action, including screening for depression.

Weight Cycling ("Yo-Yo" Dieting)

There are number of metabolic issues for which a full discussion is beyond the scope of this chapter. Nevertheless, they deserve mention due to common misperceptions. The most controversial metabolic issues center around weight cycling, often referred to as "yo-yo" dieting. For research purposes, this is defined as repetitive bouts of weight loss and regain, arbitrarily set at >20 lb. However, there is neither a standard definition of the condition nor agreement on the frequency or number of episodes and quantitative measures of weight loss that should be of concern (162). This issue has generated a great deal of controversy because results from observational epidemiologic studies and animal research have been extrapolated to claims of negative health outcomes without adequate evidence. The issues related to weight cycling are discussed below.

Cardiovascular Risk
The historical and on-going controversy about weight loss is whether there is increased mortality, particularly cardiac related, associated with weight loss and weight cycling. A detailed discussion of this topic can be found in Chapter 1. Despite a consensus conference review (163) which concluded that based on current evidence "yo-yo" dieting is not a risk in humans, and notwithstanding the position by the NIH expert panel (96) advocating weight loss to treat obesity, there are unfortunately no prospective interventional studies that address the question definitively. The NIH is embarking on the first long-term randomized weight loss trial, the SHOW trial (Study of Health Outcomes of Weight-loss) (164, 164a), but the results will not be known for a number of years and the patient population to be studied is limited to obese individuals with type 2 diabetes. In the interim, the Swedish Obesity Subjects study will provide some insight, but its conclusions will be constrained by the interventions (surgery vs. lifestyle), study design (nonrandomized), and inclusion/exclusion criteria for BMI emphasizing clinically severe (morbid) obesity while excluding BMIs in the lower 30 range as well as the overweight category (165). Thus, although there is no definitive answer yet, the current standard of practice is that weight loss should be embarked upon in those overweight and obese individuals at risk for or manifesting obesity-related illness (96).

Body Composition
The critical questions regarding body composition are:

1. What is the appropriate amount of lean body mass that should be lost with treatment?

2. Does permanent lean body mass loss (e.g., skeletal and cardiac muscle) occur with weight cycling ? (i.e., With regain, does lean body mass return to its pre-treatment level?)

3. Does weight cycling actually promote or exacerbate obesity, and consequently induce a metabolic resistance to future attempts at weight loss?

There is an extensive body of literature assessing the effects of various nutritional conditions and interventions on nitrogen balance, including the effects of weight loss on lean body mass. Of particular concern is the loss of protein, especially that derived from muscle, which occurs with weight loss. Often overlooked in the debate is that, unlike most animal models of obesity, overweight and obese humans have not only increased fat mass but increased lean body mass, so much so that the latter can account for up to 40% of excess weight (166). Therefore negative nitrogen balance with its attendant protein loss is inevitable in the initial stages of weight loss (6, 159).

At least 0.8 g protein/kg body weight is recommended to prevent negative nitrogen balance under most physiologic conditions (167, 168). However, simply increasing protein intake above these levels during weight loss to counteract negative nitrogen balance may not be adequate. Carbohydrate, among other factors including vitamins, minerals, exercise, protein quality, and caloric deficit, has a protein-sparing effect, probably by modulating ketosis/acidosis (57, 147, 157, 169). Thus, despite the popularity of low carbohydrate weight reducing regimens, carbohydrate intake in concert with protein intake to preserve muscle mass is important. Protein intake greater than needed is simply burned for fuel and provides no significant additional benefit. Moreover, there exists at least a theoretical, if not actual, risk to patients with impaired renal function of consuming too much protein, particularly those with diabetes and hypertension. In general, at least 70 g protein intake/d is needed during active weight loss (159). Based on these studies and other data, a consensus on these questions was reached by a recent task force panel (170). Although an appropriate amount of loss of lean body mass has not been identified, typically a 25% of weight loss is lean body mass and, as reviewed in Chapter 7, this can be attenuated with resistance exercise. Unlike animals, a significant majority of human studies indicate that fluctuations in body composition associated with weight cycling do not induce a metabolic resistance to future attempts at weight loss. Thus, the effects of weight cycling on body composition are probably health neutral, being neither particularly beneficial nor significantly harmful.

Metabolic Rate
There is a common misperception that obese individuals have significantly lower metabolic rates, predisposing them to obesity and, with further declines during weight loss, a propensity for regain. On a whole-body basis,

it has been demonstrated unequivocally that in absolute terms obesity is associated with higher energy expenditure than is the case for nonobese individuals (171). Also, evidence from carefully performed interventional metabolic studies shows that there is an appropriate and proportionate, not disproportionate, decline in metabolic rate with weight loss (172-174). Nevertheless, prospective studies suggest there may be small differences in total energy expenditure and fat oxidation rates, modulated by gender and ethnicity, that contribute to a propensity for developing obesity and regaining weight after weight loss (174-180). However, these differences are highly variable and on an individual basis it is hard to determine their importance and how to use this information in treating patients (181). Furthermore, it is estimated that environment influences ~60% of weight (182), and biological differences cannot account for the obesity epidemic and impact of lifestyle factors that overwhelm these metabolic issues (183). Thus, even though slightly lower metabolic rates may play a role in obesity, there are numerous environmental influences that patients can alter to have a favorable impact on their weight despite a possible underlying predisposition towards obesity.

Bone Mass Density

Although there is heightened awareness about the impact of osteoporosis on morbidity and mortality, because it is well known that bone mass density is higher in obese individuals (184), it might be assumed that this is not a major concern compared with other obesity-related risks. It should be noted, however, that weight loss can be associated with significant negative calcium balance (159, 185), and thus some investigators have begun studying changes in bone mineral density with weight loss (186-189). Furthermore, a small study suggests that obese children and adolescents have a relative decrease in bone mineral density, which portends problems in later adulthood (190). Moreover, besides the issue of inadequate calcium intake as a general problem in the population (187), ketosis/chronic acidosis, a metabolic state associated with weight loss, promotes negative calcium balance as well (190a). The few studies measuring bone mineral density with weight loss suggest that significant decreases in bone density, particularly at the greater trochanter, occur with intentional weight loss (186, 188). However, one small study demonstrated recovery of bone mineral density with regain (188) and that the health outcome of interest, fracture rate, is not increased with intentional weight loss (189).

Calcium balance and osteoporosis is an issue that needs to be approached in a manner similar to body composition and nitrogen balance. The key question is whether there is a disproportionate loss of bone mass density with weight loss, over and above what is appropriate for the decrease in overall body mass. More importantly are the potential consequences of the loss of bone mass. Does it place individuals at higher risk for fracture, and does bone mass recover with weight regain? Although simply providing adequate calcium intake/supplementation counteracts the negative calcium balance associated with weight loss (143,159), more focused research would be useful to determine whether other modalities, such as bicarbonate supplementation (191), are useful, and whether even a short cycle of calcium imbalance has a negative impact on the critical health outcome, fracture rate. Given the data available, because the other medical risks associated with obesity are greater than not intervening, it is important to promote treatments, including weight-bearing exercise (as tolerated) and adequate vitamin and mineral intake, to maintain appropriate bone mass during weight loss therapy.

Recommendations

The expert NIH panel recommends the rate of weight loss using conventional treatment modalities should be $^1/_2$ to 2 lb/week to achieve 10% weight loss over a period of six months (1). This recommendation is based primarily on efficacy data. Additional and/or more rapid weight loss has generally not been shown to be effective long term. Thus, based on the evidence available, slow but sustained weight loss is as effective, if not more effective, long term, and on average this requires about six months to reach the 10% goal. Furthermore, this is the level at which most people plateau. To lose more weight is challenging because there are so many redundant metabolic pathways and physiologic mechanisms to maintain weight, and this is further complicated by behavioral barriers.

Ten percent weight loss is clinically efficacious and is a conservative goal that by most standards would be considered safe. Nevertheless, there are few studies available to support or refute the safety of this recommendation. The most extensive data available are for gallbladder-related complications. As noted above, overweight/obese people are at higher risk *a priori* for cholelithiasis. Studies indicate that the underlying risk of gallbladder disease increases substantially when weight loss exceeds greater than 1.5 kg/wk (~3 lb/wk) (110). Thus it is clear that rates higher than this should be avoided. Another criterion for safe weight loss could also be based on minimizing nitrogen loss to preserve protein. This also is difficult to ascertain but weight loss of 0.3 lb/1000 cal deficit/d or approximately 1%/wk is generally safe (6, 7, 192).

Particularly problematic is the initial diuresis. It may be difficult to limit initial weight loss. Based on anecdotal evidence, weight loss at a rate greater than 2%/week probably warrants laboratory testing to rule out electrolyte imbalance, particularly if medication is being prescribed concomitantly that may promote diuresis. A basic metabolic panel including sodium, potassium, and BUN is the minimum to monitor under these conditions. Appropriate patient counseling to reiterate the hazards of rapid weight loss and the importance of adhering to a balanced meal plan is essential.

To properly monitor patients, not only is safety an issue but adequate feedback is just as important. Even with conventional intervention conducted in a monitored environment, patients need encouragement as well as minor treatment adjustments to assist them. The NIH recommended schedule is a prudent approach to accomplish all goals. At least one visit should occur within two to four weeks and sooner (at one week) if there is concern about a potential rapid diuresis or side effects from antiobesity medication. This can be followed by monthly visits for three months, quarterly for the remainder of the first year, and as needed after that. Not all visits need to be conducted by the physician to facilitate achieving goals. In fact, visits supervised by allied health professionals (e.g., RN, RD) can potentially be more effective because more time is available for interaction than with the physician, as long as medical monitoring occurs and parameters set to trigger physician intervention.

■   ■   ■

Key Points

- Diuresis is a normal consequence of all weight reduction treatments, with the most significant diuresis occurring within the first two weeks of dieting.

- Obesity-related illnesses, such as type 2 diabetes mellitus and hypertension, may contribute to the medical complications of weight loss, particularly during the early phase of weight loss.

- Complications of weight reduction that can occur as late as months into treatment include cholelithiasis, pancreatitis, hepatic dysfunction, and complications associated with obesity-related cardiac disease and hyperuricemia.

- Although obesity itself is a risk factor for cholelithiasis, weight loss increases the risk to 15 to 25 times that incurred by obesity without weight loss.

- Weight cycling ("yo-yo" dieting) has been a subject of much controversy.

- The expert NIH panel recommends a rate of weight loss (using conventional treatments) of $1/_2$ to 2 lb/wk to achieve a 10% weight loss over six months.

■   ■   ■

REFERENCES

1. **NHLBI Obesity Education Expert Panel.** Clinical Guidelines on the Identification, Evaluation, and Treatment of Overweight and Obesity in Adults: The Evidence Report. NIH Publication 98-4083. Bethesda, MD: National Institutes of Health/National Heart, Lung, and Blood Institute; 1998:95-7.

2. **National Task Force on the Prevention and Treatment of Obesity.** Very low-calorie diets. JAMA. 1993;270:967-74.

3. **Harris J A, Benedict FG.** A biometric study of basal metabolism in man. Washington, DC: Carnegie Institute of Washington; 1919:279.

4. **Welle S, Forbes GB, Statt M, et al.** Energy expenditure under free-living conditions in normal-weight and overweight women. Am J Clin Nutr. 1992;55:14-21.

5. **Schulz LO, Schoeller DA.** A compilation of total daily energy expenditures and body weights in healthy adults. Am J Clin Nutr. 1994;60:676-81.

6. **Yang M-U, VanItallie TB.** Effect of energy restriction on body composition and nitrogen balance in obese individuals. In: Treatment of the Seriously Obese Patient. Wadden TA, VanItallie TB, eds. New York: Guilford Press; 1992:83-106.

7. **VanItallie TB, Yang M-U.** Current concepts in nutrition: diet and weight loss. N Engl J Med. 1972;297:1158-61.

8. **Butterfield A, South J, Fitz R.** Marie Osmond collapses in deadly diet drama. The National Enquirer. 16 April 2000:32-3..

9. **Nilsson LH.** Liver glycogen content in man in the postabsorptive state. Scand J Clin Lab Invest. 1973;32:317-23.

10. **Mayes PA.** Metabolism of glycogen. In: Harper's Biochemistry. Murray R, Granner DK, Mayes PA, Rodwell V, eds. Stamford, CT: Appleton and Lange; 1996:185-93.

11. **Nilsson LH, Hultman E.** Liver glycogen in man: the effect of total starvation or a carbohydrate-poor diet followed by carbohydrate refeeding. Scand J Clin Lab Invest. 1973;32:325-30.

12. **Krotkiewski M, Landin K, Mellstrom D, Tolli J.** Loss of total body potassium during rapid weight loss does not depend on the decrease of potassium concentration in muscles: different methods to evaluate body composition during a low energy diet. Int J Obes. 2000;24:101-7.

13. **Russell DM, Walker PM, Leiter LA, et al.** Metabolic and structural changes in skeletal muscle during hypocaloric dieting. Am J Clin Nutr. 1984;39:503-13.

14. **Wilder RM, Winter MD.** The threshold of ketogenesis. J Biol Chem. 1922;393-401.

15. **Mayes PA.** Integration of metabolism and the provision of tissue fuels. In: Harper's Biochemistry. Murray R, Granner DK, Mayes PA, Rodwell V, eds. Stamford, CT: Appleton and Lange; 1996:284-91.

16. **Sigler MH.** The mechanism of the natriuresis of fasting. J Clin Invest. 1975;55:377-87.

17. **DeHaven J, Sherwin R, Hendler R, Felig P.** Nitrogen and sodium balance and sympathetic-nervous-system activity in obese subjects treated with a low-calorie protein or mixed diet. N Engl J Med. 1980;302:477-82.

18. **Cahill GF Jr.** Starvation in man. N Engl J Med. 1970;282:668-75.

19. **Gougeon-Reyburn R, Leiter LA, Yale J-F, Marliss EB.** Comparison of daily diets containing 400 kcal (1.67 MJ) of either protein or glucose, and their effects on the response to subsequent total fasting in obese subjects. Am J Clin Nutr. 1989;50:746-58.

20. **Phinney SD, Bistrian BR, Wolfe RR, Blackburn GL.** The human metabolic response to chronic ketosis without caloric restriction: physical and biochemical adaptation. Metabolism. 1983;32:757-68.

21. **Schloeder FX, Stinebaugh FJ.** Studies on the natriuresis of fasting. II. Relationship to acidosis. Metabolism. 1966;15:838-46.

22. **Hall JE.** Renal and cardiovascular mechanisms of hypertension in obesity. Hypertension. 1984;23:381-94.

23. **Hall JE, Brands MW, Henegar JR, Shek EW.** Abnormal kidney function as a cause and a consequence of obesity hypertension. Clin Exp Pharmacol Physiol. 1998;25:58-64.

24. **Stoffel M, Donckier J, Ketelslegers JM, Kolanowski J.** Changes in blood pressure and in vasoactive and volume regulatory hormones during semistarvation in obese subjects. Metabolism. 1998;47:592-7.

25. **Leiter LA, Grose M, Yale JF, Marliss EB.** Catecholamine responses to hypocaloric diets and fasting in obese human subjects. Am J Physiol. 1984;247: E190-E197.

26. **Graudal NA, Galloe AM, Garred P.** Effects of sodium restriction on blood pressure, renin, aldosterone, catecholamines, cholesterol, and triglyceride: a meta-analysis. JAMA. 1998;279:1383-91.

27. **Reisin C, Abel R, Modan M, et al.** Effect of weight loss without salt restriction on the reduction of blood pressure in overweight hypertensive patients. N Engl J Med. 1978;298:1-5.

28. **Kolanowski J.** Obesity and hypertension: from pathophysiology to treatment. Int J Obes. 1999;23(suppl 1):42-6.

29. **Gougeon R, Mitchell T, Lariviere F, et al.** Effects of sodium supplementation during energy restriction on plasma norepinephrine levels in obese women. J Clin Endocrinol Metab. 1991;73:975-81.

30. **US Department of Agriculture, Agricultural Research Service.** Data tables: results from USDA's 1994-96 Continuing Survey of Food Intakes by Individuals and 1994-96 Diet and Health Knowledge Survey. ARS Food Surveys Research Group. Riverdale, MD: US Department of Agriculture; 1997:1-58 (www.barc.usda. gov/bhnrc/foodsurvey/home.htm).

31. **Taubes G.** The (political) science of salt. Science. 1998;281:898-907.

32. **McCarron DA.** The dietary guideline for sodium: should we shake it up? Yes! Am J Clin Nutr. 2000;71:1013-9.

33. **Kaplan NM.** The dietary guideline for sodium: should we shake it up? No. Am J Clin Nutr. 2000;71:1020-6.

34. **National Heart, Lung, and Blood Institute.** NHLBI study shows large blood pressure benefit from reduced dietary sodium. National Heart, Lung, and Blood Institute Web site.

35. **Niels GA, Galloe AM, Garred P.** Effects of sodium restriction on blood pressure, renin, aldosterone, catecholamines, cholesterols, and triglyceride: a meta-analysis. JAMA. 1998;279:1383-93.

36. **DeFronzo RA.** The effect of insulin on renal sodium metabolism: a review with clinical implications. Diabetologia. 1981;21:165-71.

37. **Golay A, Felber JP, Dusmet M, et al.** Effect of weight loss on glucose disposal in obese and obese diabetic patients. Int J Obes. 1985;9:181-90.

38. **Freidenberg GR, Reichart D, Olefsky JM, Henry RR.** Reversibility of defective adipocyte insulin receptor tyrosine kinase activity in non-insulin-dependent diabetes mellitus: effects of weight loss. J Clin Invest. 1988;82:1398-1406.

39. **Welle S, Statt M, Barnard R, Amatruda J.** Differential effect of insulin on whole-body proteolysis and glucose metabolism in normal-weight, obese, and reduced-obese women. Metabolism. 1994;43:441-5.

40. **Atkinson RL, Pi-Sunyer FX.** Very-low-calorie diets. Am J Clin Nutr. 1992; 56(suppl 1):175S-305S.

41. **Gumbiner B, Polonsky KS, Beltz WF, et al.** Effects of weight loss and reduced hyperglycemia on the kinetics of insulin secretion in obese non-insulin-dependent diabetes mellitus. J Clin Endocrinol Metab. 1990;70:1594-1602.

42. **Polonsky KS, Gumbiner B, Ostrega D, et al.** Alterations in immunoreactive proinsulin and insulin clearance induced by weight loss in NIDDM. Diabetes. 1994;43:871-7.

43. **Letiexhe MR, Scheen AJ, Gerard PL, et al.** Postgastroplasty recovery of ideal body weight normalizes glucose and insulin metabolism in obese women. J Clin Endocrinol Metab. 1995;80:364-9.

44. **Phinney SD, Horton ES, Sims EA, et al.** Capacity for moderate exercise in obese subjects after adaptation to a hypocaloric, ketogenic diet. J Clin Invest. 1980;66:1152-61.

45. **Gupta AK, Clark RV, Kirchner KA.** Effects of insulin on renal sodium excretion. Hypertension. 1992;19(suppl 1):I-78-I-82.

46. **Saudek CD, Boulter PR, Arky RA.** The natriuretic effect of glucagon and its role in starvation. J Clin Endocrinol Metab. 1973;36:761-5.

47. **Spark RF, Arky RA, Boulter PR, et al.** Renin, aldosterone and glucagon in the natriuresis of fasting. N Engl J Med. 1975; 292:1335-40.

48. **Farah AE.** Glucagon and circulation. Pharmacol Rev. 1983;35:181-217.

49. **Starke A, Starke G, Jorgens V, et al.** Raised plasma glucagon levels in obesity. Dtsch Med Wochenschr. 1982;107:1125-8.

50. **Starke AA, Erhardt G, Berger M, Zimmerman H.** Elevated pancreatic glucagon in obesity. Diabetes. 1984;33:277-80.

51. **Larsson H, Ahren B.** Islet dysfunction in obese women with impaired glucose tolerance. Metabolism. 1996;45:502-9.

52. **Fery F, Balasse EO.** Glucose metabolism during the starved-to-fed transition in obese patients with NIDDM. Diabetes. 1994;43:1418-25.

53. **Larsson H, Ahren B.** Islet dysfunction in insulin resistance involves impaired insulin secretion and increased glucagon secretion in postmenopausal women with impaired glucose tolerance. Diabetes Care. 2000;23:650-7.

54. **Ipp E.** Impaired glucose tolerance: the irrepressible alpha cell? Diabetes Care. 2000;23:569-70.

55. **Savage PJ, Bennion LJ, Flock EV, et al.** Diet-induced improvement of abnormalities in insulin and glucagon secretion and in insulin receptor binding in diabetes mellitus. J Clin Endocrinol Metab. 1979;48:999-1007.

56. **Kanaley JA, Haymond MW, Jensen MD.** Effects of exercise and weight loss on leucine turnover in different types of obesity. Am J Physiol. 1993;264:E687-E692.

57. **Vazquez JA, Adibi SA.** Protein sparing during treatment of obesity: ketogenic versus nonketogenic very low calorie diet. Metabolism. 1992;41:406-14.

58. **Ravussin E, Burnand B, Schutz Y, Jequier E.** Energy expenditure before and during energy restriction in obese patients. Am J Clin Nutr. 1985;41:753-9.

59. **Gumbiner B, Wendel JA, McDermott MP.** Effects of diet composition and ketosis on glycemia during very-low-energy-diet therapy in obese patients with non-insulin-dependent diabetes mellitus. Am J Clin Nutr. 1996;63:110-5.

60. **Low CC, Grossman EB, Gumbiner B.** Potentiation of effects of weight loss by monounsaturated fatty acids in obese NIDDM patients. Diabetes. 1996;45:569-71.

61. **McGarry JD.** What if Minkowski had been ageusic? An alternative angle on diabetes. Science. 1992;258:766-70.

62. **Unger RH, Orci L.** Physiology and pathophysiology of glucagon. Physiol Rev. 1976;56:778-826.

63. **Lewis SB, Wallin JD, Kane JP, Gerich JE.** Effect of diet composition on metabolic adaptations to hypocaloric nutrition: comparison of high carbohydrate and high fat isocaloric diets. Am J Clin Nutr. 1977;30:160-70.

64. Therapeutic category index. In: PDR for Herbal Medicines. Gruenwald J, Brendler T, Jaenicke C, eds. Montvale, NJ: Medical Economics; 1998:201-27.

65. **Daniels TC, Jorgensen EC.** Central nervous systems stimulants. In Wilson and Grisvold's Textbook of Organic Medicinal and Pharmaceutical Chemistry. Doerge RF, ed. Philadelphia: JB Lippincott; 1982:383-400.

66. **Neuhauser-Berthold BS, Verwied SC, Luhrmann PM.** Coffee consumption and total body water homeostasis as measured by fluid balance and bioelectrical impedance analysis. Ann Nutr Metab. 1997;41:29-36.

67. **Bellet S, Roman L, DeCastro O, et al.** Effect of coffee ingestion on catecholamine release. Metabolism. 1969;18:288-91.

68. **Rachima-Maoz C, Peleg E, Rosenthal T.** The effect of caffeine on ambulatory blood pressure in hypertensive patients. Am J Hypertens. 1998;11:1426-32.

69. **Romoff MS, Keusch G, Campese VM, et al.** Effect of sodium intake on plasma catecholamines in normal subjects. J Clin Endocrinol Metab. 1979;48:26-31.

70. **Marliss EB.** Protein diets for obesity: metabolic and clinical aspects. CMAJ. 1978;119:1413-21.

71. **Genuth SM.** Supplemented fasting in the treatment of obesity and diabetes. Am J Clin Nutr. 1979;32:2579-86.

72. **Astrup A, Vrist E, Quadde F.** Dietary fibre added to very low calorie diet reduces hunger and alleviates constipation. Int J Obes. 1989;14:105-12.

73. **Bistrian BR.** Clinical use of a protein-sparing modified fast. JAMA. 1978;240: 2299-2302.

74. **Amatruda JM, Richeson JF, Welle SL, et al.** The safety and efficacy of a controlled low-energy ('very-low-calorie') diet in the treatment of non-insulin-dependent diabetes and obesity. Arch Intern Med. 1988;148:873-7.

75. **Seely BL, Olefsky JM.** Potential cellular and genetic mechanisms for insulin resistance in the common disorders of diabetes and obesity. In: Insulin Resistance. Moller DE, ed. London: John Wiley; 1993:187-252.

76. **DeFronzo RA.** The triumvirate: beta-cell, muscle, liver—a collusion responsible for NIDDM. Diabetes. 1988;37:667-87.

77. **Polonsky KS.** The B-cell in diabetes: from molecular genetics to clinical research. Diabetes. 1995;44:705-17.

78. **Cahill GF Jr.** Beta-cell deficiency, insulin resistance, or both? N Engl J Med. 1988;318:1268-9.

79. **Gumbiner B.** The treatment of obesity in type 2 diabetes mellitus. Prim Care. 1999;26:869-93.

80. **Henry RR, Gumbiner B.** Benefits and limitations of very-low-calorie diet therapy in obese NIDDM. Diabetes Care. 1991;14:802-23.

81. **Kelley D.** Effects of weight loss on glucose homeostasis in NIDDM. Diabetes Reviews. 1995;3:366-77.

82. **Henry RR, Scheaffer L, Olefsky JM.** Glycemic effects of intensive caloric restriction and isocaloric refeeding in noninsulin-dependent diabetes mellitus. J Clin Endocrinol Metab. 1985; 61:917-25.

83. **Kelley DE, Wing R, Buonocore C, et al.** Relative effects of calorie restriction and weight loss in noninsulin-dependent diabetes mellitus. J Clin Endocrinol Metab. 1993;77:1287-93.

84. **Wing RR, Koeske R, Epstein LH, et al.** Long-term effects of modest weight loss in type II diabetic patients. Arch Intern Med. 1987;147:1749-53.

85. **Wing RR, Blair EH, Bononi P, et al.** Caloric restriction per se is a significant factor in improvements in glycemic control and insulin sensitivity during weight loss in obese NIDDM patients. Diabetes Care. 1994;17:30-6.

86. **Wing RR, Epstein LH, Nowalk MP, et al.** Does self-monitoring of blood glucose levels improve dietary compliance for obese patients with type II diabetes? Am J Med. 1986; 81:830-6.

87. **Hollander PA, Elbein SC, Hirsch IB, et al.** Role of orlistat in the treatment of obese patients with type 2 diabetes: a 1-year randomized double-blind study. Diabetes Care. 1998;21:1288-94.

88. **Minuk HL, Vranic M, Hanna AK, et al.** Glucoregulatory and metabolic response to exercise in obese non-insulin-dependent diabetes. Am J Physiol. 1981;240: E458-E464.

89. **Wasserman DH, Zinman B.** Fuel homeostasis. In: The Health Professional's Guide to Diabetes and Exercise. Ruderman N, Devlin JT, eds. Alexandria, VA: American Diabetes Association; 1995:27-48.

90. **Bogardus C, Ravussin E, Robbins DC, et al.** Effects of physical training and diet therapy on carbohydrate metabolism in patients with glucose intolerance and non-insulin-dependent diabetes mellitus. Diabetes. 1984;33:311-8.

91. **Trovati M, Carta Q, Cavalot F, et al.** Influence of physical training on blood glucose control, glucose tolerance, insulin secretion, and insulin action in non-insulin-dependent diabetic patients. Diabetes Care. 1984;7:416-20.

92. **Dela F, Ploug T, Handberg A, et al.** Physical training increases muscle GLUT4 protein and mRNA in patients with NIDDM. Diabetes. 1994;43:862-5.

93. **Kemmer FW, Tacken M, Berger M.** Mechanism of exercise-induced hypoglycemia during sulfonylurea treatment. Diabetes. 1987;36:1178-82.

94. **American Diabetes Association.** Clinical practice recommendations—2001. Diabetes Care. 2001;24(suppl 1):S1-S137.

95. **JNC VI:** The Sixth Report of the Joint National Committee on Prevention, Detection, Evaluation, and Treatment of High Blood Pressure. Arch Intern Med. 1997;157:2413-46.

96. **NHLBI Obesity Education Expert Panel.** Clinical guidelines on the identification, evaluation, and treatment of overweight and obesity in adults: the evidence report. NIH Publication 98-4083. Bethesda, MD: National Institute of Health/National Heart, Lung, and Blood Institute; 1998.

97. **MacMahon S, Cutler J, Brittain E, Higgins M.** Obesity and hypertension: epidemiological and clinical issues. Eur Heart J. 1987;8(suppl B):57-70.

98. **Wassertheil-Smoller S, Blaufox MD, Oberman AS, et al.** The Trial of Antihypertensive Interventions and Management (TAIM) study: adequate weight loss, alone and combined with drug therapy in the treatment of mild of hypertension. Arch Intern Med. 1992;152:131-6.

99. **Wassertheil-Smoller S, Langford HG, Blaufox MD, et al.** Effective dietary intervention in hypertensives: sodium restriction and weight reduction. J Am Diet Assoc. 1985;85:423-30.

100. **Langford HG, Davis BR, Blaufox MD, et al.** Effect of drug and diet treatment of mild hypertension on diastolic blood pressure. The TAIM Research Group. Hypertension. 1991;17:210-7.

101. **Whelton PK, Appel LJ, Espeland MA, et al.** Sodium reduction and weight loss in the treatment of hypertension in older persons: a randomized controlled trial of nonpharmacologic interventions in the elderly (TONE). JAMA. 1998;279:839-46.

102. **The Trials of Hypertension Prevention Collaborative Research Group.** Effects of weight loss and sodium reduction intervention on blood pressure and hypertension incidence in overweight people with high-normal blood pressure. Arch Intern Med. 1997;157:657-67.

103. **Espeland MA, Whelton PK, Kostis JB, et al.** Predictors and mediators of successful long-term withdrawal from antihypertensive medications. TONE Cooperative Research Group. Trial of Nonpharmacologic Interventions in the Elderly. Arch Fam Med. 1999;8:228-36.

104. **Stampfer MJ, Maclure KM, Colditz GA, et al.** Risk of symptomatic gallstones in women with severe obesity. Am J Clin Nutr. 1992;55:652-8.

105. **Everhart JE.** Contributions of obesity and weight loss to gallstone disease. Ann Intern Med. 1993;119:1029-35.

106. **Hofmann AF.** Primary and secondary prevention of gallstone disease: implications for patient management and research priorities. Am J Gastro. 1993;165:541-8.

107. **Marks JW, Bonorris GG, Schoenfield LJ.** Effects of ursodiol or ibuprofen on contraction of gallbladder and bile among obesity patients during weight loss. Dig Dis Sci. 1996;41:242-9.

108. **Weinsier RL, Ullmann DO.** Gallstone formation and weight loss. Obes Res. 1993;1:51-5.

109. **Sugerman HJ, Brewer WH, Shiffman ML, et al.** A multicenter, placebo-controlled, randomized, double-blind, prospective trial of prophylactic ursodiol for the prevention of gallstone formation following gastric-bypass-induced rapid weight loss. Am J Surg. 1995;169:91-7.

110. **Weinsier RL, Wilson LJ, Lee J.** Medically safe rate of weight loss for the treatment of obesity: a guideline based on risk of gallstone formation. Am J Med. 1995;98:115-7.

111. **Hoy MK, Heshka S, Allison DB, et al.** Reduced risk of liver-function-test abnormalities and new gallstone formation with weight loss on 3350-kJ (800-kcal) formula diets. Am J Clin Nutr. 1994;60:249-54.

112. **Festi D, Colecchia A, Orsini M, et al.** Gallbladder motility and gallstone formation in obese patients following very low calorie diets: use it (fat) to lose it (well). Int J Obes. 1998;22:592-600.

113. **Gebhard RL, Prigge WF, Ansel HJ, et al.** The role of gallbladder emptying in gallstone formation during diet-induced rapid weight loss. Hepatology. 1996; 24:544-8.

114. **Reuben A, Qureshi Y, Murphy GM, Dowling RH.** Effect of obesity and weight reduction on biliary cholesterol saturation and the response to chenodeoxycholic acid. Eur J Clin Invest. 1985;16:133-42.

115. **Broomfield PH, Chopra R, Sheinbaum RC, et al.** Effects of ursodeoxycholic acid and aspirin on the formation of lithogenic bile and gallstones during loss of weight. N Engl J Med. 1988;319:1567-72.

116. **Shiffman ML, Kaplan GD, Brinkman-Kaplan V, Vickers FF.** Prophylaxis against gallstone formation with ursodeoxycholic acid in patients participating in very-low-calorie diet program. Ann Intern Med. 1995;122:899-905.

117. **Shoheiber O, Biskupiak JE, Nash DB.** Estimation of the cost savings resulting from the use of ursodiol for the prevention of gallstones in obese patients undergoing rapid weight reduction. Int J Obes. 1997;21:1038-45.

118. **Marks JW, Stein T, Schoenfield LJ.** Natural history and treatment with ursodiol of gallstones formed during rapid loss of weight in man. Dig Dis Sci. 1994;39:1981-4.

119. **Lee SP, Nicholls JF, Park HZ.** Biliary sludge as a cause of acute pancreatitis. N Engl J Med. 1992;326:589-93.

120. **Keane FB, Fennell JS, Tomkin GH.** Acute pancreatitis, acute gastric dilation and duodenal ileus following refeeding in anorexia nervosa. Ir J Med Sci. 1978;147: 191-2.

121. **Gryboski J, Hillemeier C, Kochoshis S, et al.** Refeeding pancreatitis in malnourished children. J Pediatr. 1980;97:441-3.

122. **Foster DW.** Anorexia nervosa and bulimia. In: Harrison's Principles of Internal Medicine. Isselbacher KJ, Braunwald E, Wilson JD, eds. New York: McGraw-Hill; 1994:452-5.

123. **Neuschwander-Terti B, Bacon BR.** Nonalcoholic steatohepatitis. Med Clin North Am. 1996;80:1147-66.

124. **Sheth SG, Gordon FD, Chopra S.** Nonalcoholic steatohepatitis. Ann Intern Med. 1997;126:137-45.

125. **James OFW, Day CP.** Non-alcoholic steatohepatitis (NASH): a disease of emerging identity and importance. J Hepatol. 1998;29:495-501.

126. **Ratziu V, Giral P, Charlotte F, et al.** Liver fibrosis in overweight patients. Gastroenterology. 2000;118:1117-23.

127. **Marceau P, Biron S, Hould F-S, et al.** Liver pathology and the metabolic syndrome X in severe obesity. J Clin Endocrinol Metab. 1999;84:1513-7.

128. **Hotamisligil GS, Spiegelman BM.** Tumor necrosis factor alpha: a key component of the obesity-diabetes link. Diabetes. 1994;43:1271-8.

129. **Berliner JA, Navab M, Fogelman AM, et al.** Atherosclerosis: basic mechanisms oxidation, inflammation, and genetics. Circulation. 1995;91:2488-96.

130. **Andersen T, Gluud C, Franzmann M-B, Christoffersen P.** Hepatic effects of dietary weight loss in morbidly obese subjects. Hepatology. 1991;12:224-9.

131. **Luyckx FH, Desaive C, Thiry A, et al.** Liver abnormalities in severely obese subjects: effect of drastic weight loss after gastroplasty. Int J Obes. 1998;22:222-6.

132. **Frank S, Colliver JA, Frank A.** The electrocardiogram in obesity: statistical analysis of 1,029 patients. J Am Coll Cardiol. 1986;7:295-9.

133. **Messerli FH, Nunez BD, Ventura HO, Snyder DW.** Overweight and sudden dealth: increased ventricular ectopy in cardiopathy of obesity. Arch Intern Med. 1987;147:1725-8.

134. **Park J-J, Swan PD.** Effect of obesity and regional adiposity on the QT_c interval in women. Int J Obes. 1997;21:1104-10.

135. **Drenick EJ, Fisler JS.** Sudden cardiac arrest in morbidly obese surgical patients unexplained after autopsy. Am J Surg. 1988;155:720-6.

136. **Isner JM, Sours HE, Paris AL, et al.** Sudden, unexpected death in avid dieters using the liquid-protein modified-fast diet: observations in 17 patients and the role of the prolonged QT interval. Circulation. 1979;60:1401-12.

137. **Sours HE, Frattali VP, Brand CD, et al.** Sudden death associated with very low calorie weight reduction regimens. Am J Clin Nutr. 1981;34:453-61.

138. **Frank A, Graham C, Frank S.** Fatalities on the liquid-protein diet: an analysis of possible causes. Int J Obes. 1981;5:243-8.

139. **Brown JM, Yetter JF, Spicer MJ, Jones JD.** Cardiac complications of protein-sparing modified fasting. JAMA. 1978;240:120-2.

140. **Moss AJ.** Caution: very-low-calorie diets can be deadly. Ann Intern Med. 1985;102:121-3.

141. **Center for Disease Control.** Liquid protein diets. EPI-78-11-2. Atlanta, US Public Health Service; 1979.

142. **Seim HC, Mitchell JE, Pomeroy C, deZwaan, M.** Electrocardiographic findings associated with very low calorie dieting. Int J Obes. 1995;19:817-9.

143. **Amatruda JM, Biddle TL, Patton ML, Lockwood DH.** Vigorous supplementation of a hypocaloric diet prevents cardiac arrhythmias and mineral depletion. Am J Med. 1983;74:1016-22.

144. **Phinney SD, Bistrian BR, Kosinski E, et al.** Normal cardiac rhythm during hypocaloric diets of varying carbohydrate content. Arch Intern Med. 1983;143: 2258-61.

145. **Doherty JU, Wadden T, Zuk L, et al.** Long-term evaluation of cardiac function in obese patients treated with a very-low-calorie diet: a controlled clinical study of patients without underlying cardiac disease [Abstract]. Am J Clin Nutr. 1991;53:854-8.

146. **Devereux RB.** Appetite suppressants and valvular heart disease. N Engl J Med. 1998;339:765-7.

147. **Klein AL, Burstow DJ, Tajik AJ, et al.** Age-related prevalence of valvular regurgitation in normal subjects: comprehensive color flow examination of 118 volunteers. J Am Soc Echocardiogr. 1990;3:54-63.

148. **Reid CL, Gardin JM, Yunis C, et al.** Prevalence and clinical correlates of aortic and mitral regurgitation in a young adult population [Abstract]. Circulation. 1994;90:1520.

149. **Khan MA, Herzog CA, St. Peter JV, et al.** The prevalence of cardiac valvular insufficiency assessed by transthoracic echocardiography in obese patients treated with appetite-suppressant drugs. N Engl J Med. 1998;339:713-8.

150. **Jick J, Vasilakis C, Weinrauch LA, et al.** A population-based study of appetite-suppressant drugs and the risk of cardiac-valve regurgitation. N Engl J Med. 1998;339:719-724.

151. **Weissman NJ, Tighe JF, Gottdiener JS, Gwynne JT, for the Sustained-Release Dexfenfluramine Study Group.** An assessment of heart-valve abnormalities in obese patients taking dexfenfluramine, sustained-release dexfenfluramine, or placebo. N Engl J Med. 1998;339:725-32.

152. **Bach DS, Rissanen AM, Mendel CM, et al.** Absence of cardiac valve disease dysfunction in obese patients treated with sibutramine. Obes Res. 1999;7:363-9.

153. **Karason K, Wallentin I, Larsson B, Sjostrom L** Effects of obesity and weight loss on cardiac function and valvular performance. Obes Res. 1998;6:422-9.

154. **Matsuura F, Yamashita S, Nakamura T, et al.** Effect of visceral fat accumulation on uric acid metabolism in male obese subjects: visceral fat obesity is linked more closely to overproduction of uric acid than subcutaneous obesity. Metabolism. 1998;47:929-33.

155. **Fox IH, Halperin ML, Goldstein MB, Marliss EB.** Renal excretion of uric acid during prolonged fasting. Metabolism. 1976;25:551-9.

156. **Henry RR, Wiest-Kent TA, Scheaffer L, et al.** Metabolic consequences of very-low-calorie diet therapy in obese non-insulin-dependent diabetic and nondiabetic subjects. Diabetes. 1986;35:155-64.

157. **Vazquez JA, Kazi U, Madani N.** Protein metabolism during weight reduction with very-low-energy diets: evaluation of the independent effects of protein and carbohydrate on protein sparing. Am J Clin Nutr. 1995;62:93-103.

158. **Yamashita S, Matsuzawa Y, Tokunaga K, et al.** Studies on the impaired metabolism of uric acid in obese subjects: marked reduction of renal urate excretion and its improvement by a low-calorie diet. Int J Obes. 1986;10:255-64.

159. **Fisler JS, Drenick EJ.** Starvation and semistarvation diets in the management of obesity. Annu Rev Nutr. 1987;7:465-84.

160. **Spaulding SW, Chopra IJ, Sherwin RS, Lyall SS.** Effect of caloric restriction and dietary composition on serum T3 and reverse T3 in man. J Clin Endocrinol Metab. 1976;42:197-200.

161. **Davies HJA, Baird IM, Fowler J, et al.** Metabolic response to low- and very-low-calorie diets. Am J Clin Nutr. 1989;49:745-51.

162. **Fisler JS.** Cardiac effects of starvation and semistarvation diets: safety and mechanisms of action. Am J Clin Nutr. 1992;56:230S-234S.

163. **National Task Force on the Prevention and Treatment of Obesity.** Weight cycling. JAMA. 1994;272:1196-1202.

164. **Blackburn GL.** Benefits of weight loss in the treatment of obesity. Am J Clin Nutr. 1999;69:347-9.

164a. Study of Health Outcomes of Weight-loss (SHOW) Trial. http://www.niddk.nih.gov/patinet/SHOW/showhmpg.htm.

165. **Sjostrom L, Larsson B, Backman L, et al.** Swedish obese subjects (SOS): recruitment for an intervention study and a selected description of the obese state. Int J Obes. 1992;16:465-79.

166. **Forbes GB, Welle SL.** Lean body mass in obesity. Int J Obes. 1983;7:99-107.

167. **Brylinsky C.** The nutritional care process. In: Krause's Food, Nutrition, and Diet Therapy. Mahan K, Escott-Stump S, eds. Philadelphia: WB Saunders; 2000:431-51.

168. **Ettinger S.** Macronutrients: carbohydrates, proteins, and lipids. In: Krause's Food, Nutrition, and Diet Therapy. Mahan K, Escott-Stump S, eds. Philadelphia: WB Saunders; 2000;31-66.

169. **Vazquez JA, Morse EL, Adibi SA.** Effect of dietary fat, carbohydrate and protein on branched-chain amino acid catabolism during caloric restriction. J Clin Invest. 1985;76:737-43.

170. **National Task Force on the Prevention and Treatment of Obesity.** Weight cycling. JAMA. 1994;272:1196-202.

171. **James WP, Davies HL, Bailes J, Dauncey MJ.** Elevated metabolic rates in obesity. Lancet. 1978;1:1122-5.

172. **Amatruda JM, Statt MC, Welle SL.** Total and resting energy expenditure in obese women reduced to ideal body weight. J Clin Invest. 1993;92:1236-42.

173. **Weinsier RL, Nelson KM, Hensrud DD, et al.** Metabolic predictors of obesity: contribution of resting energy expenditure, thermic effect of food, and fuel utilization to four-year weight gain of post-obese and never-obese women. J Clin Invest. 1995;95:980-5.

174. **Weinsier RL, Hunter GR, Zuckerman PA, et al.** Energy expenditure and free-living physical activity in black and white women: comparison before and after weight loss. Am J Clin Nutr. 2000;71:1138-46.

175. **Ferraro R, Lillioja S, Fontvieille AM, et al.** Lower sedentary metabolic rate in women compared with men. J Clin Invest. 1992;90:780-4.

176. **Swinburn BA, Nyomba BL, Saad MF, et al.** Insulin resistance associated with lower rates of weight gain in Pima Indians. J Clin Invest. 1991;88:168-73.

177. **Ballor DL, Harvey-Berino JR, Ades PA, et al.** Decrease in fat oxidation following a meal in weight-reduced individuals: a possible mechanism for weight recidivism. Metabolism. 1996;45:174-8.

178. **Larson DE, Ferraro RT, Robertson DS, Ravussin, E.** Energy metabolism in weight-stable postobese individuals. Am J Clin Nutr. 1995;62:735-9.

179. **Gannon B, DiPietro L, Poehlman ET.** Do African Americans have lower energy expenditure than Caucasians? Int J Obes. 2000;24:13.

180. **Ravussin E, Bogardus C.** A brief overview of human energy metabolism and its relationship to essential obesity. Am J Clin Nutr. 1992;55:242S-245S.

181. **Weyer C, Pratley RE, Salbe AD, et al.** Energy expenditure, fat oxidation, and body weight regulation: a study of metabolic adaptation to long-term weight change. J Clin Endocrinol Metab. 2000;85:1094.

182. **Bouchard C, Perusse L.** Genetics of obesity. Annu Rev Nutr. 1993;13:337-54.

183. **Hill JO, Peters JC.** Environmental contributions to the obesity epidemic. Science. 1998;280:1371-4.

184. **National Institute of Arthritis and Musculoskeletal and Skin Diseases Consensus Development Panel.** Osteoporosis Prevention, Diagnosis and Therapy. NIH Consensus Statement Online 17(2), 1-36. National Institutes of Health. Ref Type: Electronic Citation.

185. **Licata AA, Lantigua RA, Amatruda JM, Lockwood DH.** Adverse effects of liquid protein fast on the handling of magnesium, calcium and phosphorus. Am J Med. 1981;71:767-72.

186. **Andersen RE, Wadden TA, Herzog RJ.** Changes in bone mineral content in obese dieting women. Metabolism. 1997; 46:857-61.

187. **Salamone LM, Cauley JA, Black DM, et al.** Effect of a lifestyle intervention on bone mineral density in premenopausal women: a randomized trial. Am J Clin Nutr. 1999;70:97-103.

188. **Compston JE, Laskey MA, Croucher PI, et al.** Effect of diet-induced weight loss on total body bone mass. Clin Sci. 1992;82:429-32.

189. **Ensrud KE, Cauley J, Lipschutz R, Cummings SR, for the Study of Osteoporotic Fractures Research Group.** Weight change and fractures in older women. Arch Intern Med. 1997;157:857-63.

190. **Goulding A, Taylor RW, Jones IE, et al.** Overweight and obese children have low bone mass and area for their weight. Int J Obes. 2000;24:627-32.

190a. **Kraut JA, Coburn JW.** Bone, acid and osteoporosis. N Engl J Med. 1994;330: 1821-2.

191. **Gougeon-Reyburn R, Lariviere F, Marliss EB.** Effects of bicarbonate supplementation on urinary mineral excretion during very low energy diets. Am J Med Sci. 1991;302:67-74.

192. **VanItallie TB.** Treatment of obesity: can it become a science? Obes Res. 2000;7: 605-6.

KEY REFERENCES

Everhart JE. Contributions of obesity and weight loss to gallstone disease. Ann Intern Med. 1993;119:1029-35.

Fisler JS. Cardiac effects of starvation and semistarvation diets: safety and mechanisms of action. Am J Clin Nutr. 1992;56:230S-234S.

Fisler JS, Drenick EJ. Starvation and semistarvation diets in the management of obesity. Annu Rev Nutr. 1987;7:465-84.

Henry RR, Gumbiner B. Benefits and limitations of very-low-calorie diet therapy in obese NIDDM. Diabetes Care. 1991;14:802-23.

National Task Force on the Prevention and Treatment of Obesity. Very low-calorie diets. JAMA. 1993;270:967-74.

National Task Force on the Prevention and Treatment of Obesity. Weight cycling. JAMA. 1994;272:1196-1202.

NHLBI Obesity Education Expert Panel. Clinical Guidelines on the Identification, Evaluation, and Treatment of Overweight and Obesity in Adults: The Evidence Report. NIH Publication 98-4083. Bethesda, MD: National Institutes of Health/National Heart, Lung, and Blood Institute; 1998:95-7.

VanItallie TB, Yang M-U. Current concepts in nutrition: diet and weight loss. N Engl J Med. 1972;297:1158-61.

Weinsier RL, Ullmann DO. Gallstone formation and weight loss. Obes Res. 1993;1:51-5.

Weinsier RL, Wilson LJ, Lee J. Medically safe rate of weight loss for the treatment of obesity: a guideline based on risk of gallstone formation. Am J Med. 1995;98:115-7.

5

■ ■ ■

Medical Assessment and Treatment of the Obese Patient

Leonard I. Mastbaum, MD

Barry Gumbiner, MD

eview articles and book chapters on how to perform the medical assessment of the obese patient are among the most challenging to compose. This is a reflection of obesity's impact on nearly every major organ system and the pervasiveness of the condition. Invariably, the review or chapter reads more like a basic medical school text on how to conduct a comprehensive history and physical exam rather than one focused on the obese patient. The complexity of obesity, however, requires a more comprehensive approach than the typical challenges of primary care medicine. Within that context this chapter, emphasizing the unique issues encountered in the obese patient, has been purposely placed after the chapter on medical complications. By doing so, it is hoped that practitioners can apply this information when performing their assessment and formulate a treatment plan tailored to anticipated problems. Thus the practitioner's basic, already-mastered medical skills can be utilized in a new context to provide a systematic and safe treatment regimen for the obese patient.

Effective management must be based on a thorough understanding of both the medical condition and the psychosocial milieu of the individual patient. For many patients with clinical obesity, this evaluation, as well as subsequent treatment, are most effectively carried out by a coordinated team of professionals experienced in obesity treatment. The team approach blends the skills of a physician experienced in obesity management with the dietitian, behaviorist, and exercise physiologist. The availability of a consulting staff in the related disciplines (e.g., physical therapy, psychology/psychiatry, cardiology) is also essential. The critical role of the primary care physician is to coordinate care of the obese patient under the auspices of a multidisciplinary health care team and to ensure the medical safety of the patient during treatment.

The objectives of the medical assessment are to

- Characterize the overweight or obese condition of the patient
- Determine the level of health risk associated with the patient's overweight or obese condition
- Delineate the co-morbidities that are caused and/or exacerbated by the obesity and may interfere or even contraindicate treatment
- Identify reversible conditions contributing to the patient's excess weight or potential to reduce weight (e.g., secondary etiologies of obesity such as hypothyroidism, Cushing syndrome, and pharmacotherapies that promote weight gain)
- Determine the patient's level of motivation
- Design the most appropriate strategy for weight management

As noted in Chapters 8 and 12, studies support the anecdotal experience of nearly all practitioners that a patient's expectations for weight loss are usually unrealistic and often focus on cosmetic rather than health concerns. Nevertheless, the evidence discussed in Chapters 1, 3, and 4 and summarized in the National Institutes of Health (NIH) report clearly indicates that only a sustained, approximately 10% weight loss is required for significant improvement of health. Moreover, clinical trials have proven that this is a reasonable and achievable goal for most patients. Therefore the major challenge for the practitioner may be reorienting the patient's expectations, or in psychology terms, *cognitive restructuring*.

After the patient achieves and sustains the 10% weight reduction goal, the need for further weight loss can be reassessed. Weight loss beyond 10% is not recommended for most patients until they successfully practice, apply, and reinforce their new lifestyle skills for a significant period. This is far more difficult than losing more weight and warrants the additional attention needed to optimize long-term weight maintenance. Anecdotally, continually reminding the patient that the scale is simply a medical monitoring tool and not an end in itself can be an effective way to help the patient overcome this major psychological obstacle.

Characterization of Excess Weight

Whole-Body Assessment

Body mass index (BMI) and related anthropometrics should be given a status equal to vital signs. These measures are key predictive and monitoring tools. BMI is the most practical way to define the significance of excess body weight in an individual patient. More sophisticated measurements (described in the Methods of Characterization section below) are unnecessary and cost prohibitive in the clinical setting.

BMI is the measurement of weight "normalized" to height:

$$BMI = Weight\ (in\ kilograms)/Height\ (in\ meters)^2$$

or

$$BMI = [Weight\ (in\ pounds)/Height\ (in\ inches)^2] \times 703$$

The actual calculation is cumbersome, but numerous tables, nomograms, and even slide rules exist to assist the clinician in rapidly obtaining this information (Fig. 5.1). Furthermore, because height, unlike weight, is essentially constant over time, BMI mathematically correlates directly with weight. Thus weight can be used to monitor clinical progress and attainment of a BMI goal.

BMI is now unequivocally the standard method for determining obesity. The term *ideal body weight* (IBW) should be removed from the practitioner's lexicon when communicating with patients and health professionals. (IBW is still useful for some purposes, such as determining certain nutritional needs, but otherwise this term is obsolete.) IBW incorrectly conveys a goal that is not only unrealistic but unnecessary for achieving healthy outcomes. Even the term *desirable weight*, a designation many consider more acceptable, suffers from this pitfall. As part of the cognitive restructuring process, the term *healthy weight* has more legitimacy because of its positive connotation and its ability to be customized to the needs and goals of individual patients.

Although the terms *overweight* and *obesity* are often used interchangeably, recent clinical guidelines published by NIH differentiate the terms (Table 5.1). The overweight category, in particular, is commonly misunderstood by both patients and health care professionals. It is meant to connote an "at risk" category rather than an absolute medical condition and is not intended to be pejorative, even though it is commonly perceived as such. Thus some overweight individuals can be extremely healthy, so their medical risk is minimal as long as they remain weight stable. The classic example is athletes who can have a BMI in the overweight range but do not have excess fat. However, the typical patient encountered in the clinical

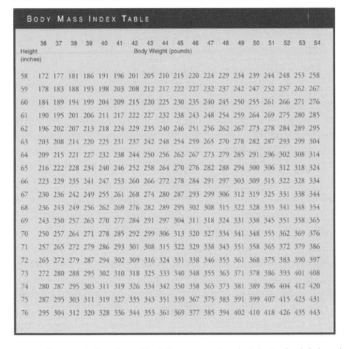

Figure 5.1 Body mass index chart. Find the appropriate height in the left-hand column. Move across to the appropriate weight. The number at the top of the column is the BMI for that height and weight. Pounds have been rounded off. (From NHBLI, Obesity Guidelines—Executive Summary—BMI Chart; *http://www.nhlbi.nih.gov/guide-lines/obesity/bmi_tbl.htm.*)

Table 5.1   NIH Definitions of Weight Classifications

Classification	BMI (kg/m²)
Underweight	<18.5
Normal	18.5–24.9
Overweight	25.0–29.9
Obesity*	30.0–39.9
Extreme obesity†	≥40.0

Modified from NHLBI Obesity Education Expert Panel. Clinical Guidelines on the Identification, Evaluation, and Treatment of Overweight and Obesity in Adults: the Evidence Report. NIH Publication 98-4083. Bethesda, MD: National Institutes of Health/National Heart, Lung, and Blood Institute; 1998.
* The NIH further subdivides both *obesity* and *extreme obesity* into three subclasses.
† The more common term *morbid obesity* is generally synonymous with *extreme obesity* and is still used in the clinical setting and research literature.

setting does not fit this description, and based on risk assessment (described below), most overweight patients benefit from weight loss. Furthermore, even athletes with BMIs in the obese range almost always have excess adiposity that places them at risk (e.g., a football lineman).

Regional Distribution of Fat

A preponderance of adipose tissue distributed in the abdominal region is associated with severe metabolic disturbances and increased morbidity and mortality. This obese condition is referred to by various terms: *central, upper body, upper segment,* or *android obesity.* This is in contrast to *lower body, lower segment,* or *gynoid obesity* in which the risks for morbidity and mortality are intermediate to those with normal BMI versus upper body obesity. Therefore, when characterizing obesity, fat distribution is an important parameter to determine overall risk in overweight and obese individuals.

Historically, the waist-to-hip ratio is the most studied established measurement of fat distribution. Those with a high ratio were deemed to have upper body obesity. However, as reviewed in the NIH report, it has been determined that waist circumference alone without hip measurement correlates better with biomarkers of health risk (e.g., hyperlipidemia, hyperglycemia, hypertension) and presumably health outcomes (actual disease manifestation and mortality). The waist circumference cut-offs established by the NIH to identify those at increased risk are

Men: >102 cm (>40 in.)
Women: >88 cm (>35 in.)

These cutoffs are valid for BMIs $\leq$ 35 kg/m²; waist circumference loses predictive power for BMI > 35 so obtaining this measurement is of questionable medical value at the highest BMI ranges. More importantly, these cut-points are very conservative and underestimate risk in many non-Caucasian populations (1, 2). (The NIH report further subclassifies risk using a combined categorization of BMI and waist circumference but in the clinical setting; the aforementioned cut-offs will achieve the same objective.)

Methods of Characterization

Several other methods are used to classify patient weight and adiposity, but in the vast majority of patients BMI and waist circumference correlate adequately with fat accumulation and are the most practical and economical measurement for clinical purposes. Thus these measurements are now the standard of practice for the medical assessment and monitoring of obesity. However, to help the practitioner address the queries of more knowledgeable patients, some other methods are summarized below.

Ideal Body Weight

Ideal body weight is a product of the classic Metropolitan Life Tables (3), but this method of classification has proven to be quite limited. Unlike BMI, IBW requires a judgement about body habitus (small, medium, or large frame), whereas BMI automatically incorporates this characteristic into its formula. Furthermore, IBW is of narrow utility because it was initially established in upper-middle-class Caucasian males and designed for very limited purposes (i.e., mortality as the only health outcome). Numerous studies have demonstrated that IBW cannot be accurately applied to women or to other ethnic groups. Finally, as noted above, IBW is an unfortunate choice of terminology with connotations that are detrimental to the communication of clinical goals.

Underwater Weighing (Hydrodensity)

Underwater weighing (hydrodensity), an indirect method used to measure total body fat, is considered the gold standard for measuring body composition (4,5). Underwater weighing determines body density based on water displacement and the underwater weight of the patient using strain gauges in conjunction with regular body weight measured on a scale. This method of measurement requires specialized equipment and is highly dependent on the patient's cooperation (e.g., the patient must completely expire and hold breath under water; the patient must have no fear of water). Like all indirect measures, underwater weighing requires use of mathematical models with inherent assumptions to make a final determination of body composition. Nevertheless, under most research conditions, it is considered the best measure of whole-body composition. In the clinical setting, however, it does not have a practical purpose and the equipment needed to conduct the test is not readily available.

Bioelectrical Impedance
Bioelectrical impedance, an indirect method of determining body composition, relies on disparities in the electrical conductance of different tissues, fat and bone being poor conductors compared with aqueous tissues (e.g., muscle) (4-6). Again, like all indirect methods, bioelectrical impedance must use mathematical models with inherent assumptions to determine percent body fat rather than biophysical principles, the validity of which is in question (7). Bioelectrical impedance has the potential to be an effective method but is currently unreliable because of a lack of manufacturing and procedural standardization. The outcome of bioelectrical impedance can be affected by the degree of hydration, a constraint in methodology for weight loss measurements caused by the fluid and electrolyte shifts that occur with treatment (8-10). Moreover, biological impedance is not accurate in determining body composition of severely obese patients (4). Unfortunately, despite the potential for misleading results, bioelectrical impedance is quite popular because the instrument is inexpensive and easy to operate.

Skinfolds
By using special calipers to measure key areas of subcutaneous fat (e.g., triceps, subscapular, pectoral), body composition can be determined after applying mathematical models with inherent assumptions (4, 5). This method is limited by the high level of technical expertise required; even with well-trained, experienced technicians, it is still considered among the least reliable measures of body composition (5).

Dual Energy X-Ray Absorptometry
Dual energy x-ray absorptometry (DEXA) can measure tissue density by determining the attenuation of the intensity of an x-ray or photon source through tissue (4). It is related to the density, thickness, and composition of the tissue and has been most successfully applied to measuring bone mineral density to diagnose osteoporosis. However, when programmed with proper software, DEXA has proven to be quite effective in determining total body composition when a complete body scan is performed. It is relatively inexpensive, no risk to the patient, and an easy test to perform. DEXA has proven to be very useful in a variety of disorders that may affect hydration and body composition (11). Only if the patient is too large to fit on the standard table is there a problem, but even in that situation doubling a half-body measurement has proven to be valid (12). Therefore, if future research proves that measuring body composition in the clinical setting is useful, and as the DEXA technology improves enough to reliably determine both whole-body and regional tissue measurements (e.g.,

intra-abdominal fat), DEXA may prove a cost-effective evaluation in some obese patients. But it has not reached that level of sophistication, and because most bone and radiology centers do not have the software to conduct this procedure it remains relatively inaccessible.

Computed Tomography and Magnetic Resonance Imaging

Besides tissue sampling, computed tomography (CT) and magnetic resonance imaging (MRI) measure body composition with the most accuracy of any method (4, 5). These scans can differentiate between adipose and other tissue types, making them powerful methods for determining not only regional fat distribution but very specific depots as well (13). However, to determine total body composition is expensive and, in the case of a CT scan, requires radiation exposure that is hard to justify for clinical purposes. On the other hand, CT and MRI scans are invaluable tools for measuring regional fat distribution in the research setting, particularly visceral adipose tissue using limited abdominal cuts. In addition, measuring thigh composition to determine intramuscular fat (triglyceride) content may be useful because of the growing appreciation of its metabolic impact (14).

Potassium 40

Potassium 40, a naturally occurring radioisotope, comprises approximately 1% of the body's total potassium (4, 5). Because virtually no potassium is found in triglycerides, fat-free mass can be determined by measuring the body's potassium 40 in a special lead-lined chamber for approximately 45 minutes and applying certain assumptions to a mathematical model. There are very few of these special chambers in the world, but this method has served as a valuable research tool.

24-Hour Urinary Creatinine and 3-Methylhistidine

Ninety-eight percent of total body creatinine is located in skeletal muscle (5). Thus its urinary excretion theoretically can be extrapolated to determine muscle mass. 3-Methylhistidine is a marker of skeletal muscle breakdown, and it too is a tool for determining skeletal muscle mass. Both are relatively inexpensive tests, but as most practitioners know from experience, 24-hour urine collections are notoriously difficult to collect properly. An error of only 15 minutes in the collection can result in up to a 2% error. There is a significant amount of daily variation, partly because of renal physiology and partly because of diet composition. Nevertheless, within the well-controlled environment of a metabolic research unit, 24-hour urinary creatinine has proven to be another useful research tool.

Air Plethysmography

Air plethysmography, a relatively new methodology, is becoming very popular in commercial fitness centers. Similar to the underwater weighing method, air plethysmography relies on principles of volume displacement, in this case air (4, 15). To conduct the test, the individual sits in a special airtight, egg-shaped shell in which air pressure is slightly increased during the procedure. Because pressure is mathematically related to volume, with the help of a reference chamber within in the apparatus, the results can be applied to a mathematical model (with the same caveats alluded to previously when using mathematical models) to determine body composition. Unless the patient is claustrophobic, air plethysmography poses minimal problems or risk. It is easily performed, can be done quickly, and allows repetitive measurements. Although promising (16, 17), the use of air plethysmography is ahead of its validation as an accurate measure of obesity, particularly under the dynamic conditions of weight loss. More studies published in peer-reviewed journals are needed.

Summary

Overall, though all of the foregoing methods have a valuable role in the research setting, it is questionable whether their use will change medical assessments, treatment plans, and implementation of therapy, let alone be cost-effective. Furthermore, these are quantitative measurements that can set up unrealistic expectations and goals for patients. At this time, the only standard of practice is determining the BMI and waist circumference.

Clinical Evaluation of the Obese Patient

Medical assessment must include obesity-specific questions, physical examination, and laboratory evaluation. Completion of a food and activity diary at home before the visit is strongly recommended. This will facilitate developing and integrating the other major components of the treatment plan (nutrition, physical activity, and behavioral therapy) as well as gauge the patient's willingness to use one of the basic and effective tools in weight management .

Obesity-Specific Medical History

The following questions will help elicit obesity-specific information of interest:

1. *When did the patient first consider himself/herself overweight?*

Early onset of obesity, coupled with a strong family history, suggest a strong genetic component to the obesity (see Chapter 2) and reduce the likelihood of secondary endogenous causes (e.g., Cushing syndrome).

2. *When were the periods of major weight gain?*

Patients often say that their weight gain was gradual, but careful questioning may identify periods of major weight gain, often related to significant medical or psychosocial events. Most patients can remember their approximate weight and/or weight gain at milestones in their lives (e.g., high school or college graduation, marriage, military discharge, postpartum). These periods in turn are often associated with major changes in lifestyle (e.g., cessation of high levels of physical activity such as organized sports) and physiological contributors such as pregnancy. Childhood onset can often be elicited through queries about being teased. Again, this can be useful information to determine whether further evaluation for secondary causes of obesity is warranted.

3. *Are there any medications the patient associates with weight gain or with difficulty in losing weight?*

Reviewing current and past medications may provide additional insight (Table 5.2). Some medications are particularly notorious for promoting weight gain (18). Tricyclic antidepressants can result in as much as a 4 kg/month weight gain. Lithium is associated with long-term weight gain of more than 10 kg (independent of its association with hypothyroidism). Anticonvulsants can cause significant and rapid weight gain, particularly valproic acid and carbamazepine. Certain steroids can result in significant weight gain. Corticosteroids are the classic medication here, with a 2 to 13 kg increase in more than 50% of patients treated with prednisone. Moreover, there is a redistribution of fat from the periphery to the central abdominal area. Ovarian hormone derivatives can cause weight gain, although with the current lower-dose formulations they are no longer a common cause of significant weight gain. Antidiabetic agents, particularly those with insulin-promoting effects (e.g., pancreatic secretagogues such as sulfonylureas, thiazolidinediones, and insulin itself) can cause 5 to 10 kg weight gain in very short periods. Of importance is that some of the rapid weight gain can be caused by edema, which needs to be addressed independently. Therefore these medications, even if no longer in the patient's

---

Table 5.2   Major Classes of Medications Promoting Weight Gain

Antidepressants	Anticonvulsants
• Tricyclics	• Valproic acid
• Monamine oxidase inhibitors	• Carbamazepine
Antipsychotics	Steroids
• Clozapine	• Corticosteroids
• Chlorpromazine	• Ovarian steroids
• Perphenazine	Antidiabetics
• Chlorprothixene	• Insulin
• Thiothixene	• Sulfonylureas
• Olanzapine	• Thiazolidinediones
Lithium	Antineoplastics

current pharmacotherapy profile, can have a profound effect on weight that must be taken into consideration when determining realistic treatment goals, choice of plan, and expectations. Even when discontinued, anecdotally it appears that it is harder to lose weight after significant exposure to these medications if they were associated with weight gain. Because discontinuing such agents usually is not an option, a more realistic goal for these patients is to minimize weight gain. Again, the psychological impact of this (e.g., disappointment, frustration) needs to be addressed by the health care team.

4. *What are the highest (nonpregnant) and lowest weights as an adult, and how many times has the patient intentionally lost more than 20 pounds?*

This two-part question will help ascertain if the individual weight cycles ("yo-yo" dieting), generally defined for research purposes as ±20 lb. As discussed in Chapter 4, despite the public's perceptions, inherent medical risk has yet to be established. However, identifying weight cycling can help focus the discussion on the patient's past weight-loss strategies, resistance to certain interventions and recommendations, motivation and attitude, and appropriate goals.

5. *What is the nature of the patient's current life style?*

Information regarding eating habits, meals associated with business or social activities, activity level at work and in leisure activities, active or sedentary hobbies, stress factors, alcohol and tobacco usage, and presence of depression or evidence of binge eating (i.e., consumption of a large amount of food in a brief period of time accompanied by a feeling of loss of control) should be sought to help identify potential barriers to success. A minimum three-day diary of food intake, activity, and emotions occurring at the time of these activities is particularly helpful for gaining insight into lifestyle factors contributing to the patient's current weight problem.

6. *What treatment methods has the patient tried, and what were the results?*

a. Traditional Methods—A patient with chronic obesity and/or progressive weight gain with a history of previous unsuccessful or transient weight loss efforts will more likely be a candidate for aggressive structured medical and/or pharmacotherapeutic intervention and, in some cases, surgery. Documenting past attempts is extremely useful to determine inadequacies in previous treatment plans, failed strategies not worth attempting again, and recurrent obstacles that would benefit from specific attention (e.g., excessive eating out, work-related travel). Although the NIH guidelines recommend at least 6 months of lifestyle intervention before more aggressive treatment, if the patient has had reasonable exposure to the nutrition, exercise, and behavior components of treatment in the past (quite often there is a history of multiple six-month periods) to allow him/her to struggle through another prolonged attempt at lifestyle change is unwise. For example, a patient who has participated in Weight Watchers, a self-directed walking regimen, or a structured exercise program (e.g., the YMCA's) has already demonstrated lack of success. Thus, more aggressive treatment in conjunction with a higher level of intervention should be considered early in the new treatment plan. In the example above, the patient has had some nutrition intervention and behavior support from Weight Watchers. Consequently, after a medical assessment is completed, RD counseling should be initiated and another type of support group should be instituted, followed by a more aggressive treatment plan, which might include pharmacotherapy (if not contraindicated) within a few weeks rather than months if the patient demonstrates a willingness to make an effort with the other components of the treatment plan.

b. Nontraditional Methods—Of particular concern are methods that are unmonitored and dangerous. A history of a behavioral disorder, including binging, purging, anorexia, bulimia, abuse of over-the-counter (OTC) or prescription medications (including laxatives, diuretics, amphetamines, thyroid medication), and excessive or inappropriate use of meal replacement products are among the many methods about which the patient should be queried. There are a number of products that can be dangerous and that have required FDA warnings about their use (see FDA Web site: *www.fda.gov*). A recent FDA warning has been for OTC compound/ingredient phenylpropanolamine; plans to remove it from the nonprescription market were announced in a Public Health Advisory on 6 November 2000 (19). In addition, prepublished reports on the *New England Journal of Medicine* Web site (*www.nejm.org*) about the dangers of *Ephedra* and phenylpropanolamine were available. More often, these products are ineffective and ultimately detract from the basic treatment issues that are the cornerstone to weight management.

7. *What co-morbidities are present that may affect the choice of weight loss treatment?*

Co-morbidities may limit the treatment choices because of a predisposition for medical complications associated with weight loss, as described in Chapter 4. For example, a recent myocardial infarction, angina, severe arthritis, pulmonary disease, severe congestive heart failure, liver disease, renal failure, or recent traumatic injury may affect the patient's ability to exercise as well as limit the degree of caloric restriction.

To more thoroughly assess treatment options, some particular areas of concern should be discussed with patients because of the complications and side effects that can occur with intentional weight loss, as outlined in Chapter 4. These areas include

- *Pulmonary*—limitations in exercise tolerance, such as asthma; symptoms of sleep apnea (Table 5.3)

- *Cardiovascular*—limitations in exercise tolerance and/or caloric restriction, such as angina, dyspnea on exertion, claudication, palpitations, syncope, or other symptoms of arrhythmia

Table 5.3   Sleep Apnea Screening

Snoring and Gaspimg
Usually individuals with obstructive sleep apnea snore (but most people who snore
do not have sleep apnea); patients are often aware of gasping that can interrupt
sleep

Classic Symptoms
Morning headaches, restless sleep, daytime drowsiness when trying to concentrate
and remain awake (e.g., at work), depression

Associated Signs
Systemic hypertension (right-sided heart failure in severe cases that have progressed)

Large Neck
>17 in. circumference

Pharyngeal Examination
Poor upper palate excursion

Witnessed Apneic Episodes
Aggressively pursue other sources of information (e.g., family members)

- *Gastrointestinal*—symptoms of food intolerance or symptoms that indicate gallbladder disease
- *Endocrine*—symptoms of diabetes, thyroid dysfunction, ovarian dysfunction including hirsutism
- *Musculoskeletal*—limitations in exercise tolerance; symptoms of gout
- *Neurologic*—limitations in exercise tolerance, such as dysequilibrium; dysesthesia, particularly in hands suggesting carpal tunnel syndrome
- *Psychiatric*—symptoms of depression, major disorders; general anxiety level; sexual or physical abuse; unusual eating behaviors or frank eating disorders; situational issues (e.g., recent divorce, death, job change) (see Chapter 8 for more details)
- *Lifestyle Habits*—smoking, substance abuse, particularly alcohol intake; frequency and intensity of exercise as well as general (unstructured) physical activity, with related attitude queries; general consumption habits, including high-calorie drinks (soda, fruit juice, milk), frequency of eating out (including work-site cafeteria), snacking patterns, fruit and vegetable intake

8. *What is the patient's family history?*
Patterns of obesity as well as fat distribution are often familial (see

Chapter 2) (20, 21). Other conditions, including thyroid dysfunction, frequency of cardiovascular disease, hypertension, cancer, diabetes, dyslipidemia, and longevity, should be assessed because all are likely to be familial.

9. *What is the patient's motivation to lose weight at this time?*

Determining motivation is the most challenging component of the obesity history. Unfortunately, studies have yet to identify reliable predictors of motivation that are linked to success or failure. As reviewed by the NIH, specific factors to assess are

- Reason for wanting weight loss
- Previous attempts and attitude toward setbacks
- Family, friend, and work-site support and obstacles
- Awareness of medical issues
- Attitude towards physical activity
- Time availability
- Barriers to success
- Financial constraints

This information is extremely useful in *a)* customizing the patient's treatment plan, *b)* identifying deficiencies in key areas that can be addressed early in treatment, *c)* providing an opportunity to educate and reorient a patient's perspective (i.e., cognitive restructuring), and *d)* identifying patients who, in the judgement of the treatment team, are not ready to embark on a comprehensive program.

Obesity-Specific Physical Examination

The physical examination should be attentive to characterizing obesity, its possible causes, and its recognizable complications.

Anthropometrics

Height (in stocking feet) and weight (in light indoor clothing rather than gown because, typically, long-term weight monitoring will be performed with clothing) should be carefully measured and recorded; self-reports by patients are notoriously inaccurate. (Anecdotally, patients invariably report being at least 1 in. taller and 5 lb lighter than measured height and weight!) As noted previously, these measurements are then used to determine the BMI, the key parameter to designing a safe and effective treatment plan.

Per the NIH report, the waist circumference is measured to help determine fat distribution. A variety of methods are described in the literature. The NIH recommends measuring at the superior margin of the right iliac crest with the patient standing. This is approximately at the level of the umbilicus and therefore is not the same as the waist measurement used for purposes of tailoring clothes. (Do not use a man's stated waist size, which is invariably smaller and at a level below the circumference of interest.) Although the NIH indicates the waist circumference at BMI > 35 is not predictive of morbidity, it is still a useful nonweight parameter that provides powerful positive feedback to the patient, particularly when overall weight loss progress slows.

Vital Signs

Determination of blood pressure in the obese patient requires the proper equipment and technique. Although most health professionals learned this technique during their education, the correct bladder cuff size is often overlooked (22). If too narrow, blood pressure will be falsely elevated and lead to an erroneous diagnosis of hypertension or inadequate tapering of antihypertensive medication. The bladder width should be 40% to 50 % of the upper arm circumference. A large adult cuff (15 cm wide) is generally appropriate for overweight and moderately obese patients, but a thigh cuff (18 cm wide) may be necessary for larger patients, especially if the arm circumference exceeds 16 in. Occasionally, obese patients have a short upper arm with a large circumference that makes use of an appropriate width cuff impossible. In such cases, measurement of blood pressure in the forearm may be more accurate.

General Physical Examination

Symptoms and diseases associated with obesity affect almost every organ system, and all of these systems require careful evaluation to determine the patient's prognosis and guide therapy. On average, 70% of clinically obese patients (BMI $\geq$ 30) suffer from at least one obesity-related illness (23). Further complicating the general physical is the fact that many obese patients avoid having routine preventive care, such as breast exam, pelvic exam, Pap smears, rectal exam, and stool guaiacs, often for years, because of embarrassment or previous negative encounters with physicians. The general physical provides an opportunity to perform these routine health care needs in a positive, supportive, and nonthreatening way.

Diagnostic Laboratory Evaluation

The NIH report does not provide absolute guidelines on pretreatment laboratory and diagnostic screening and testing. To balance the need for thoroughly understanding the patient's medical condition with cost considerations, the evaluation should *a*) screen appropriate age-related and/or obesity-related risks factors, and *b*) test for conditions that provide a baseline for future monitoring of potential complications from the treatment plan (as described in Chapter 4) or health outcomes of interest (Tables 5.4 and 5.5). Recently performed tests may be available that are adequate for screening purposes if there has been no major intervening illness or significant medication change that could have caused interim changes. Based on these principles, the following diagnostic laboratory evaluations are generally justified:

1. *Fasting Plasma Glucose*—Per the American Diabetes Association recommendations (24) for adults with any risk factor, including obesity, screening should be undertaken at three-year intervals. Fasting plasma glucose obtained by venipuncture (not capillary blood sample from fingerstick) is the preferred test. HbA_{1c} is not recognized as a screening test.

2. *Fasting Lipid Panel*—The minimal screening guidelines established by the National Cholesterol Education Program expert panel state that all adults starting at age 20 should be screened with a total and HDL cholesterol every five years (25). Non-HDL cholesterol is a useful predictor of risk (26), but because the American Heart Association has reclassified obesity as a major, modifiable cardiovascular risk factor for coronary heart disease (27), and because of the increasing evidence for the atherogenicity of hypertriglyceridemia (25, 28) (a condition more prevalent in obesity), a complete pretreatment fasting lipid panel is warranted. Thus concurrent measurement of plasma triglycerides and HDL also allows determination of LDL cholesterol levels, a test with which many patients are familiar. (If TG > 400, the equation for the calculated LDL is inaccurate and a direct LDL as-

Table 5.4 Diagnostic Laboratory Evaluation in the Management of Patients with Obesity

Obesity-Specific Testing	*Other Testing (Not Obesity-Specific)*
• Fasting plasma glucose	• CBC
• Fasting lipid panel	• Urinalysis
• TSH	• Calcium, phosphorus
• ALT, AST, alkaline phosphatase, total bilirubin	
• Electrolytes	*Testing That Should Not Be Performed Routinely*
• Renal function	• Plasma cortisol
• Uric acid	• Plasma insulin
• Resting ECG	• Basal metabolic rate
• Disease- and medication-appropriate tests (e.g., HbA_{1c})	

Table 5.5 Recommended Minimal Pretreatment Tests*

- Fasting plasma glucose

- Fasting lipid panel: total cholesterol, LDH, HDL, triglycerides

- TSH

- Liver tests: AST, ALT, alkaline phosphatase, total bilirubin

- Electrolytes: sodium, potassium, chloride, bicarbonate

- Renal function: BUN, creatinine

- Disease- or medication-related test (e.g., HbA_{1c} for diabetes mellitus)

- Resting ECG

---

* Tests performed within ~3 months, and in some cases within 1 year, of starting treatment are generally acceptable.

say must be used.) If abnormal, the response to therapy should be evaluated periodically to determine if further (pharmacologic) intervention is needed. An added benefit of monitoring lipids is that it serves as another powerful nonweight parameter that can help reorient a patient's perspective about his or her treatment goals.

3. *Thyroid-Stimulating Hormone*—Although hypothyroidism causes weight gain, there is a general misconception that it can account for the clinically obese condition. Nevertheless, because thyroid function modulates weight and thyroid dysfunction is such a prevalent problem, screening has been shown to be cost-effective. New guidelines established by the American Thyroid Association recommend screening for thyroid disease by measuring thyroid-stimulating hormone every five years beginning at age 35 (29).

4. *Liver Tests*—As discussed in detail in Chapter 4, steatosis is a nearly universal condition associated with obesity, and its more serious outcome, NASH, is quite common. Moreover, gallbladder disease is quite prevalent. Consequently, ALT, AST, alkaline phosphatase, and total bilirubin should be checked. If abnormal, an appropriate evaluation for liver and/or gallbladder disease should be conducted. If other causes of liver disease are ruled out, NASH should be considered. Whether a biopsy-proven diagnosis is warranted should be determined on a case-by-case

basis. At a minimum, follow-up lab testing is indicated, but testing must be conducted at appropriate intervals. As discussed in Chapter 4, it can be anticipated that liver enzymes will increase initially with weight loss. Therefore, unless there is another indication, routine follow-up should occur months later after weight loss has reached a plateau (e.g., 6 months), and a diagnostic evaluation should be pursued with the assistance of a gastroenterologist if liver enzymes remain abnormal.

5. *Electrolytes, Renal Function, Uric Acid*—These lab determinations are important not only for general medical screening but also as comparators if complications occur.

6. *Disease-and Medication-Appropriate Labs*—The general principles of practicing medicine should be applied to determine which tests are indicated. Any complications or changes in a condition that can occur with weight loss warrant testing. For example, HbA_{1c} is important to monitor in patients with type 2 diabetes. (Again, Chapter 4 on medical complications can serve as a guide.)

7. *Resting ECG*—The usefulness of obtaining a resting ECG in people without symptoms or known cardiac disease is questionable. However, as discussed in the previous chapter, the higher prevalence of prolonged QT_c interval in obesity (30) and the controversy over its relationship to serious complications during weight loss warrant conducting this test. If the QT_c is normal, whether follow-up ECGs should be done periodically after significant weight loss is debatable. Because there are no guidelines, good medical judgment, as always, takes precedence.

The following lab evaluations are often obtained as part of medical assessment consistent with good medical practice but not necessarily obesity-specific:

1. *Complete Blood Count*—Anemia, which is typically associated with more serious medical problems, can also be nutritionally related in etiology. It would be unwise to embark on a treatment under such conditions.

2. *Urinalysis*—There are a number of obesity-related conditions in which early renal problems can be identified by urinalysis.

3. *Calcium, Phosphorus*—There is generally no direct relationship with abnormalities in these parameters and obesity. However, it is often more cost-effective to obtain a general chemistry panel that includes these parameters than to order individual labs that exclude them. (Because both of the authors are endocrinologists, a bias in favor of obtaining these labs should be noted.)

Baseline Evaluations Not Justified for Routine Use

There are some evaluations that are not justified on a routine basis, but unfortunately some physicians may perform them because of misconceptions about the etiology of obesity:

1. *Plasma Cortisol*—Despite the well-described effects of cortisol on body weight and fat distribution, random plasma cortisol measurements are generally not useful. Furthermore, tests specifically designed to screen for Cushing syndrome are also not warranted on routine basis. Screening should be reserved for individuals with signs and symptoms suggesting its presence.

2. *Plasma Insulin*—Although many commercial diet books claim hyperinsulinemia is the culprit underlying obesity, this view is at best oversimplified and at worst a marketing ploy. The current standard of practice is that plasma insulin levels serve neither a diagnostic nor a monitoring purpose in the general treatment of obesity. In addition, there are no clinical assay standards or even a consensus on a normal range. Finally, it is predictable that fasting plasma insulin levels will decrease with weight loss (see Chapter 3). Thus plasma insulin results are uninterpretable in the clinical setting, do not serve a monitoring purpose, and do not justify the cost.

3. *Basal Metabolic Rate (BMR)*—For a small investment, indirect calorimeters can be purchased to determine metabolic rate. The theory and methodology dates back almost a century, but modern technology has made it easier to determine BMR in humans. Metabolic rate is directly related to O_2 consumption and CO_2 production. Test parameters can be quantitated and applied to standard equations to determine the BMR (31). The clinical utility of measuring BMR remains to be established. Making such a determination suffers from the same deficiencies as measuring plasma insulin levels. Furthermore, BMR cannot be justified for designing a management plan because there are more cost-effective approaches to devising nutrition and exercise plans. Finally, BMR is always high because of its correlation and physiologic link to BMI (more specifically, increased lean body mass associated with obesity). In the academic community, defining an appropriate BMR and its proportional decrease in response to weight loss is still being debated, but this debate has yet to be translated into clinical practice guidelines with acceptable ranges and standards.

Common Pretreatment Diagnostic Evaluations

Quite often after completing the medical assessment, medical problems are unmasked. Generally, standards of medical practice dictate the need for further evaluation, but in the context of the obese patient some common problems always need to be evaluated because they may affect the treatment plan and/or identify an obstacle to success.

Cardiovascular Problems

The American Heart Association recently upgraded obesity from a contributing to a major modifiable risk factor for coronary heart disease, independent of its co-morbidities (e.g., diabetes, hypertension, hyperlipidemia) (27). Physical activity and structured exercise are critical components to treatment and the major predictor of long-term success (32, 33). Therefore a thorough assessment of risk is warranted in some patients before embarking on an exercise program.

Several patient advocate groups have published exercise recommendations (e.g., the American Diabetes Association (34) recommends exercise testing for any patient with diabetes over age 35), but none have yet incorporated obesity *per se* into their decision algorithms. Among the most useful are the recommendations by the American College of Sports Medicine, which provide a reasonable, albeit conservative, approach that covers most situations encountered in the obese patient (Table 5.6). Although it appears that the guidelines recommend a stress test for almost every obese patient, in practice this is not the case. Good clinical judgement and an exercise prescription that does not immerse the patient in a program that tries to accomplish too much too soon will help avoid excessive screening of all patients. Nevertheless, when in doubt, a stress test is warranted, particularly if the physician is concerned that a patient will self-initiate a vigorous program too soon and without proper monitoring. Finally, if there is any possibility of underlying coronary heart disease based on typical risk factors, unexplained chest pain, or symptoms or signs of an arrhythmia, an evaluation is warranted (Table 5.7).

Obstructive Sleep Apnea

Hypoventilation syndromes are more common in obesity, and of specific concern is obstructive sleep apnea. Unfortunately, there is an underappreciation for the need to diagnose this problem in the weight-management setting because it is wrongly assumed that weight loss will adequately address the condition. There are number of reasons it is important to pursue the diagnosis and then treat with modalities other than weight loss (e.g., C-PAP, home O_2).

COMPLICATIONS

The complications associated with sleep apnea, including systemic and pulmonary hypertension, arrhythmias, and depression, are quite serious and place individuals at higher mortality risk. In addition, if in the future the patient needs a surgical procedure, this information will be extremely useful to the surgeon and anesthesiologist.

Table 5.6   ACSM Recommendations for (A) Medical Examination and Clinical Exercise Test Before Participation in Exercise Program and (B) Physician Supervision of Exercise Test

(A) Medical Examination and Clinical Exercise Test Recommended Before Participation?

	Apparently Healthy Individuals		Individuals at Increased Risk*		
	Younger[‡]	Older	No Symptoms	Symptoms	Known Disease[†]
Moderate exercise[§]	No[‖]	No	No	Yes	Yes
Vigorous exercise[¶]	No	Yes[#]	Yes	Yes	Yes

(B) Physician Supervision Recommended During Exercise Test?

	Apparently Healthy Individuals		Individuals at Increased Risk		
	Younger	Older	No Symptoms	Symptoms	Known Disease
Submaximal testing	No	No	No	Yes	Yes
Maximal testing	No	Yes	Yes	Yes	Yes

*Persons with two or more risk factors or one or more signs or symptoms.
[†]Persons with known cardiac, pulmonary, or metabolic disease.
[‡]*Younger* implies ≤40 years for men, ≤50 years for women.
[§]*Moderate exercise* is defined as an intensity of 40% to 60% Vo_{2max}. If intensity is uncertain, *moderate exercise* may be defined as an intensity well within the individual's current capacity; such exercise can be comfortably sustained for a prolonged period (e.g., 60 min), has a gradual initiation and progression, and is generally noncompetitive.
[¶]*Vigorous exercise* is defined as an exercise intensity >60% Vo_{2max}. If intensity is uncertain, *vigorous exercise* may be defined as exercise intense enough to represent a substantial cardiorespiratory challenge or exercise that results in fatigue within 20 min.
[‖]A "No" response means that an item is deemed "not necessary." The "No" response does *not* mean that the item should not be done.
[#]A "Yes" response means that an item is recommended. *In Part B this means that a physician is in close proximity and readily available should there be an emergency.*
Adapted from Kenney WL, Humphrey RH, Bryant CX eds. ACSM's Guidelines for Exercise Testing and Prescription, 5th ed. Baltimore: Williams & Wilkins; 1995:25; with permission.

CHOICE OF TREATMENT

Less aggressive weight loss plans should be considered until the patient is diagnosed and treated for sleep apnea. (A common logistical problem is the long waiting list at most sleep centers for scheduling studies.) Any plan that facilitates rapid weight loss can cause a number of side effects, particularly fluid and electrolyte imbalance, that may place the individual at higher risk for cardiac and other complications (see Chapter 4).

Table 5.7   Contraindications to Exercise Testing

Absolute Contraindications

1. Recent significant change in resting ECG that suggests infarction or other acute cardiac event

2. Recent complicated myocardial infarction (unless patient is stable and pain free)

3. Unstable angina

4. Uncontrolled ventricular arrhythmia

5. Uncontrolled atrial arrhythmia that compromises cardiac function

6. Third-degree AV heart block without pacemaker

7. Acute congestive heart failure

8. Severe aortic stenosis

9. Suspected or known dissecting aneurysm

10. Active or suspected myocarditis or pericarditis

11. Thrombophlebitis or intracardiac thrombi

12. Recent systematic or pulmonary embolus

13. Acute infections

14. Significant emotional distress (psychosis)

Relative Contraindications

1. Resting diastolic blood pressure > 115 mm Hg or resting systolic blood pressure > 200 mm Hg

2. Moderate valvular heart disease

3. Known electrolyte abnormalities (hypokalemia, hypomagnesemia)

4. Fixed-rate pacemaker (rarely used)

5. Frequent or complex ventricular ectopy

6. Ventricular aneurysm

7. Uncontrolled metabolic disease (e.g., diabetes, thyrotoxicosis, myxedema)

8. Chronic infectious disease (e.g., mononucleosis, hepatitis, AIDS)

9. Neuromuscular, musculoskeletal, or rheumatoid disorders exacerbated by exercise

10. Advanced or complicated pregnancy

From Kenney WL, Humphrey RH, Bryant CX eds. ACSM's Guidelines for Exercise Testing and Prescription. 5th ed. Baltimore: Williams & Wilkins; 1995:42; with permission.

QUALITY OF LIFE

Upon diagnosis and treatment, patients can gain immediate relief or improvement in a variety of symptoms, including headache, fatigue, and depression. This can be a profoundly life-altering treatment.

EFFICACY OF WEIGHT LOSS

It is often assumed that weight loss will cure obstructive sleep apnea. Unfortunately, this is not true in at least one third of the cases in individuals who lose and sustain significant weight loss (35). Moreover, given the significant rate of recidivism (weight regain), the problem will recur. To identify high-risk patients who should be evaluated, there are number of signs and symptoms to consider (see Table 5.3).

Any level of sleep apnea suspicion warrants a referral for a pulmonary and/or ENT evaluation in conjunction with polysomnography (sleep study). Even if the case is only mild, nighttime O_2, if indicated, can have a significant impact on the patient's life as well as potentially arrest complications of the disease.

Psychiatric Illness

Although it is not clear whether psychiatric illness is caused by or is more prevalent in obesity, it can be a major obstacle, even a relative contraindication, to treatment. It should be emphasized that some psychiatric illnesses, including major depression, are life-threatening, and psychiatric treatment takes precedenace over weight management. The more common and problematic situation, however, is the presence of mild-to-moderate depression. Screening for depression is useful in all patients, and simple instruments are available to assist the practitioner (e.g., Beck Inventory Depression). In conjunction with the assessment by other team members, particularly the behaviorist, a more thorough evaluation by a psychiatrist should be considered to determine if medication is indicated. Even patients already diagnosed for depression may benefit from further evaluation, particularly those already being treated with antidepressants that still manifest significant signs and symptoms.

Alcohol Abuse

Because of the calories associated with alcohol intake, the medical assessment provides the opportunity to discuss past and current abuse of alcohol. Alcohol abuse may be identified during the history, in the diet records, or by the behaviorist's evaluation. It can be quite difficult to make progress on weight control issues when alcohol problems are present. Alcohol abuse complicates nearly every component of treatment. It also must be determined whether the patient with an alcohol problem will detract from the treatment of others if a group treatment program for obesity is being used. Thus serious consideration needs to be given to deferring weight management until the alcohol problem is adequately addressed, and then only when an independent treatment plan is in place that will clearly demonstrate progress in controlling the problem.

Substance Abuse

The same concerns with alcohol abuse apply to substance abuse. Ironically, in conjunction with overall improvement in health and, in some cases, elimination of metabolic and physiologic influences (e.g., appetite suppression by stimulants), many former substance abusers gain weight, often turning to food to fill an emotional need.

Tobacco

Smoking cessation often results in significant weight gain. As reviewed in detail in the NIH report, the average weight gain is 4 to 7 lb but can exceed 28 lb in 10% of tobacco quitters. Regrettably, some patients use smoking as a weight control method because tobacco use increases metabolic rate. Thus weight gain is inevitable after cessation. Unfortunately, various smoking cessation therapies will only delay the weight gain unless comprehensive therapy for weight control is implemented. To quit smoking and attempt weight loss simultaneously is not recommended by the NIH. Goals should be tailored towards preventing weight gain during smoking cessation; other weight issues can be addressed after smoking cessation is successful.

Orthopedic Problems

Some patients with orthopedic problems may benefit from an evaluation by a physical therapist to focus on areas of concern and set limitations on exercise that could be harmful and exacerbate an underlying condition. After the evaluation, exercise supervision can be continued by the physical therapist or exercise physiologist if needed.

Goals and Recommendations for Treatment

Treatment goals, risk status determination, and contraindications to weight loss are summarized in this section.

General Goals

The NIH expert panel has identified three treatment goals:
1. Prevent further weight gain.
2. Initiate program to reduce body weight by 10% at a rate of 1 to 2 lb/wk during a period of 6 months.
3. Maintain weight after 6 months of weight loss rather than attempt further weight loss. (Weight maintenance is defined by the NIH as sustained weight reduction within 3 kg and waist circum-

ference within 4 cm for at least 2 years; however, re-evaluation for additional weight loss sooner than 2 years may occur if determined to be appropriate by the treatment team.)

Risk Status

To determine appropriate goals and treatment plan, risk status due to weight is determined using the following parameters:

1. Severity of overweight/obesity (BMI)
2. Abdominal obesity (waist circumference)
3. Absolute risk factors (cardiovascular, co-morbidities)
4. Fitness (activity/exercise frequency and intensity)

Individualized Treatment Goals

Although the NIH report utilizes a complex and exhaustive list of risk factors (degree of absolute risk, relative vs. absolute, a detailed treatment algorithm), it focuses on the above four parameters to determine which of the treatment goals are appropriate. Based on classication, the goals are:

1. *Normal Weight:* Prevent weight gain and reinforce a healthy lifestyle.
2. *Overweight:*
   a. Prevent weight gain if waist circumference is not enlarged, no absolute risk factors are present, and fitness level is adequate
   b. Weight loss indicated if patient has large waist circumference, absolute risk factor(s), and/or sedentary lifestyle, or patient desires to lose weight.
3. *Obese:* Weight loss indicated regardless of risk assessment unless patient is not ready, in which case weight gain prevention is the goal.

The NIH report reviews data that indicate it is unlikely these overweight and obese individuals will attain an average "normal" body weight (BMI < 25) and maintain that weight for an extended period. Therefore, the manner in which these goals are communicated to the patient is critical. Again, the unrealistic expectations and misguided goals of patients are immediate obstacles. Flatly stating the aforementioned goals will not only disappoint patients but sometimes dissuade them from seeking help in a setting composed of qualified professionals. Each physician must devise his or her own style and approach, keeping the patient hypersensitivity associated with this issue in mind.

Some strategies that are useful include

- Focus on behavioral outcomes (e.g., increase fruit and vegetable intake, walk 10 min × 3 sessions daily). Avoid discrete quantitative goals.

- Query the patient on his or her goals, then modify the goals by implementing a step-by-step approach into attainable multiple goals (e.g., patient's goal to lose 100 lb in 6 months can be modified by starting with 10 lb in 2 months). Attempting too much will overwhelm the individual and usually lead to frustration.

The specifics of designing a program are described in the other chapters. It is the job of the physician to oversee a systematic, methodical, safe approach that provides structure and progresses at a realistic and reasonable rate.

Contraindications

There are situations in which weight loss is contraindicated. Most are conditions in which the risk from potential complications is too great to consider treatment until the condition stabilizes. These include pregnancy or lactation, serious psychiatric illness, a recent major illness, type 2 diabetes mellitus in which the patient is under poor metabolic control, myocardial infarction, or a cerebrovascular event.

There are also high-risk medical conditions that benefit from weight loss but are better treated in the context of a comprehensive program staffed by specialists. Examples include pretransplant weight loss, heart failure, type 1 diabetes mellitus, conditions that require frequent monitoring which may not be feasible in the primary care setting (e.g., insulin-requiring type 2 diabetes, hypertension treated with multiple medications), and interventions best handled by an experienced staff (e.g., a very low calorie diet).

Contraindications to weight loss are discussed in detail in Chapter 4.

Treatment Plan

Based on the assessment outlined in this chapter and bearing in mind the medical complications associated with weight loss (as discussed in Chapter 4), it should be feasible to design an individualized treatment. As long as it incorporates all the major components of therapy (nutrition, physical activity, social support, and medical monitoring) and the implementation is a staged (step-by-step) approach that avoids overwhelming the patient, there are no strict guidelines on how to begin. There is a paucity of research to guide the practitioner in determining which component should be implemented first or simultaneously with another. Thus a discussion with each patient should be conducted to assist in directing the plan. Anecdotally, despite resistance by many patients to address nutrition issues (because of their claims of adequate knowledge, previous attempts, or low calorie consumption), initiating exercise first can be difficult and frustrating until some weight reduction occurs to allow ease of movement. This can only be accomplished by decreasing caloric intake (see Chapter 6). Physician-guided implementations of the nonmedical components are also important (see Chapters 7 and 8). Finally, if aggressive therapy is being considered (i.e., any treatment regimen that could result in rapid weight loss), if there are complex medical problems, or if rigorous monitoring is required, referring to a specialist in weight management affiliated with a structured program should be considered.

■   ■   ■

Key Points

- Evaluation and treatment of clinical obesity is best managed by a team of health professionals, including a physician with experience in obesity management, a dietitian, a behaviorist, and an exercise physiologist.

- When assessing the degree of obesity, determining the body mass index and characterizing the regional distribution of fat (lower body vs. upper body obesity) by measurement of waist circumference are the two most practical and economical means for clinical purposes.

- The medical assessment should be focused on customizing the treatment plan to the individual patient, based on that patient's level of health risk related to the degrees of obesity and weight loss, associated conditions, previous success or failure with weight loss regimens, weight gain history, etiologic factors, and current lifestyle.

- Laboratory testing should include screening for obesity-related risk factors and baseline testing to assist future monitoring of potential complications of weight loss.

- The general goals of treatment are to prevent further weight gain, to achieve an initial weight loss of 10% during the first 6 months at a rate of 1 to 2 lb/wk, and to maintain weight after the first 6 months rather than attempt further weight loss.

■   ■   ■

REFERENCES

1. **Molarius A, Seidell JK.** Selection of anthropometric indicators for classification of abdominal fatness: a critical review. Int J Obes. 1998;22:719-27.

2. **World Health Organization.** Defining the Problem of Overweight and Obesity. WHO/NUT/NCD/98.1, 5-16, 1998; and Obesity: Preventing and Managing the Global Epidemic. Report of a WHO Consultation on Obesity; 1997.

3. Height and weight tables. Stat Bull Metrop Insur Co. 1983;64:2-2.

4. **Ellis KJ.** Human body composition: in vivo methods. Physiol Rev. 2000;80:649-80.

5. **Lukaski HC.** Methods for the assessment of human body composition: traditional and new. Am J Clin Nutr. 1987;46:537-56.

6. Bioelectrical impedance analysis in body composition measurement. National Institutes of Health Technology Assessment Conference Statement. 12-14 Dec. 1994. Am J Clin Nutr. 1996;64:524S-532S.

7. **Forbes GB, Simon W, Amatruda JM.** Is bioimpedance a good predictor of body-composition? Am J Clin Nutr. 1992;56:4-6.

8. **Vazquez JA, Janosky JE.** Validity of bioelectrical-impedance analysis in measuring changes in lean body mass during weight reduction. Am J Clin Nutr. 1991;54:970-5.

9. **Deurenberg P, Weststrate JA, Hautvast JG.** Changes in fat-free during weight loss measured by bioelectrical impedance and by densitometry. Am J Clin Nutr. 1989;49:33-6.

10. **Carella MJ, Rodgers CD, Anderson D, Gossain VV.** Serial measurments of body composition in obese subjects during a very-low-energy diet (VLED) comparing bioelectrical impedance with hydrodensitometry. Obes Res. 1997;5:250-6.

11. **Van Loan MD.** Is dual-energy x-ray absorptiometry ready for prime time in the clinical evaluation of body composition? Am J Clin Nutr. 1998;68:1155-6.

12. **Tataranni PA, Ravussin E.** Use of dual-energy x-ray absorptiometry in obese individuals. Am J Clin Nutr. 1995;62:730-4.

13. **Abate N, Garg A, Coleman R, et al.** Prediction of total subcutanous abnominal, intraperitoneal, and retroperitoneal adipose tissue masses in men by a single axial magnetic resonance imaging slice. Am J Clin Nutr. 1997;65:403-8.

14. **Kelley DE, Mandarino LJ.** Perspectives in diabetes: fuel selection in human skeletal muscle in insulin resistance: a re-examination. Diabetes. 2000;49:683.

15. **Dempster P, Aitkens S.** A new air displacement method for the determination of human body composition. Med Sci Sports Exer. 1995;7:1692-7.

16. **Biaggi RR, Vollman MW, Nies MA, et al.** Comparison of air-displacement plethysmography with hydrostatic weighing and bioelectrical impedance analysis for the assessment of body composition in healthy adults. Am J Clin Nutr. 1999;69:898-903.

17. **McCrory MA, Gomez TD, Bernauer EM, Mole PA.** Evaluation of a new air displacement plethysmograph for measuring human body composition. Med Sci Sport Exer. 1995;27:1686-91.

18. **Pijl H, Meinders AE.** Body weight change as an adverse effect of drug treatment: mechanisms and management. Drug Safety. 1996;4:329-42.

19. **Center for Drug Evaluation and Research (CDER).** Safety of phenyl-propanolamine. Food and Drug Administration Public Health Advisory. FDA/Center for Drug Evaluation and Research; 6 November 2000.

20. **Stunkard AJ, Harris JR, Pedersen NL, McClearn GE.** The body-mass index of twins who have been reared apart. N Engl J Med. 1990;322:1483-7.

21. **Lemieux S.** Genetic susceptibility to visceral obesity and related clinical implications. Int J Obes. 1977;21:831-8.

22. **Kushner RF, Weinsier RL.** Evaluation of the obese patient: practical considerations. Med Clin North Am. 2000;84:387-99.

23. **Must A, Spadano J, Coakely EH, et al.** The disease burden associated with overweight and obesity. JAMA. 1999;282:1523-9.

24. **American Diabetes Association.** Screening for type 2 diabetes. Diabetes Care. 2000;23:S20-S23.

25. Second Report of the Expert Panel on Detection, Evaluation, and Treatment of High Blood Cholesterol in Adults (Adult Treatment Panel II). NIH Publication 93-3096. Bethesda, MD: U.S. Department of Health and Human Services, Public Health Service, National Institutes of Health, National Cholesterol Education Program; 1993.

26. **Frost PH, Havel RJ.** Rationale for use of non-high-density lipoprotein cholesterol rather than low-density lipoprotein cholesterol as a tool for lipoprotein cholesterol screening and assessment of risk and therapy. Am J Cardiol. 1998;81:26B-31B.

27. **Eckel RH, Krauss RM.** American Heart Association call to action: obesity as a major risk factor for coronary heart disease. Circulation. 1998;97:2099-100.

28. **Austin MA, Hokanson JE, Edwards KL.** Hypertriglyceridemia as a cardiovascular risk factor. Am J Cardiol. 1998;81:7B-12B.

29. **Ladenson PW, Singer PA, Ain KB, et al.** American Thyroid Association guidelines for detection of thyroid dysfunction. Arch Intern Med. 2000;160:1573-5.

30. **Seip RL, Mair K, Cole TG, Semenkovich CF.** Induction of human skeletal muscle lipoprotein lipase gene expression by short-term exercise is transient. Am J Physiol. 1997;272:E255-61.

31. **Ferrannini E.** The theoretical bases of indirect calorimetry: a review. Metabolism. 1998;37:287-301.

32. **Pronk NP, Wing RR.** Physical activity and long-term maintenance of weight loss. Obes Res. 1994;2:587-99.

33. **Ravussin E, Gautier JF.** Metabolic predictors of weight gain. Int J Obes. 1999; 23(suppl 1):37-41.

34. **American Diabetes Association.** Diabetes mellitus and exercise. Diabetes Care. 2000;23:S50-S54.

35. **Kral JG.** Surgical treatment of obesity. In: Handbook of Obesity. Bray G, Bouchard C, James WP, eds. New York: Marcel Dekker; 1997;977-93.

6

■ ■ ■

Nutrition Intervention in the Medical Management of Obesity

Patricia A. Stewart, PhD, RD
Celia Topping, MNS, RD, CDE
Nellie Wixom, RD

Role of the Physician

Physicians have the opportunity to play a critical role in facilitating a patient's pursuit of long-term lifestyle changes. Foremost among these is appropriate nutrition intervention for weight management. Unfortunately, physician training historically has not emphasized nutrition education, and many physicians feel they are ineffective, unsuccessful, and/or frustrated in helping patients lose weight (1, 2). Nevertheless, the American College of Physicians–American Society of Internal Medicine, the US Preventive Services Task Force, and others have recommended that clinicians routinely provide nutrition assessment and counseling to their patients (3). This is important because consumers cite their physician, rather than a dietitian, as the top credible source for nutrition information (4, 5).

Patient demand for nutrition advice continues to rise in parallel with the increasing prevalence of obesity and the emergence of new weight loss products, supplements, and diets. It is important that the clinician feels comfortable with, and is effective in, nutrition intervention strategies. Generic approaches, such as handing out diet sheets and simplistic messages to reduce caloric intake, have proven to be ineffective methods of weight reduction (6). Underlying this issue is a sense on the part of the practitioner that patients lack motivation for obesity treatment, a perception not always justified and which clearly undermines attempts by both parties to address the problem (7). Most patients know they are overweight or obese, and many have tried unsuccessfully to lose weight. Patients become disillusioned, if not angry, with an approach that, rightly or wrongly, they often perceive lacks efficacy and, more importantly, empathy. Exacerbating these perceptions are reports by many overweight and obese persons of disrespectful and insensitive treatment by health care providers (8). Thus the two major barriers to physician-instituted weight management are the physician's unfamiliarity with appropriate nutrition interventions and a deficiency in counseling skills. It is the object of this chapter to provide the physician with a basic foundation in nutrition knowledge related specifically to weight management in conjunction with a collective set of behaviorally based skills to initiate, implement, and reinforce interventions for overweight and obese individuals.

Screening

As emphasized throughout this text, obesity is a heterogeneous disease and, although the final desired outcome is weight loss, there is no one foolproof "one size fits all" intervention strategy. Therefore screening for specific nutrition problems will help the physician customize weight loss intervention for each patient. In addition, screening for readiness to make long-term lifestyle changes, depth of support systems, and presence of eating disorders will identify specific obstacles that need to be addressed to successfully implement the weight management plan. There are a number of useful, validated instruments and key questions that, when administered before meeting with the patient (e.g., in the waiting area), will facilitate the process.

Nutrition Screening

An essential screening instrument for weight management is one that ultimately assists in nutrition education. Most nutrition-screening instruments are oriented towards, and validated for, consumption of fat, saturated fat, and cholesterol, not for overall dietary intake (9). However, these instruments can be adapted for weight control because fat is so calorically dense and among the high-calorie foods that should be targeted for decreased consumption. One popular and effective self-assessment questionnaire, "Rate Your Plate", provides qualitative nutrition information related to typical food choices (Table 6.1) (10). Rather than use a quantitative tool to measure a specific nutrient (e.g., fat), the authors support the use of this qualitative educational tool that patients can use to focus on gradual food-specific behavioral changes.

The questionnaire addresses 16 food categories plus a question on food preparation methods and one on the serving size of animal protein foods. Each category is formatted into three columns: fat, saturated fat, and cholesterol content. For example, in the Dairy category, whole milk, 2% low-fat milk, and skim milk appear in Columns 1, 2 and 3, respectively. Higher point values are assigned to healthier choices that are lower in both fat and calories. By choosing a phrase or food that best describes the way he or she eats in a typical week, the patient can total up the points and see how the score ranks from least to most heart-healthy, which almost always reflects a good weight control plan as well. Thus this questionnaire serves as a template for healthier eating. The goal is for the physician and patient to target items in columns 1 and 2 and move towards items in columns 2 and 3. This questionnaire can be used in variety of ways, from initiating a plan to augmenting other take-home nutrition/education interventions (e.g., as a shopping aid).

Behavior-Oriented Nutrition Screening

As emphasized in many chapters, certain key behaviors influence weight management, some of which are focused on eating habits, such as skipped meals, eating out, and alcohol consumption. Therefore it is recommended that seven additional questions be included in the screening process to address these issues (Table 6.2). As with "Rate Your Plate", the three columns depict the least healthy, moderately healthy, and most healthy behaviors. Although the physician may identify many areas that need to be changed, initially targeting only one or two can prevent overwhelming both the patient and the practitioner. Involving the patient in these decisions when tailoring the approach based on his or her preferences is essential.

Nutritionally Related Psychopathology

Learning whether a patient has binge eating habits can be helpful in identifying specific areas for additional behavioral intervention. Some key questions are (11)

1. Do you ever wake up at night to eat?
2. Do you eat what is considered more than an average serving of food at one time?
3. When this happens, do you sometimes feel overridden with guilt?
4. How often does this occur?
5. Do you ever purge (vomiting, laxatives, excessive exercise)? How often? For how long?

Table 6.1   The "Rate Your Plate" Questionnaire (Typical Weekly Consumption)

Food Group	Column 1 (1 Point)	Column 2 (2 Points)	Column 3 (3 Points)	Points
Meat, Fish, Poultry, etc.				
Meats such as beef, pork, lamb, veal	*Usually eat:* high-fat cuts such as regular hamburger, spareribs, sausage, hot dogs (all kinds)	*Usually eat:* lean cuts such as pork (loin, leg), veal (most cuts), and beef (round, sirloin, extra-lean hamburger)	*Always eat:* lean cuts or *rarely eat* meat	
Organ meats such as liver, brain, kidney	*Usually eat:* 1–2 times a week	*Usually eat:* 1–2 times a month	*Rarely or never eat*	
Chicken, turkey	*Usually:* cook with skin and eat skin	*Usually:* cook with skin but discard before eating	*Usually:* cook without skin	
Seafood	*Rarely or never eat*	*Usually eat:* 1 serving or less a week	*Usually eat:* 2 servings or more a week	
Breakfast and luncheon meats	*Usually eat:* high-fat varieties such as bologna, sausage, salami, bacon	*Usually eat:* lean varieties such as Canadian bacon, turkey breast, roast beef, ham	*Always eat:* lean varieties or *rarely eat* breakfast and luncheon meats	
Serving sizes of cooked meat, poultry, seafood, organ, breakfast and luncheon meats	*Usually eat:* large servings (7 oz or more)	*Usually eat:* medium servings (4–6 oz)	*Usually eat:* small servings (3 oz or less)	
Split peas, lentils, dried beans such as kidney, lima, garbanzo	*Rarely or never eat*	*Usually eat:* at least twice a month	*Usually eat:* once a week or more	
Eggs	*Usually eat:* 7 or more a week	*Usually eat:* 5–6 a week	*Usually eat:* 4 or less a week or use cholesterol-free egg substitute	
Dairy Products				
Milk	*Usually use:* whole-milk or never use milk at all	*Usually use:* 2% low-fat milk	*Usually use:* 1% low-fat or skim milk	

Cheese such as cheddar, American, and Swiss (1 serving = 1 oz)	*Often eat:* cheese	*Sometimes eat:* cheese	*Rarely eat:* cheese or *do eat* low-fat or calorie-reduced cheese
Frozen dairy desserts (1 serving = $^1/_2$ cup)	*Often eat:* ice cream	*Sometimes eat:* ice cream	*Rarely eat:* ice cream or *do eat* ice milk, frozen low-fat yogurt, or sherbet
Fats, Oils, Sweets, and Snacks			
Fats, oils (for cooking and eating)	*Usually use:* butter, butter blends, shortening and/or lard	*Usually use:* margarine and/or vegetable oil	*Always use:* margarine and/or vegetable oil
Food preparation	*Usually eat:* deep-fried foods	*Sometimes eat:* deep-fried foods	*Usually eat:* foods cooked by other methods such as baking, steaming, broiling
Snacks	*Often eat:* chips, nuts, crackers	*Sometimes eat:* chips, nuts, crackers	*Usually eat:* fruit, low-fat crackers, plain popcorn, pretzels
Sweets such as donuts, cookies, cakes pies, sweet rolls, chocolate	*Often eat:* sweets	*Sometimes eat:* sweets	*Rarely or never eat*
Breads, Cereals, and Pasta			
Breads, cereals, and pasta (1 serving = 1 slice or $^1/_2$ cup)	*Rarely or never eat*	*Usually eat:* 5 servings or less a day	*Usually eat:* 6 servings or more a day
Whole-grain products such as whole-wheat bread, brown rice, oatmeal, other high-fiber cereal	*Rarely or never eat*	*Sometimes eat*	*Usually eat*
Fruits and Vegetables			
Fruits and vegetables (1 serving = 1 piece or $^1/_2$ cup)	*Rarely or never eat*	*Usually eat:* 4 servings or less a day	*Usually eat:* 5 servings or more a day

From Gans KM, Sundaram SG, McPhillips JB, et al. "Rate Your Plate": an eating pattern assessment and educational tool used at cholesterol screening and education programs. Journal of Nutrition Education. 1993;25:29–36; with permission.

Table 6.2   Additional Questions to the "Rate Your Plate" Questionnaire

Food/Behavior	Column 1 (1 Point)	Column 2 (2 Points)	Column 3 (3 Points)	Points
Snacking pattern	Usually more than 4 snacks per day	Usually 3 snacks per day	Average 1–2 snacks per day	____
Skip breakfast	Frequently (two or more times per week)	Sometimes (once a week)	Rarely (less than once a week)	____
Eating out or take-out food	Average 4 or more meals per week	Usually 2–3 times per week	Average once a week or less	____
Empty-calorie beverages (non-diet soda, fruit drink/punch, sweetened tea, "designer" drinks)	Drink more than 16 oz per day	Average 8–16 oz per day	Typically less than 8 oz per day	____
Alcohol intake (one drink = 12 oz beer, 5 oz wine, one shot of hard liquor, or a mixed drink with one shot)	Drink more than 1–2 alcoholic drinks per day	Average 1 drink per day	Average less than 1 drink per day	____
Physical activity (e.g., walking briskly, gardening, jogging, swimming, biking, dancing)	<15 total minutes of activity 3 days per week	≥15 total minutes of activity 3 days per week	≥30 total minutes of activity 3 or more days per week	____
Television or video time per day	Watch more than 2 hours per day	Watch 1–2 hours per day	Average less than 1 hour per day	____

The first question screens for a syndrome described by Albert Stunkard as the "night eating syndrome"; this syndrome is highly refractory to treatment (12). Questions 2, 3, and 4 may indicate binge eating disorder (BED), a condition requiring additional intervention by a psychologist and other team members. Typically, the approach is to normalize eating patterns without focusing on weight reduction. Antidepressants are sometimes found to be helpful in the treatment of BED as well (13, 14). If the patient is purging (Question 5), other complex eating disorders, such as bulimia, may be present. Referral to a team of specialists for any of the above problems is usually warranted, and often essential. Most such problems cannot be adequately addressed in the primary care setting.

Motivation

It is critical to determine the patient's readiness for intervention. In an age of managed care and cost containment, it is obviously wiser to use more resources and energy for those individuals who are interested in pursuing weight management. Prochaska's stages of change is the classic model for determining readiness for any condition that has a lifestyle intervention as a key component to therapy (15). By asking specific time-oriented questions and listening to the patient's comments, the physician can assess readiness for change and choose the most appropriate intervention. Tailored messages are more likely to result in consistent long-term lifestyle changes compared with generic messages based on dietary guidelines such as eating fewer calories or less fat.

Table 6.3 can be used to identify a patient's stage of change and determine the most appropriate nutrition intervention. This table defines each stage of change, identifies patient characteristics in each stage, and provides some examples of the appropriate physician statements. If patients are in the precontemplation or contemplation stage, the physician should stress the benefits of weight loss, discuss individual risk, and inquire about dietary habits. At this stage, helping to raise the patient's awareness is more effective than action-oriented strategies (e.g., defer a discussion on reducing intake of high-fat foods). In the preparation stage patients begin to take steps toward action such as self-reevaluation and stimulus control (e.g., cues that trigger the desire to eat). Simple behavioral goals, such as eating lower fat snacks after work, can be effective. In the action stage patients use social support and feel they have the autonomy to change their life. Long-term, successful maintenance is associated with the belief that one is becoming the person one wants to be. Techniques to prevent relapse, limit stimulus control, and maintain behavior change are appropriate for discussion.

Table 6.3   Identifying Patient Readiness for Intervention

Stage	Definition/ Characteristics	Statements Patients May Use	Statements Physicians May Use
Precontemplation	Person is unaware of problem or uninterested in making changes in next 6 months.	I can't change. It's in my genes. There is nothing I can do about it.	You gained 5 pounds since your last visit. I am concerned because of your family history of CHD and DM. What are your thoughts on your weight?
Contemplation	Person is hoping problem behavior will solve itself or is waiting for the magic moment to start. Thinking about making changes in next 6 months.	I know I should, but it's not the right time.	It sounds as if you are thinking about your weight. By losing 5 to 10 pounds, do you realize how much your blood pressure *or* blood sugar will improve?
Preparation	Person is motivated and planning to make changes in the next 30 days or has tried making changes inconsistently.	Where can I go? How can I start? What should I do?	Why don't we start by recording what you eat and identifying foods that are high in fat and calories?
Action	Person believes change is possible. Has changed a behavior within the past 6 months and is becoming more consistent with it.	It's getting easier for me to _____. I feel I can do it.	It's great that you have reduced your portions *or* snacking at work. Have you noticed any difference in the way you feel since you reduced your caloric intake by 500 calories a day?
Maintenance	Person has maintained a new behavior longer than 6 months and is confident about ability to maintain change.	I don't have to think about it as much anymore. I just do it.	It's great that you walk with your neighbor every morning. How confident are you that meal planning will continue to be a priority *or* that you will avoid bringing high-calorie, high-fat snacks/foods into the home *or* that you will select low-fat/low-calorie foods when eating out?

Adapted from Prochaska JO, Velicer WF. Transtheoretical model of health behavior change. Am J Health Promo. 1997;12:38-48.

Targeting Treatment Approaches

Needs Assessment

Based on the information obtained from the screening instruments and the patient's medical and family histories, it is highly probable that the obese individual will have multiple nutrition-related issues requiring attention (16). The most familiar to physicians are the common medical issues, including hypertension, dyslipidemia, and diabetes. Addressing all of these concerns at once may be overwhelming. Therefore a needs assessment is necessary to prioritize the approaches to treatment. The assessment can be used as a focal point for discussion with the patient to identify where he or she is able to make changes.

When devising an approach, it should be emphasized that generic messages about weight loss (you need to eat less, cut down on your fat, your portion sizes are too large) or a long list of multiple goals is destined for failure. Generic diet sheets have been shown *not* to result in behavior change (17). Designing a nutrition intervention program tailored to the individual is essential. Some patients with multiple nutrition concerns, newly diagnosed medical problems with nutrition-based components to their intervention (e.g., diabetes), or minimal nutrition knowledge would be managed best by referral to a Registered Dietitian and/or through enrollment in a comprehensive weight management program. Still, even if the patient is referred to a dietitian or program, the physician needs to address nutrition concerns and support the actions of the allied health team. Constant reinforcement of the importance of nutrition to the patient is crucial and, when presented properly, demonstrates the supportive role the physician has in the treatment of obesity.

Goal Setting

For patients beyond the precontemplative stage, goal setting is essential for behavior change. Goal setting needs to be a collaborative effort between the patient and physician. Only two or three goals should be set at a time. Goals can be set using the acronym SMART (Specific, Measurable, Achievable, Realistic, and Time-frame–oriented) (18). Table 6.4 compares vague, nebulous goals to SMART goals.

Once a few goals are decided upon, it is important to inquire how confident the patient feels about his or her ability to achieve these goals. (In behavioral therapy, this is termed *self-efficacy*.) If the patient does not feel confident about being able to make the change(s), then different goals should be set that have a higher probability of success. Conversely, care should be taken to resist the establishment of a multitude of goals by

Table 6.4   SMART Goals*

Food-Specific Goals

Vague Goals
- Eat more vegetables and less meat.
- Eat low-fat dairy products.
- Snack less; when you do snack, make it healthy.

SMART Goals
- Include at least 1 green vegetable each day.
- Limit meat/poultry/fish portions to the size of a deck of cards at main meals.
- Order broiled fish in place of fried when eating out.
- Substitute skim or 1% milk for 2% milk.
- Limit snacks to 1–2/d and each to <150 calories

Behavior-Specific Goals

Vague Goals
- Do not eat when stressed; do something else.
- Eat out less often.
- Avoid parties.

SMART Goals
- Substitute walking or (a particular activity of the patient's liking) when arriving home from work, feeling stressed, and/or wanting to eat.
- Reduce number of times eating out from _____ to ____/wk.
- Plain ahead when going to a party. Offer to bring a vegetable tray with low-fat dip or a low-calorie appetizer to limit your caloric intake.

Activity-Specific Goals

Vague Goals
- Exercise more frequently.
- Increase physical activity.

SMART Goals
- To start, walk for ____ minutes 3 times per week.
- Take at least 1 flight of stairs at least 2 times per day.
- Park at the farthest corner of the parking lot each time you go shopping.

*SMART = Specific, Measurable, Achievable, Realistic, Time-frame–oriented.
From Rinkle WJ. The Winning Foodservice Manager, 2nd ed. Achievement Publishers, page 49.

overzealous patients who are highly motivated and ready for change. This too is a likely recipe for failure.

Once goals are set, ongoing progress toward these goals needs to be monitored. The physician should attempt a problem-solving approach with creative strategies to assist patients through difficult areas. Some effective strategies and solutions are listed below.

Small Gradual Changes

Helping the patient limit the number and/or magnitude of goals is the first step toward achieving moderation in intake. Gradual, steady, and slow weight loss is recommended. Because it is difficult to determine the exact number of calories a person expends daily or to develop a meal plan that provides a specified number of calories for weight loss, a safe approach is to assist the patient in achieving a 300 to 1000 cal/d deficit tailored to his or her initial weight (per NIH recommendations, a calorie deficit of 300 to 500 cal/d for patients with a body mass index [BMI] of 25 to 35, and a deficit of 500 to 1000 cal/d for patients with a BMI > 35) (19). To enter into a discussion about the number of calories required for weight loss is often frustrating and counterproductive. It is best to help the patient identify where he or she can easily modify food choices to achieve this goal (Table 6.5).

Self-Monitoring

Because satiety mechanisms may work differently in obese individuals and these individuals may be more sensitive to external cues (20), an external monitoring system of intake and expenditure to achieve a calorie deficit has been repeatedly demonstrated to be beneficial to many patients (21). Despite the fact that food records are fraught with errors of underestimation, they are a highly effective instrument for patients and can be used to promote discussion of places, people, or events that lead to overeating (21). Although physicians feel they lack the time and expertise to review food diaries thoroughly, some problem areas can be quickly identified:

- Patterns of eating that result in excessive intake
- Large portion sizes
- Specific foods that are high in fat and calories
- Alcohol intake
- Eating out frequently (22)

If the patient is extremely resistant to record keeping, the physician can ask him or her to record only problem food groups or specific time periods of concern. For example, if the patient consumes a routine breakfast that he/she is unwilling to change, and has the most difficulty controlling his or her intake in the evening, then asking the patient to only record what is consumed throughout the evening may be helpful. The physician can also ask the patient to make a note of servings consumed in each group of the Food Guide Pyramid (23) in order to see which areas are over- or underconsumed. It may be helpful to purchase a few food models to show patients what a typical serving size is for each category in the Food Guide Pyramid because standard portion sizes are frequently smaller than most

Table 6.5   Calorie Savings Food List

Meal	Instead of:	Kcals	Choose:	Kcals	Savings
Breakfast	3-egg omelet with 1 oz regular cheese	387	3-egg white omelet plain	50	337
	2 eggs with 3 slices of bacon	335	1 cup oatmeal with $1/2$ cup skim milk	145	190
	Chocolate chip muffin (4 oz)	370	1 English muffin with 2 teaspoons of jam	170	200
	2 creme-filled doughnuts (3 oz)	612	1 bagel (3.5 in.) with 2 tablespoons fat-free cream cheese	208	404
Lunch	Burger King Double-Whopper with cheese	960	Burger King single cheeseburger	380	580
	Taco Bell Taco Salad	850	Soft Taco	220	630
	Subway 6-in. tuna salad sub	542	Subway 6-in. turkey breast sub	289	253
	Wendy's baked potato with chili and cheese	630	Wendy's baked potato with 1 packet of margarine	370	260
	Sandwich: 3 oz bologna with 2 oz American cheese on 2 slices of white bread with 2 tablespoons of mayonnaise	725	Sandwich: 3 oz turkey with 2 oz low fat cheese on 2 slices of whole-wheat bread with 2 tablespoons fat-free mayonnaise	394	331
Dinner	Pizza Hut Pepperoni Pan Pizza (4 slices)	1120	Pizza Hut Veggie Lover's Thin and Crispy Pizza (3 slices)	510	610
	Dozen chicken wings with blue cheese dressing	1320	2 servings of a chicken fajita	520	800
	Lasagna with meat sauce (12 oz)	531	1 cup spaghetti with marinara sauce	250	281
	Fish fry (6 oz) with a larger order of French fries	1028	Broiled fish (6 oz) with baked potato with 2 tablespoons of sour cream and packet of margarine	535	493
Desserts	Cherry cheese cake ($1/12$ of 9 in. cake)	407	Angel food cake with $1/2$ cup strawberries	163	244
	Chocolate ice cream sundae (medium)	400	Nonfat frozen yogurt ($1/2$ cup)	100	300
	Chocolate cake with icing ($1/12$ of 9 in. cake)	357	Half of portion	178.5	178.5
Snacks	Dry roasted mixed nuts (4 oz)	673	Pretzel twists (10 each) (2.12 oz)	228	445
	Butterfingers candy bar (2.16 oz)	292	Tootsie Roll (1 oz)	112	180
	Lays potato chips (2 oz)	300	Popcorn (air popped) (2 cups)	82	218
	Ritz crackers (8 each) and 4 oz cheese	700	Air crisps (4 oz)	240	460
Beverages	Regular soda (16 oz)	205	Diet soda	0	205
	Chocolate whole milk (8 oz)	230	Skim milk (8 oz)	90	140
	Beer (4 glasses) (8 oz each)	480	Beer (2 glasses) (8 oz each)	240	240

people envision. (Various sets can be purchased from NASCO Nutrition Teaching Aids [800-558-9595/*www.eNASCO.com*] or the National Dairy Council's Customer Service Department [800-426-8271/*www.national-dairycouncil.org*].) There are also more sophisticated approaches available for monitoring food intake for highly motivated patients including Web sites (Table 6.6) and a personal digital assistant version of a diet analysis program.

Positive Reinforcement

Rather than focus on weight change, the physician should make every effort to recognize and comment on positive changes in health status and behaviors made by the patient, particularly since changes in lifestyle are not always measured on the scale (e.g., body composition, waist size). For example, it is beneficial to commend changes such as eating less fat or increasing physical activity. Improved blood pressure and glycemic control can result from such modifications and should be emphasized. An often neglected but important part of the physician's role in any patient's success is sincerely accentuating the positive.

Support

Social support, a behavioral strategy that is effective in assisting patients make and sustain long-term lifestyle changes, is an important component in nutrition intervention (24). Support will help many patients stay motivated and manage difficult situations, while also providing positive reinforcement of behavior changes. Many weight management programs are structured in a group format so as to provide social support to patients. This can be a very effective way to strengthen support systems. In the primary care setting health practitioners are in a unique position to provide additional support to patients by

- Evaluating current sources of support
- Encouraging patients to recruit support from spouses, family members, friends, colleagues, others

---

Table 6.6   Web Sites for Self-Monitoring

• www.cyberdiet.com	• www.ag.uiuc.edu
• www.dietlog.com	• www.dietsite.com
• www.caloriecontrol.org	• http://dawp.anet.com
• www.shapeup.org	

- Identifying and reinforcing the positive behavior changes made by the patient
- Assisting the patient in identifying barriers and in developing problem-solving skills
- Demonstrating understanding and sensitivity to the challenges that are involved in weight management

Independent, outside support is quite effective for some patients, particularly because support at home and in the workplace is often suboptimal. Besides traditional psychotherapy, a variety of reputable "do-it-yourself" and nonprofessional group programs are available, including Weight Watchers, Overeaters Anonymous (OA), and TOPS (Take Off Pounds Sensibly) (Tables 6.7 and 6.8), as well as programs of local churches, YMCAs, and health clubs. ("Gold standard" and very low calorie diet programs are discussed below.) Moreover, virtually every town has at least one hospital with support programs or referral mechanisms. Each of these programs has different approaches, and the character of individual chapters is often unique. In addition, commercial programs can be helpful but, because there are so many, identifying a reputable program can be difficult. Recognizing this problem, a conference that included government, industry, consumer advocate, and professional representatives has established guidelines and ongoing monitoring to assist the consumer (25). It is important for the patient to be aware of these resources and to try different programs, even different chapters within these programs, until one is found that is compatible with his or her needs and personality. Regardless of the program the patient chooses, social support is essential to long-term success.

Role of the Registered Dietitian

When To Refer to a Registered Dietitian

Although it is essential to address nutrition in the medical visit, at times it may be necessary to refer to a registered dietitian (RD) for further assistance (26). There are no standards of practice for RD referrals; however, there are some situations when it will be helpful, if not essential:

- Lack of progress in achieving the desired health outcome
- Complex nutrition needs (e.g., diagnoses that affect nutrition needs)
- Multiple food and eating habits requiring considerable change
- In conjunction with more involved therapies (essential for weight

Table 6.7 "Do-It Yourself" Programs*

Name	Approach	Staff	Expected Weight Loss	Cost/Year	Length	Components	Comments
Overeaters Anonymous	Patterned after 12-step Alcoholics Anonymous program; weight loss not a goal	Nonprofessional volunteers	No claims	<$100	Unlimited	Emotional, spiritual, and physical recovery	Provides group support
TOPS (Take Off Pounds Sensibly)	Does not endorse or prescribe any particular eating or exercise regimen; endorses slow, gradual changes	Nonhealth professionals; organization consults with medical adviser	No claims	<$100	Unlimited	Members encouraged to consult health care provider for exercise plan	Groups vary widely in approach

*Primary approach is group support.

Table 6.8   Nonprofessional Programs*

Name	Approach	Staff	Expected Weight Loss	Cost/Year	Length	Components	Comments
Diet Center	Focuses on achieving healthy body composition through diet and exercise; emphasizes body composition, not weight; minimum calorie level: 1200 kcal/day	Clients consult with nonprofessional staff trained by program; RDs may consult with upper-level management	1.5-2 lb/wk	$1000–$3000	Varies but 1-year maintenance program encouraged	Nutrition, exercise, behavior, maintenance	Does not require purchase of program food; little group support available; program's vitamin supplement required; lacks professional guidance at client level
Jenny Craig	Menu plans based on the purchase of program's cuisine with additional store-bought food; after clients lose half their weight they begin planning meals using their own food; calorie level: 1000-2600 kcal/day	Company consults with advisory board of MDs and RDs on program design; nonprofessional consultants trained by program; RDs available to consult with clients	1-2 lb/wk	$1000–$3000	Weekly meetings mandatory; separate 1-year maintenance program offered	Nutrition, exercise, behavior, maintenance	Must rely on program cuisine for participation; lacks professional guidance at client level
NutriSystem	Menu plans based on the purchase of program's cuisine with additional store-bought food; calorie level: 1000-2200 kcal/day; personal counseling and group sessions available	Staff dietitians, health educators, and PhDs develop program at corporate level; certified personal trainers employed	1.5-2 lb/wk	$1000–$3000	Varies with weight loss goals	Wellness and personal trainer services developed in conjunction with Johnson & Johnson Health Management	Relatively rigid diet with company food; little contact with health professionals
Weight Watchers	Emphasis on portion control and healthy lifestyle habits; clients choose from regular supermarket food, program cuisine, or both; health professionals include RDs and MDs at corporate-level direct program; calorie levels: women average 1250 kcal/day, men average 1600 kcal/day	Group leaders are trained nonprofessional graduates of the program	Up to 2 lb/wk	$1000–$3000	Unlimited length; maintenance plan is 6 wk	Emphasizes making lifestyle changes in diet and exercise; also includes maintenance phase	Weekly group meetings with mandatory weigh-ins; offers group support; encourages long-term participation; lacks professional guidance at client level; no personalized counseling except in select markets

*Major nonprofessional programs. Local programs may be modeled on them. All provide nutrition, exercise, and behavior education as well as a maintenance phase.

loss surgery and extremely helpful in conjunction with anti-obesity agents)

Identifying Reputable Nutritionists

Registered dietitians have a minimum of a bachelor's degree in food and nutrition sciences or a closely related field from an American Dietetic Association accredited university or college. In addition, RDs must complete a post-baccalaureate program (internship or other certified program) and pass the Association's registration exam. Lastly, they must maintain competency in the field through continuing education.

Often the terms *nutritionist* and *registered dietitian* are used interchangeably. Be cautious using the former. It is a general term that does not necessarily guarantee education or credentialing in the area of nutrition. However, some dietitians prefer the term *nutritionist* because the public perceives it more positively. Whether the health care provider refers to himself or herself as a dietitian or a nutritionist, only the abbreviation "RD" following his or her name guarantees appropriate and certified training.

Evaluation Performed by a Registered Dietitian

Dietitians screen and assess nutrition status, identify specific nutrition needs, and provide individualized interventions. An adequate initial assessment with an RD requires 45 to 60 min. Obviously this is usually longer than a physician or nurse practitioner is able to spend with a patient addressing nutrition concerns. Thus one sign for a referral is when the physician cannot accommodate the patient without an extended visit. Typically a physician order is required for the evaluation and implementation of an RD-supervised treatment plan. Some of the key components to look for to determine if the RD conducted an adequate and comprehensive nutrition assessment are

- *Screening*—identifying characteristics often associated with nutrition problems that may indicate nutrition risk
- *Assessment*—identifying the presence, nature, and extent of impaired nutrition status. In the obese patient, obtaining information that affects a patient's food choices is imperative, such as cultural background, emotional connections to food, economic considerations, life stressors, and coping skills.
- *Goal Setting* (as described above but more detailed)
- *Interventions:*

    EDUCATION—providing specific nutrition information on food choices and preparation and recommendations on dining-out based on individual needs. Dietitians take general dietary guidelines and tailor them to the patient's unique situation. (For example, selecting an appropriate brand of margarine or snack food for the patient based on diagnosis, preference, and cost.)

MONITORING—by using standard methods (e.g. food diaries, 24-h recall), reviewing food records, scheduling follow-up

COUNSELING—identifying barriers to behavior changes and working with the patient to develop strategies to overcome them. Counseling includes assisting patients in increasing self-awareness surrounding their dietary intake and emotional connections to food. Dietitians also assist patients in identifying high-risk situations, developing self-monitoring strategies, and improving problem-solving skills.

SUPPORT—providing positive reinforcement to patients who have made behavior changes and encouraging patients who struggle with behavior change by helping them identify barriers.

Locating Registered Dietitians

Typically, local community hospitals and universities have a comprehensive weight management program that provides group and/or individual counseling, some of which are listed in the Yellow Pages. A reputable program must have an RD affiliated with it. For weight management, the most effective way to use the services of a dietitian is through a comprehensive weight management program. The "gold standard" weight management program is given in Table 6.9. These professional programs are generally hospital or university based.

If there are no "gold standard" weight management programs, patients can be referred to a specific dietitian for individual nutrition counseling. The health practitioner can refer either to a hospital-based dietitian who does outpatient care or to a dietitian in private practice. Most hospitals have an outpatient dietitian who has experience with weight management programs. Private dietitians can be found in the local telephone directory or through the American Dietetic Association Hotline (1-800-366-1655).

It is important to develop a rapport with the dietitian you use. Many health practitioners develop partnerships with dietitians based on the nutrition needs of their patient population. If the decision to refer to a dietitian has been made, a brief phone interview may be helpful in determining which dietitian would best meet the needs of your practice. Some important information to obtain during this interview includes

- Past experience in treating obesity

Table 6.9   "Gold Standard" Program*

Name	Approach	Staff	Expected Weight Loss	Cost/Year	Length	Components	Comments
"Gold Standard"	Comprehensive and individualized, focusing on long-term lifestyle changes; primary objectives are teaching patients skill building, problem-solving techniques, and behavioral strategies along with providing education in all disciplines	Health professionals with degrees in dietetics, exercise physiology, and behavioral counseling; each program has a medical director; the team uses an interdisciplinary approach	1% of weight per week	$1000–$3000	Intensive phase should be minimum of 6 months, with on-going maintenance phase	Medical, nutrition, behavior, and exercise components and built-in maintenance phase; weekly classes as well as one-to-one counseling in each discipline; frequency of visits is increased in the initial phase, decreased in the maintenance phase	Experts in all disciplines; a healthy balanced diet is used for caloric reduction not under 1200 calories using regular food; no purchase of program food or other products is required; antiobesity medications may be used when appropriate

*"Gold standard" programs can be found in medical centers for other clinical outpatient settings. Health care professionals in the various disciplines are used in the treatment team with on-going patient contact. The program uses a multidisciplinary team approach that includes a maintenance phase. An individualized treatment plan is developed for healthy meals with a minimum of 1200 calories per day.

- General weight management approach used (e.g., focus on lifestyle and healthy eating habits as opposed to restrictive dieting)
- Cost and insurance coverage
- Ability to coordinate care with others (e.g., mental and exercise health care professionals) when necessary
- Regular communications about treatment with primary health care provider

To assist a dietitian in making the most efficient use of his or her time with the patient, the referring practitioner should provide the following information:

- Diagnoses and relevant medical history
- Focus of the visit
- Chief complaint related to diet
- Pertinent laboratory data (e.g., cholesterol, FBS)
- Pertinent medications
- Pertinent physical exam data (e.g., weight loss/gain, blood pressure changes)
- Insight into any lifestyle information related to nutrition (e.g., truck driver, chef, night-shift nurse)
- Life stressors (e.g., recent divorce, loss of loved one, change in employment)

Common Nutrition Issues

Diet Composition and Weight Loss

The Unified Dietary Guidelines, an evidence-based synopsis reported by the leading professional and patient advocate organizations for nutritionally related diseases (American Heart Association, American Cancer Society, American Dietetic Association, American Academy, Division of Nutrition Research Coordination of the National Institutes of Health, American Society of Clinical Nutrition), established unanimity by canvassing a cross section of nutrition experts on their recommendations for maintaining a healthy lifestyle (27). Nevertheless, the plethora of diet books attests to popular interest in weight loss approaches that often deviate from the basic principles of nutrition therapy (e.g., a diet composition that induces and sustains the most weight loss in the shortest amount of time).

Despite years of carefully performed research on the safety and efficacy of various nutrition plans, numerous myths persist. Clinical investigators have rigorously investigated different diet compositions that could be effective in enhancing weight loss including very low fat, low fat, high fiber, low carbohydrate, and high protein weight-reducing meal plans (28-34). The overriding conclusions from these studies are that *under free-living conditions* caloric intake is the major determinant for weight loss and that variations in macronutrient (i.e., fat, carbohydrate, protein) composition do not have a significant impact on weight and moreover raise safety concerns. Thus, although diet composition is important in terms of overall health promotion and disease prevention, during the weight loss phase it has little influence on overall weight loss compared with the caloric deficit (35-38).

Fat

Energy balance is the most important factor in successful weight loss. However, there is suggestive evidence that fat may place obese individuals or those prone to obesity at greater risk for weight gain for the following reasons:

- *Satiety*—Satiety is the reduction of hunger and termination of eating. Among the physiologic effects of fat is delayed gastric emptying and release of the gastric hormone cholecystokinin (CCK). Both of these should induce satiety, yet studies have demonstrated that high fat intake has a diminished effect on satiety (39-45). Obese and postobese individuals (patients who have reduced their weight into the normal BMI range) eating a high fat meal not only overeat but fail to compensate for these extra calories in subsequent meals in contrast to the compensation that occurs following high carbohydrate or high protein meals (46-48).

- *Preference (food of choice)*—Obese and postobese individuals have a greater preference for fat, which places them at greater risk of weight gain given a high fat environment (49).

- *Palatability (pleasing to taste)*—The palatability of fat also has an impact on passive overconsumption of calories on a high fat diet in both lean and obese individuals (50-52). In a survey regarding favorite foods of obese men and women, protein-fat sources (meat dishes) were listed as favorites for men and carbohydrate-fat sources (ice cream, doughnuts, cookies, cake) as favorites for women (53, 54). If applicable, these types of foods may be best targeted in the respective sexes.

- *Caloric Density*—Fat, at 9 cal/g compared with 4 cal/g for carbohydrate and protein, is the most calorically dense nutrient. Both obese and lean individuals eat more when exposed to a high energy density diet (one high in fat and simple sugars and low in fiber) than when exposed to a low energy density diet (one low in fats and sugars and high in fiber) (55-57).

Given that the appetite control mechanism in obese individuals may fail to respond to high fat foods and the high caloric density of fat, it is wise to emphasize decreasing fat intake. Therefore the intake of high fat foods should be decreased within the context of the reduction of 300 to 1000 cal/d as noted above. To the dismay of food manufacturers who produce thousands of low fat/nonfat products, weight loss will occur only if a reduction of fat leads to a caloric deficit. Numerous studies have demonstrated that reduction of fat intake without attention to overall decreases in caloric intake is not an effective weight loss strategy when weight loss, as opposed to disease prevention, is the primary goal (58). However, diets too low in fat can, at least in the short term, increase plasma triglycerides and if not properly designed can lack essential fatty acids and micronutrients (59). Moreover, the type of fat consumed is important, with an emphasis on monounsaturated fats and fish oils probably being metabolically and medically more favorable than polyunsaturated fats, and certainly saturated fats (60, 61). In fact, in their recently revised dietary guidelines, the American Heart Association took the unprecedented step of recommending consumption of two servings of fish at least twice weekly (61). Only small changes in fat consumption are required to attain these benefits (61-63). Thus these findings reaffirm that a vague goal and simplistic messages do not provide adequate treatment for the obese patient.

To be most effective, fat reduction should be accompanied by an increase in fiber, not simple sugars or other sources of calories. Under free-living conditions, the decreased total and LDL cholesterol as well as the secondary weight loss that occurs with high fiber diets is most likely due to the replacement of dietary saturated fat and cholesterol with fiber (as reviewed and recommended by the American Heart Association's Nutrition Committee (64)). After weight loss a low fat *ad libitum* diet may be more helpful in the maintenance phase because patients have rated this type of diet as more palatable and easier to follow. This type of approach has also been associated with a decrease in binge-eating scores (11).

Carbohydrates

Despite innumerable studies demonstrating that low fat, high carbohydrate, portion-controlled diet plans reduce weight and promote cardiovascular health, carbohydrates have recently been targeted as the villain nutrient. A revival of the anticarbohydrate campaign is reflected in the number of low carbohydrate diet books on the bestseller list. As a class, carbohydrates include simple carbohydrates (sugars) and complex carbohydrates (starches and fiber). A common misconception is that carbohydrate causes insulin resistance that in turn promotes obesity. Supporters of this postulate cite the coincident rise in the prevalence of obesity with the decline in fat consumption and the increase in carbohydrate consumption. They also claim that, because carbohydrate is a potent insulin secretagogue, it promotes hyperinsulinemia, which in turn facilitates fat synthesis. However, what these studies do not acknowledge is that there are no studies proving or disproving this postulate; what is clear is that hyperinsulinemia is the normal compensatory response to underlying insulin resistance. Moreover, while cross-sectional studies demonstrate that insulin resistance is associated with obesity, longitudinal studies suggest insulin sensitivity favors weight gain and that insulin resistance that develops with the onset of obesity is actually protective of further weight gain (65).

Unfortunately, with increased awareness of reducing fat consumption, carbohydrate has been substituted in many diets, predominantly in the form of simple sugars, not complex carbohydrates such as whole grains and other high fiber foods. Thus individuals are simply trading fat for carbohydrate calories rather than reducing overall caloric intake. On the other hand, although epidemiologic studies point to fruits and vegetables as healthful foods, they have not supported an association between sugar intake and obesity in population studies (33, 66-68). Eating sugar does not promote weight gain unless caloric intake exceeds output. There is some evidence, however, that foods high in fat and sugar may promote general overconsumption in obese individuals, particularly when they are hungry (42).

Even though population studies have shown an inverse relation between fiber intake and the prevalence of obesity (69) and low intake is more predictive of weight gain and concomitant development of risk factors than total and saturated fat intake (70), the role dietary fiber plays in weight control is unclear. The purported mechanisms for the role of fiber include

- Delayed gastric emptying, which enhances satiety
- Fullness related to the bulk of a high fiber diet, which may lead to a decrease in energy intake
- Longer chewing time, resulting in a greater effort to eat, which in turn may result in a decrease in energy intake
- Decreased efficiency of energy absorption

In general, fiber tends to decrease feelings of hunger even if it has not been shown to consistently result in decreased food intake (32). Unfortunately, research studies on both soluble (legumes, oatmeal and oat bran, citrus) and insoluble fiber (skins on fruits and vegetables, wheat bran) have been inconclusive. On the other hand, fiber intake should clearly not be ignored. It may be important in cancer prevention, reduction in blood cholesterol, and the prevention of type 2 diabetes (71). The recommended daily intake of fiber is 25 to 30 g, which is about one half the average American intake (72). Table 6.10 lists good sources of fiber.

Table 6.10   Sources of Fiber

Soluble
   Oats, oat bran, oatmeal
   Peas
   Beans
   Legumes
   Barley
   Strawberries
   Citrus fruits
   Apples
   Rice bran
Insoluble
   Wheat bran
   Whole grains (e.g., brown rice, whole-wheat bread)
   Fresh or steamed vegetables (e.g., carrots, cabbage, beets, Brussel sprouts, turnips, cauliflower)
   Whole-grain cereals
   Fresh fruits

Protein

Of all the macronutrients, protein seems to exert the most powerful effect on satiety. Subjects consuming a high protein meal report greater feelings of fullness and a greater decrease in the desire to eat compared with subjects consuming a high carbohydrate meal (73, 74). In addition, high protein diets increase thermogenesis more than the other macronutrients, although the relevance to weight loss is questionable because the thermic effect of food, which is only a minor component of total energy expenditure, is blunted in obesity (75). However, these isolated observations from small studies under the highly controlled conditions of the clinical research environment remain to be proved (or disproved) in larger studies under more realistic free-living conditions.

Nevertheless, this situation has not dissuaded some "experts" from extrapolating and generalizing these findings to untested diet plans and writing books espousing their virtues. Lured by mass-marketing techniques, many obese individuals attempt these diets, diets that are often unbalanced, and under some circumstances, dangerous (see Chapter 4). What results is often a dieter with a very high intake of unhealthy saturated fat, intake beyond the requirements of any macronutrient, particularly protein, the excess of which is converted to fat, and a deficiency in known dietary components that are healthy (fruits and vegetables with their related vitamins and fiber). Thus, particularly in those with obesity-related illnesses, it is of concern that patients with hyperlipidemia may be consuming amounts of saturated fat that counteract the benefits of weight loss or that patients with diabetes and/or hypertension may be consuming more protein than can be handled by their impaired kidneys (76).

High protein diets are characterized by an "unlimited" calorie intake focused on high protein and typically high fat foods. Diets of this composition are relatively ketogenic. Carbohydrates are initially limited to approximately 20 g/d, the amount in a large apple or in a little more than a slice of bread. Controlled research studies on this type of approach are sparse. The initial weight loss associated with this type of diet is caused by diuresis (see Chapter 4 for a complete description of mechanisms). Individuals receive positive feedback from these rapid results and are encouraged to continue this approach.

What these individuals fail to recognize is that, after the initial diuresis, weight loss is a result of the fundamental tenet of weight management—reduced caloric intake compared with expenditure. That is, as with any structured meal plan, patients will lose weight, whether on a healthy or unhealthy diet, as long as energy intake is less than energy output. Although the satiating effect of protein and the resultant ketosis may have a role in this dietary approach, the monotony of the diet is just as likely to contribute to decreasing caloric intake. Of course, the effectiveness of the monotony is also a major drawback; patients become bored with the plan and revert to previous eating habits. The overall diet, however, is very unbalanced and unhealthy, especially because the high protein foods are usually high in fat and saturated fats that are especially deleterious to the lipid profile. Other potential problems associated with this type of diet (many which are discussed in Chapter 4) include

- Enhanced progression of renal problems, which may be especially important for patients with diabetes
- Calcium loss from bones, potentially putting individuals at risk for osteoporosis
- Increased risk of heart disease as a result of high saturated fat intake
- Cancer risk, particularly for colon and prostate cancer, which is associated with high fat intake
- Gout as a result of increased uric acid levels
- Halitosis as a result of ketosis
- Constipation as a result of a low fiber intake
- Inadequate vitamin, mineral, micronutrient, and trace element intake, which has been associated with cardiac dysfunction (see Chapter 4)

Therefore this approach is not recommended, even for short duration, and certainly not in an unmonitored setting.

It should also be noted that the typical American consumes 1.5 times the amount of protein required for health (72). This is likely related to the perceived size of a serving. An appropriate serving size is approximately 3 oz of meat (looks like a deck of cards), 4 oz of tofu, 1 cup of beans, 1 cup of yogurt or milk, or 1.5 oz of cheese. On average, to meet protein requirements individuals should consume two servings from the dairy group and two servings from the meat/protein group on a daily basis.

Nevertheless, under supervised conditions, there may be a role for a modestly higher intake of protein during weight loss, as demonstrated by two small clinical trials in individuals who were overweight or obese but not manifesting obesity-related illnesses and who adhered to a plan that was otherwise well-balanced (77, 78). More protein may be useful for more active individuals. It may also help with those who have satiety problems. Under such circumstances, good sources of protein with each meal can be incorporated into their nutrition plan, especially low fat protein: fish, skinless poultry, lean meat, legumes (lentils, garbanzo beans, black beans, etc.), tofu, and low fat milk, cheese, or yogurt.

Alcohol

Besides the well-known health concerns related to excessive intake, alcohol is of particular concern in the obese patient because of its lack of effect on satiety and subsequent energy intake (79). From a metabolic perspective, alcohol at 7 kcal/g is the second most calorically dense macronutrient. In the typical American diet alcohol contributes 1% and 3% of total energy intake for women and men, respectively (72). As with other food, alcohol is usually underestimated in a dietary intake recall. Questions about alcohol intake should always be incorporated in a nutrition screening form. A decrease in alcohol intake is a prime target for creating a 300 to 1000 calorie deficit because a 12 oz beer has approximately 120 calories and 1 oz of alcohol has 100 calories. Finally, if there are indications of excess intake, it is often wise to address alcohol intake and potential alcoholism before embarking on a comprehensive weight management plan. Not addressing the emotional or behavioral issues related to alcohol intake may make it difficult to make progress in the overall lifestyle change needed for successful long-term weight control. A case-by-case assessment, including the help of an experienced therapist, is a prudent course of action.

Sugar Substitutes

The role of artificial sweeteners (also called nonnutritive and intense sweeteners) in weight management is to extend the range of palatable low fat foods and promote adherence to a low calorie diet. The FDA has approved four nonnutritive sweeteners: saccharine (Sweet'n Low, Sugar Twin, and Sweet10), aspartame (NutraSweet and Equal), AcesulfameK (Sunette, Sweet Swiss, and Sweet One), and sucralose (Splenda) (80). Aspartame is the most studied of these. In 1985 the Council on Scientific Affairs of the AMA concluded: "Available evidence suggests that consumption of aspartame by normal humans is safe and is not associated with serious adverse effects" (81).

There is a popular misconception based on some early research that consumption of intense sweeteners, like aspartame, may result in an increased appetite (82). Further research has not supported these initial studies. Intense sweeteners do not affect plasma insulin or blood glucose concentrations, and there is no known mechanism by which they would be a physiologic stimulus to increase hunger. Additional studies have confirmed that the use of aspartame does not negatively affect food intake. Depending on the study conditions, replacement of intense sweeteners for sugar results in complete, partial, or no compensation for the calories displaced (83). Although sugar sweeteners do not directly promote weight loss, they may be helpful in long-term weight maintenance. Individuals who used aspartame in a 12-month multidisciplinary weight loss program lost and sustained more weight loss than nonusers (84). In another study, women using aspartame showed better weight maintenance during the follow-up period (85). In summary, artificial sweeteners allow a greater array of intake without adding extra calories and therefore may be helpful in weight loss efforts as part of an overall nutritious, balanced diet.

Fat Substitutes

Fat intake is one of the most important factors associated with obesity. Fat significantly adds to the flavor and palatability of foods, and taste is the primary determinant of the food choices people make (86). Hence foods that are high in fat are more often selected and preferred. Nonetheless, as Americans strive for better health and weight loss there has been increased demand for reduced fat, low fat, and fat-free products that taste good. In response to that demand, food manufacturers have developed fat substitutes with sensory properties similar to dietary fat but that provide fewer calories.

Fat substitutes can be carbohydrate, protein, or fat based. They range from 0 to 5 cal/g compared with 9 cal/g for fat (87). Olestra, a fat substitute made by Procter & Gamble, was approved for use in snack foods by the FDA in 1996. It is a sucrose polyester that is neither digested nor absorbed and therefore contributes no calories. Olestra is the most studied fat substitute. Its use in place of dietary fat results in a decrease in fat intake and in some cases a decrease in energy intake (88). In studies where products containing olestra are covertly provided, young lean individuals tend to compensate for the caloric reduction whereas older nonobese or obese individuals incompletely compensate for the caloric reduction, resulting in a net caloric deficit in these older individuals (89). Fat-specific compensation does not appear to occur.

In experimental studies where subjects are made aware of the use of fat substitutes, caloric compensation occurs to a greater extent in males than in females (90, 91). This result is significant because consumers are typically aware that they are ingesting a product containing a fat substitute because it is listed on the food label and is extensively advertised. Thus if individuals are aware they are consuming a product that contains a fat substitute, they are more likely to eat more of that product, saving fewer calories. This is similar to behavioral response to low fat foods in general and the propensity to substitute other foods and calories (e.g., carbohydrate) rather than reduce total intake.

Because under proper conditions fat substitutes can decrease fat intake and overall energy intake, they potentially can help with weight loss; however, there are some safety concerns. Absorption of fat-soluble vitamins (A, D, E, and K), carotenoids, and cholesterol is decreased in products containing olestra. As a result, vitamins A, D, E, and K are supplemented in these products in amounts that are commonly found in foods (92). Beta-carotene, alpha-carotene, lycopene, and lutein, all of which are considered to have beneficial health effects, are not supplemented. The long-term impact of this problem is unknown. Side effects due to consumption of a nonabsorbed food (e.g., loose or soft stools, flatulence, diarrhea, bloating, nausea) have been reported by some subjects consuming olestra (93). However, in controlled studies the reported GI symptoms were similar in both control and fat substitute groups (94, 95). In some studies, the frequency of bowel movements in the olestra group was greater (96, 97).

In summary, the use of fat substitutes may be helpful in lowering total fat intake and possibly caloric intake. However, use of these products will not necessarily result in spontaneous weight loss and improved health, unless it is part of an overall weight management approach that focuses on limiting caloric intake, meeting current dietary guidelines, and making long-term behavior changes. Lastly, the impact of regular long-term use of these products on nutrition and health status remains to be determined.

Treatment Approaches

Calorie Restriction

As noted previously, a calorie reduction of 300 to 1000 cal/d (tailored to degree of overweightness or obesity), regardless of current intake, will result in a weight loss of 1 to 2 lb/wk. Overall NIH guidelines are summarized in Table 6.11. Consequently, a moderate reduction in calories still allows for a reasonable number of calories for consumption. There is essentially no need to determine energy needs using complicated formulas. Rather, as recommended by the NIH, a caloric deficit of 300 to 500 cal/d in patients with a BMI of 27 to 35, and a deficit of 500 to 1000 cal/d for patients with a BMI > 35, will result in a safe $^1/_2$ to 2 lb weight loss per week, achieving the recommended 10% weight loss in 6 months. This message is simple and concise, and particular foods should be targeted (see Table 6.5).

Try not to be persuaded by the individual who wants to make sweeping changes in his or her dietary habits. These will most likely not be sustainable. On the other hand, do not be deterred by those individuals who insist that they only eat 800 to 1000 cal/d and can not lose weight. As noted earlier, self-reports notoriously underestimate intake. Moreover, previous weight loss does not have a significant metabolic effect on future attempts (see the section on weight cycling ["yo-yo" dieting] in Chapter 4). Use screening instruments and eating patterns to focus nutrition intervention on food-specific behaviors.

Although the patient's particular medical diagnosis will have a significant impact on the type of dietary intervention needed, there are a number of nutrition strategies that the most prevalent obesity-related medical conditions have in common; some have been discussed earlier in this chapter.

Table 6.11   Summary of NIH Guidelines for Composition of a Weight-Reducing Meal Plan*

Fat	
Total	<30%
Saturated	8–10%
Polyunsaturated	≤10%
Monounsaturated	≤15%
Cholesterol	<300 mg
Protein	~15%
Carbohydrates	≥55%
Fiber	20–30 g
Salt (NaCl)	<6 g
Calcium	1–1.5 g
Alcohol	
Women	≤1 drink
Men	≤2 drinks

*Percent daily intake with caloric deficit of 300 to 1000 cal/d based on initial BMI.

Below are additional factors that might need attention based on diagnoses commonly found in patients with obesity. Detailed descriptions are beyond the scope of this book, and nutrition strategies may require the expertise of and referral to an RD.

- *Diabetes*—meal spacing, frequency of intake of high glycemic foods, intake of saturated fat.
- *Dyslipidemia*—fat content of the diet, in particular intake of foods high in saturated fat and even *trans*-fatty acids (hydrogenated fats), as recommended by the American Heart Association (98) (see Table 6.12 for a list of foods high in saturated fat and *trans*-fatty acids).
- *Hypertension*—intake of foods high in sodium and low in potassium and calcium.

The Food Guide Pyramid

The Food Guide Pyramid (Fig. 6.1) (23), posted on many food labels, is a fundamental and effective, yet regrettably neglected and devalued, nutrition education tool. This is unfortunate because it is a straightforward tool

Table 6.12   Foods High in Saturated Fat and *Trans*-Fatty Acids

Foods High in Saturated Fat	*Foods High in Trans-Fatty Acids*
Whole-fat dairy, e.g.	"Partially hydrogenated" or "vegetable
Whole milk	shortening" in the ingredients list
Regular cheese	Processed or "snack" foods, e.g.
Butter	Crackers
Sour cream	Cookies
Cream	
Cream cheese	Commercial baked goods, e.g.
Ice cream	Donuts
Beef	Muffins
	Pastries
Pork	Danish
Poultry with skin	Stick margarine
Lard	Deep-fried foods, e.g.
Palm and palm kernel oil	French fries
	Fried chicken
Coconut oil	Fried fish
	Natural sources, including beef, pork,
	lamb, butter, whole milk

for illustrating and assessing variety, balance, and moderation in eating. Its use as a foundation for healthy eating crosses socioeconomic lines and, with modification, it can be used in diverse cultures and for various medical conditions (106). Each of the food groups and concomitant vitamins and other components—grains (iron, B vitamins, fiber), vegetables (beta-carotene, folate, vitamin C, potassium), fruits (vitamin C, beta-carotene, potassium), dairy (protein, vitamin B_{12}, calcium), and meat/alternatives (protein, vitamin B_{12}, iron)—makes important nutrient contributions to a healthy diet.

The food groups appear in the pyramid in proportion to the number of daily servings recommended. Therefore it can be used to guide the patient in making food choices as well as to assess the adequacy of the diet. The breadth of the base, or foundation, of the pyramid shows that grains (breads, cereals, rice, pasta) deserve more emphasis in the diet. The tip is smallest to convey that fats, oils, and sweets should be used sparingly. Unfortunately, ~40% of the calories in the typical American diet come from the tip (72). Foods that fit in this section include butter, salad dressings, cakes, cookies, pies, candy, sweetened beverages, potato chips, and other caloric-dense, nutrient-sparse snack foods.

Most patients underestimate the amount of food they eat. The pyramid can be used to review appropriate portion sizes. The pyramid depicts

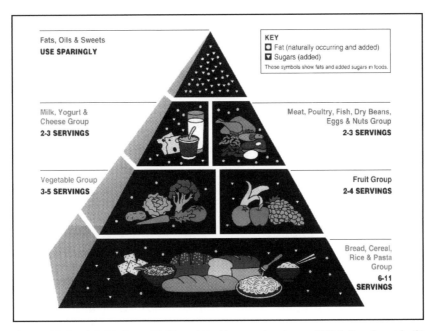

Figure 6.1 Food Guide Pyramid. (From http://warp.nal.usda.gov:80/fnic/Fpyr/pymid.gif.)

lower fat food choices in each group and provides serving sizes. If these low fat choices are selected and the lower limit of servings in each category is eaten, then approximately 1600 calories will be consumed. If the upper range of suggested servings is selected in each category, approximately 2200 cal/day will be consumed. Thus, although creating a 500-calorie daily deficit by decreasing portion size and modifying food selection is a simple and general strategy emphasized by the NIH, for some individuals this general recommendation may not be specific enough. These individuals may benefit from a more definitive plan, such as the Food Guide Pyramid approach, that uses low fat foods and limited servings.

Food Guide Pyramids can be purchased from various organizations such as the American Dietetic Association or the Dairy Council or they can be downloaded from the USDA Web site (*www.usda.gov*). In addition, the pyramid can easily be adapted for vegetarian or ethnic groups. Moreover, the American Dietetic Association has developed culturally adjusted pyramids that are available on the Internet (*www.eatright.org*).

The pyramid can also be used as a monitoring tool. Blank pyramids can be distributed for patients to record their food intake by group. A quick review by the health care provider will catch over- or under-representation in any area. Some patients eat healthily, but simply eat too much. For others, balance and moderation may need to be addressed. It may also be helpful to suggest that patients consume something from each level of the pyramid (grain and fruit or vegetable and meat/alternative or dairy) at each meal (Table 6.13). This will ensure greater variety and balance as well as discourage meal skipping, all of which are valuable for improved health status. If review of the pyramid reveals a deficiency of intake in several areas or massive overconsumption in others, referral to a dietitian may be helpful.

Meal Replacements

Meal replacements are nutrition alternatives that are substituted for a meal or snack. They are characterized by liquid formulas, powder formulations reconstituted with water or milk, or nutrition bars that are typically nutrient fortified with or without fiber. These products are quite popular; one well-known product was used by 20 million people in 1990. These products are marketed as convenient, nutritious, and relatively low in cost, and as an aid in adhering to a low calorie diet. These products have helped create a new industry, nutraceuticals, food products that claim to combine nutrition with therapeutic and/or preventive health properties. Related to this trend is the burgeoning herbal supplement industry (see Chapters 4 and 8). Regulation of these products by the FDA, as well as by the FTC, is quite different than that for prescription medications; the former are not held to the same rigorous testing for efficacy and safety nor to strict manufacturing standards.

Table 6.13   Sample Food Guide Pyramid Meal Plan (refer to Fig. 6.1)

Breakfast

1 cup cereal (grain) – 1 oz
3/4 cup juice (fruit) – 6 oz
1 cup skim milk (dairy) – 8 oz

Lunch

2 oz turkey on (meat)
2 slices whole-wheat bread (grain)
1 tbsp low fat mayonnaise (tip)
1 cup mixed salad with tomatoes, carrots, and cucumbers (vegetable) w/light salad
  dressing (tip)

Dinner

3 oz lean meat or $^1/_2$–$^3/_4$ cups of red beans (meat/alternatives)
1 cup cooked rice (grain) – 2 servings
1 cup cooked carrots (vegetable) – 2 servings
1 slice whole-wheat bread (grain)

Snacks*

1 cup yogurt (dairy) – 8 oz
1 piece fresh fruit (fruit)
6 squares graham crackers (grain) – 2 servings

Total Pyramid Servings

7 grains
2 fruits
3 vegetables
2 dairy
2 meat/meat alternatives
2 from tip of pyramid

*Snacks provide the missing quantities that help patients meet minimum requirements while addressing appetite issues.

Though new phytochemicals (plant-based molecules) important to health are being identified on a regular basis, it seems the most prudent approach to weight management remains a balanced diet that provides a variety of foods. In general, little is known about the efficacy of consuming isolated, altered, or manufactured phytochemicals outside the context of regular food consumption. Fundamental issues such as bioavailability, safety for use in certain medical conditions, and interactions with prescription medicine are rarely investigated. Unfortunately, many patients cite lack of time, expense, and lack of self-control as barriers to eating a healthy, food-based diet for weight loss.

It should be noted that although there are few studies that have tested the effectiveness of meal replacement as a weight loss strategy in the real-world setting, one recent report demonstrated that use of these types of products may not only be helpful during weight loss but also in long-term maintenance (99). In addition, providing prepared meals has also shown promise (100, 101). Thus, although more research is needed to determine whether these types of products are generally useful, their employment in some particular cases may be helpful as long as the context in which they are provided is a balanced approach and used to facilitate making less deleterious food choices.

Very Low Calorie Diets

Very low calorie diets (VLCDs) are meal plans consisting of no more than 800 cal/d (102). They are typically provided as packages of powdered supplements that need to be reconstituted and that contain 100% of the RDA. This diet is usually undertaken in the context of a comprehensive program that entails medical monitoring, weekly behavioral group support, and nutrition education. Weight loss averages 1.5 to 2.5 kg/wk, and the VLCD typically lasts 12 to 16 weeks. Protein is provided at a minimum of 1 g/kg of ideal body weight to limit lean body mass loss. This approach is generally safe in moderately or severely obese patients (BMI > 30), but because close medical supervision is essential VLCD probably should not be used in the primary care setting (102). (Safety is reviewed in the context of medical complications associated with intentional weight loss in Chapter 4.)

Short-term VLCD success is significant; a recent study refutes the previously abysmal 95% to 100% long-term failure rate (103). Nevertheless, ~70% of patients will not achieve sustained 10% weight loss over a 5-year interval, and this comprehensive approach can be expensive. Again, this intervention is not designed to be provided solely by a physician out of a private office. A well-rounded multidisciplinary health care team is needed to implement this type of therapy. Table 6.14 lists some VLCD programs.

Antiobesity Medications

As per the NIH report, antiobesity medication is to be used only after a 6-month trial of lifestyle intervention has failed. Medication is an adjunctive treatment to facilitate long-term lifestyle changes in nutrition, behavior, and physical activity in conjunction with a comprehensive weight management program. Medications can assist patients in making behavior changes. Based on clinical experience, many patients, as well as some members of the lay press, believe that medications are the "magic bullet" that will somehow decrease weight without a lifestyle change. This belief exists despite no clinical trials ever being conducted, nor antiobesity medication approved by the FDA, without a lifestyle therapy included in the study design. Given these misconceptions and expectations, patients are often impatient and determined to obtain this medication regardless of their involvement in a weight management program. Some become downright angry when a physician will not prescribe these medications without first addressing lifestyle issues. Others become frustrated when the desired results are not achieved and will continue to search for another "magic bullet".

Despite these pressures, it is imperative for health care practitioners to continually reinforce the basic principles of long-term weight management. Under those circumstances, these medications can be extremely helpful in carefully selected cases. (Some available medications are described in Chapter 9.) From a nutrition perspective, it is important for an RD to support the use of medication when both the physician and patient agree that this is the therapeutic plan of choice.

In addition to providing the general nutritional and behavioral guidance, there are some medications whose efficacy benefits from RD consultation. This would apply to medications whose mechanism of action is to block calorie absorption. Currently, orlistat is the only approved medication in this category. It acts by inhibiting the absorption of fat; therefore, to be effective with minimal side effects, specific dietary instruction is needed. Patients who have a poor concept of fat intake and cannot determine if they are consuming the 20 to 30 g per meal that would avoid side effects will benefit from the help of an RD. Specifically, an RD can help with the pharmaceutical company's recommended nutrition guidelines:*

- Use with a mildly hypocaloric diet.
- Dietary fat should be <30% of total calories per day.
- >30% total calories from dietary fat may lead to increased GI effects.
- Dosage: one 120 mg capsule tid (one with each main meal; a meal with no fat requires no medication).
- Patients should take a daily supplement containing vitamins A, D, E, and K. This should be taken 2 hours before or after taking orlistat.
- Distribute fat content of diet proportionately over three meals.

Meal Frequency

Despite the popular perception than snacking contributes to obesity, studies indicate that the relationship between frequency of eating and obesity is unclear (104). Factors such as age, caloric intake, diet composition, and

---

*Adapted from Xenical PI, Roche Laboratories, 1998.

Table 6.14   Very Low Calorie Diet Programs*

Name	Approach	Staff	Expected Weight Loss	Cost/Year	Length	Components	Comments[†]
Health Management Resources	Medically supervised VLCD of fortified, high-protein liquid meal replacements (520–800 kcals daily) or low calorie option consisting of liquid supplements and prepackaged entrées (800–1300 kcal daily)	Participants assigned "personal coaches" (RDs, exercise physiologists, health educators); dieters on VLCDs see MD or RN weekly	2–5 lb/wk	>$3000	Reducing phase lasts 12 weeks; refeeding phase lasts 6 weeks; maintenance program lasts up to 18 months	Maintenance meetings available; recommended that clients burn a minimum of 2000 kcal in physical activity per week; mandatory weekly 90-min group meetings; one-to-one counseling	BMI >30 necessary for VLCD; side effects include constipation, dry skin, and headaches; diet is very high in protein; contraindicated for clients with liver and kidney disease
Medifast	Physician-supervised VLCD of fortified meal replacements containing 450–500 kcal/day; program also provides low calorie diet of 860 kcal/day	Program supervised by physician	3–5 lb/wk	$1000–$3000	Reducing phase lasts 16 weeks; refeeding phase is 4–6 weeks; maintenance phase is up to 1 year	Comprehensive education program includes behavior modification, physical activity, and nutrition education; maintenance phase also provided	Close contact with one or more health professionals; clients must be >30% over ideal body weight; contraindicated for clients with liver and kidney disease
New Direction	Medically supervised VLCD program of fortified meal replacements of 600–840 kcal/day; moderate-calorie programs of 1000–1500 kcal/day	Health professionals with degrees in dietetics, exercise physiology; behavioral counseling; each program has medical director	2–3 lb/wk	$1000–$3000	Reducing phase lasts 12–16 weeks; adapting phase lasts 5 weeks; maintenance phase is at least 6 months	Medical, nutrition, behavioral, exercise, and maintenance phase; weekly classes and one-to-one counseling in each discipline	Clients must need to lose at least 40 lb; close contact with health care professionals; contraindicated for clients with liver and kidney disease

| Optifast | Medically supervised program of fortified meal replacements, food bars, eventually including regular food; calorie levels of 800, 950, or 1200 kcal/day; moderate-calorie programs of 1000–1500 kcal/day | Staff includes medical director, dietitians, psychologists, counselors, exercise physiologists | Limited to 2% of body weight per week | $1000–$3000 | Active weight loss phase lasts about 13 weeks; transition phase lasts 6 weeks; maintenance phase is ongoing | Medical, nutrition, exercise, behavioral, and maintenance phase; weekly group meeting and one-to-one sessions | Clients need to be at least 50 lb over ideal body weight; close contact with health professionals; emphasis placed on making long-term lifestyle changes; contraindicated for clients with liver and kidney disease |

*VLCD programs are used for a select obese population that would benefit from rapid weight loss. The long-term outcomes for VLCD, however, are similar to traditional weight management programs due to the prevalence of weight regain. All programs provide nutrition, exercise, and behavior education as well as a maintenance phase.
†See Chapter 4 for a discussion of medical complications of intentional weight loss.

physical activity probably play a more important role in the development of obesity than feeding frequency. In addition, there is no evidence that weight loss on a hypocaloric diet is affected by frequency of eating (105). The recommendation to increase meal frequency to enhance weight loss came into vogue for two reasons:

1. There was some epidemiologic evidence suggesting that those who consume fewer meals per day have lower body weight and skinfold measurements (105, 106). Unfortunately the epidemiologic evidence linking infrequent eating (<3 meals/day) to obesity is weak.

2. Studies had shown that an increase in meal frequency resulted in a decrease in total cholesterol and insulin levels (107–109). This, however, was demonstrated typically after 8 or more "meals" per day.

Under free-living conditions, the clinical usefulness of increasing meals is typically offset by the failure to reduce the size of meals. When this occurs, patients actually gain weight as a result of an increase in total caloric intake. The most common scenario observed when counseling obese individuals is this: Patients describe skipping breakfast, having a light lunch, then "binging" on a large dinner meal and frequent evening snacks. This cycle perpetuates itself when the effects of overeating the night before are felt the following morning (i.e., a decreased appetite leading to skipping breakfast). Although there are few data on only eating three meals per day versus promoting a certain number of snacks, many report anecdotally that regular eating patterns may prevent the haphazard eating that often leads to high calorie eating. In fact, one study concluded that eating breakfast helped reduce dietary fat and minimized impulsive snacking (110). At a minimum, eating breakfast has been shown to improve dietary adequacy (111). Asking the patient to keep a food diary helps to determine individual food patterns and analyze what changes would be most helpful. It may be wise to encourage patients to consume at least 3 meals per day with 1 or 2 snacks.

Nutrition Strategies for Long-Term Success

Information from the National Weight Control Registry (NWCR) has allowed us to determine strategies used by individuals who are successful at long-term maintenance of weight loss (112). On average, registrants have lost 30 kg and maintained a minimum of 13.6 kg for 5.5 years. It is helpful for practitioners to be aware of these approaches for two reasons: 1) to promote their use early on in the weight loss phase, and 2) to support their ongoing use in the maintenance phase. Those individuals successful at long-term weight loss maintenance report the following characteristics:

- Eat a low energy diet (females on average report 1306 cal/d, males 1685 cal/d)
- Eat a low fat diet (24.3% of calories for females, 23.5% for males)
- Have regular meal patterns (4.95 eating times/day for females, 4.54 for males)
- Engage in regular physical activity (equivalent of walking 28 miles/wk)

Other strategies included

- Limiting intake of certain types of foods (92% employ this strategy, 49.2% limit quantities of food, 38.1% limit energy from fat, 35.5% count calories, 30% count fat grams)
- Weighing themselves regularly (75% weigh themselves once a week)
- Preparing or eating the majority of meals at home (eat at fast-food restaurants less than once a week, eat an average of 2.5 meals/week in non-fast-food restaurant)

Nutrition intervention, primarily focused on limiting fat and calories, and increased physical activity appear to be important during both the weight loss and weight maintenance phase. In a study by Toubro (57) it was shown that an *ad libitum* low fat approach for weight maintenance was superior to restricting both fat and calories. Those in the NWCR actually consume a fat content lower than recommended by the Dietary Guidelines (<30% of calories from fat). In addition, self-monitoring (limiting certain types of foods, counting calories, counting fat grams, weighing self regularly) seems to be crucial in long-term success.

It should be emphasized that many different strategies are used by successful maintainers. Rather than professing the use of one standard set of strategies, it is best to allow individuals to select their own approach of restricting intake and increasing physical activity through your knowledge and guidance of techniques that have been beneficial to others.

Summary

The most effective weight loss approach is caloric restriction, achieved by decreasing food intake and increasing physical activity. Numerous strategies and skills have been discussed to help physicians play a key role in helping their obese patients manage their weight. Most recognize the physician's traditional clinical role in taking baseline measurements such as weight, blood pressure, blood cholesterol, and blood sugar that help track patient progress. In addition, the physician can be involved in screening for specific nutrition problems, assessing readiness to make long-term lifestyle changes, recommending the best treatment approaches, targeting realistic goals, and providing ongoing support and encouragement. With a positive, nonjudgmental attitude, it is the physician who "drives home the message" that small changes in food and physical activity behaviors can have a large impact on patient health. Physicians listen to patient concerns, acknowledge feelings and barriers, and clarify any ambivalence towards changing behaviors. Physicians can provide help, or suggest resources, for developing a plan of action. Physicians can help patients solve problems creatively, resulting in improved patient self-confidence and motivation. They can emphasize that any change is better than no change. Lastly, physicians can compliment positive steps and celebrate milestones. Overall, if the physician supports the other members of the multidisciplinary treatment team and reinforces their interventions, while at the same time educating the patient and deflecting the often disappointing feedback from the bathroom scale from him or her and focusing on the patient's improved health, the patient generally appreciates these efforts and benefits from the treatment plan. It is a challenging, and sometimes time-consuming, process, but the benefits to the overall well-being of the patient are worth the undertaking.

■   ■   ■

Key Points

- Because of the increasing prevalence of obesity, the emergence of new weight loss products and supplements, and growing patient interest in nutrition advice, it is important for clinicians to be knowledgeable about nutrition intervention strategies.

- Screening for specific nutrition problems allows the clinician to tailor the weight loss intervention for the individual patient. The information that is gathered in the screening pertains to food choices, key behaviors (e.g., binge-eating), and level of motivation to lose weight.

- Patients with obesity often have multiple nutrition-related medical problems (e.g., hypertension and diabetes) that make a needs assessment necessary to prioritize the treatment approaches.

- Referral to a registered dietitian is advisable when the patient has multiple eating habits requiring considerable change, coexisting diagnoses that affect nutrition needs, or involved therapies (e.g., weight loss surgery).

- Caloric reduction, not diet composition, is the major determinant of weight loss. Although decreasing fat intake should be emphasized, weight loss occurs only if this results in a caloric deficit.

- In conjunction with caloric reduction, treatment approaches may include use of the Food Guide Pyramid, "meal replacements", changing meal frequency, and antiobesity medications. Antiobesity medications should generally be used only after a 6-month trial of lifestyle intervention has failed.

■   ■   ▩

REFERENCES

1. **Levine BS, Wigman MM, Chapman DS, et al.** A national survey of attitudes and practices of primary care physicians relating to nutrition: strategies for enhancing the use of clinical nutrition in medical practice. Am J Clin Nutr. 1993;57:115-9.

2. **Orleans TC, George LK, Houpt JL, Brodie KH.** Health promotion in primary care: a survey of US family practitioners. Prev Med. 1985; 4:636-47.

3. **US Preventive Services Task Force.** Clinicians' Handbook of Preventive Services, 2nd ed. Washington, DC: US Public Health Service/International Medical Publishing; 1998;400-12.

4. **Margolis D.** Nutrition and policy, part 5: who should teach patients about nutrition? Ann Intern Med. 1999;131:317-20.

5. **American Dietetic Association.** Nutrition and You: Trends 2000. Available at http://www.eatright.org/feature/010100.html.

6. **Cade J, O'Connell S.** Management of weight problems and obesity: knowledge, attitudes and current practice of general practitioners. Br J Gen Pract. 1991;41:147-50.

7. **Hiddink GJ, Hautvast JGAJ, van Woerkum CMJ, et al.** Nutrition guidance by primary-care physicians: perceived barriers and low involvement. Eur J Clin Nutr. 1995;49:842-51.

8. **Stunkard AJ, Wadden TA.** Psychological aspects of severe obesity. Am J Clin Nutr. 1992;55(suppl):524S-532S.

9. **Yaroch AL, Resnicow K, Khan LK.** Validity and reliability of qualitative dietary fat index questionnaires: a review. J Am Diet Assoc. 2000;100:240-4.

10. **Gans KM, Sundaram SG, McPhillips JB, et al.** "Rate Your Plate": an eating pattern assessment and educational tool used at cholesterol screening and education programs. J Nutr Edu. 1993;25:29-36.

11. **Yanovski SZ.** Binge eating disorder: current knowledge and future directions. Obes Res. 1993;1:306-24.

12. **Birketvedt GS, Florholmen J, Sundsfjord J, et al.** Behavioral and neuroendocrine characteristics of the night-eating syndrome. JAMA. 1999;282:689-90.

13. **Mayer L, Walsh BT.** The use of selective serotonin reuptake inhibitors in eating disorders. J Clin Psychiatry. 1998;59(suppl 15):28-34.

14. **Walsh BT, Devlin M.** Pharmacotherapy of bulimia nervosa and binge eating disorder. Addict Behav. 1995;20:757-64.

15. **Prochaska JO, Velicer WF.** Transtheoretical model of health behavior change. Am J Health Promo. 1997;12:38-48.

16. **Rippe JM.** The obesity epidemic: challenges and opportunities. J Am Diet Assoc. 1998;98(suppl 2):S5.

17. **Nichols S, Waters WE, Woolaway M, Hamilton-Smith MB.** Evaluation of the effectiveness of a nutritional health education leaflet in changing public knowledge and attitudes about eating and health. J Hum Nutr Dietetics 1988;1:233-8.

18. **Rinkle WJ.** The Winning Foodservice Manager, 2nd ed. Achievement Publishers; 49.

19. **National Institutes of Health/National Heart, Lung, and Blood Institute.** Clinical Guidelines on the Identification, Evaluation, and Treatment of Overweight and Obesity in Adults. Bethesda, MD: US Department of Health and Human Services, 1998.

20. **Prentice AM, Black AE, Coward WA, Cole TJ.** Energy expenditure in overweight and obese adults in affluent societies: an analysis of 319 doubly labeled water measurements. Eur J Clin Nutr. 1996;50:93-7.

21. **Boutelle KN, Kirschenbaum DS.** Further support for consistent self-monitoring as a vital component of successful weight control. Obes Res. 1998;6:219-24.

22. **McCory MA, Fuss PJ, Hays NP, et al.** Overeating in America: association between restaurant food consumption and body fatness in healthy adult men and women ages 19 to 80. Obes Res. 1999;7:564-71.

23. The Food Guide Pyramid. Home and Garden Bulletin No. 252. Washington, DC: US Department of Agriculture, Human Nutrition Information Service; 1992.

24. **Perri MG, McAdoo WG, McAllister DA, Lauer JB.** Effect of peer support and therapist contact on long-term weight loss. J Consul Clin Psychol. 1987;55:615-7.

25. Commercial weight loss products and programs: what consumers stand to gain and lose. Available at www.ftc.gov/os/1998/9803/weightlo.rpt.htm.

26. **White JV, Young E, Lasswell AB.** Position of the American Dietetic Association. Nutrition: an essential component of medical education [Editorial]. J Am Diet Assoc. 1993.

27. **Deckelbaum RJ, Fisher EA, Winston MKS, et al.** AHA Conference Proceedings. Summary of a scientific conference on preventive nutrition: pediatrics to geriatrics. Circulation. 1999;100:450-6.

28. **Prentice AM, Poppitt SD.** Importance of energy density and macronutrients in the regulation of energy intake. Int J Obes. 1996:20(suppl 2);S18-S23.

29. **Hill JO, Drougas H, Peters JC.** Obesity treatment: can diet composition play a role? Ann Intern Med. 1993;119:694-7.

30 **Rolls BJ, Hammer VA.** Fat, carbohydrate, and the regulation of energy intake. Am J Clin Nutr. 1995;62(suppl 5):1086S-1095S.

31. **Hirsch J, Hudgins LC, Leibel RL, Rosenbaum M.** Diet composition and energy balance in humans. Am J Clin Nutr. 1998;67(suppl):551S-555S.

32. **Doucet E, Tremblay A.** Food intake, energy balance and body weight control. Eur J Clin Nutr. 1997;51:846-55.

33. **Hill JO, Prentice AM.** Sugar and body weight regulation. Am J Nutr. 1995;62(suppl):264S-274S.

34. **Lissner L, Levitsky DA, Strupp BJ, et al.** Dietary fat and the regulation of energy intake in human subjects. Am J Clin Nutr. 1987;46:886-92.

35. **Shah M, Garg A.** High-fat and high-carbohydrate diets and energy balance. Diabetes Care. 1996;19:1142-52.

36. **Golay A, Allaz A, Morel Y, et al.** Similar weight loss with low- or high-carbohydrate diets. Am J Clin Nutr. 1996;63:174-8.

37. **Low CC, Grossman EB, Gumbiner B.** Potentiation of effects of weight loss by monounsaturated fatty acids in obese NIDDM patients. Diabetes. 1996;45:569-71.

38. **Gumbiner B, Low CC, Reaven PD.** Effects of a monounsaturated fatty acid-enriched hypocaloric diet on cardiovascular risk factors in obese patients with type 2 diabetes. Diabetes Care. 1998; 21:9-15.

39. **Bray GA, Popkin BM.** Dietary fat intake does affect obesity. Am J Clin Nutr. 1998;68:1157-73.

40. **Blundell JE, MacDiarmid JI.** Fat as a risk factor for overconsumption: satiation, satiety, and patterns of eating. J Am Diet Assoc. 1997;97(suppl 7):S63-9.

41. **Blundell JE, Lawton CL, Cotton JR, MacDiarmid JI.** Control of human appetite: implications for the intake of dietary fat. Annu Rev Nutr. 1996;16:285-319.

42. **Rolls BJ.** Carbohydrates, fats, and satiety. Am J Clin Nutr. 1995;61(suppl 4):960S-967S.

43. **Blundell JE, Burley VJ, Cotton JR, Lawton CL.** Dietary fat and the control of energy intake: evaluating the effects of fat on meal size and postmeal satiety. Am J Clin Nutr. 1993;57(suppl):772S-8S.

44. **Blundell JE, King NA.** Overconsumption as a cause of weight gain: behavioral-physiological interactions in the control of food intake (appetite). Ciba Found Symp. 1996;201:138-54.

45. **Blundell JE, Cotton JR, Delargy H, et al.** The fat paradox: fat-induced satiety signals versus high fat overconsumption. Int J Obes. 1995;19:832-5.

46. **Golay A, Bobbioni E.** The role of dietary fat in obesity. Int J Obes 1997;21(suppl 3):S2-11.

47. **Astrup A.** Dietary composition, substrate balances and body fat in subjects with a predisposition to obesity. Int J Obes. 1993;17(suppl 3):S32-6.

48. **Drewnoski A, Brunzell JD, Sande K, et al.** Sweet tooth reconsideration: taste responsiveness in human obesity. Physiol Behav. 1985;35:617-22.

49. **Drewnowski A.** Why do we like fat? J Am Diet Assoc. 1997;97(suppl 7):S58-62.

50. **Stubbs RJ, Ritz P, Coward WA, Prentice AM.** Covert manipulation of the ratio of dietary fat to carbohydrate and energy density: effect on food intake and energy balance in free-living men eating ad libitum. Am J Clin Nutr. 1995;62:330-7.

51. **Proserpi C, Sparti A, Schutz Y, et al.** Ad libitum intake of a high-carbohydrate or high-fat diet in young men: effects on nutrient balances. Am J Clin Nutr. 1997;66:539-45.

52. **Lawton CL, Burley VJ, Wales JK, Blundell JE.** Dietary fat and appetite control in obese subjects: weak effects on satiation and satiety. Int J Obes Relat Metab Disord. 1993;17:409-16.

53. **Duncan KH, Bacon JA, Weinsier RL.** The effects of high and low energy density diets on satiety, energy intake, and eating time of obese and nonobese subjects. Am J Clin Nutr. 1983;37:763-7.

54. **Jeffery RW, Hellerstedt WL, French SA, Baxter JE.** A randomized trial of counseling for fat restriction versus calorie restriction in the treatment of obesity. Int J Obes. 1995;19:132-7.

55. **Green SM, Blundell JE.** Effect of fat- and sucrose-containing foods on the size of

eating episodes and energy intake in lean dietary restrained and unrestrained females: potential for causing overconsumption. Eur J Clin Nutr. 1996;50:625-35.

56. **Rolls BJ, Bell EA, Castellanos VH, et al.** Energy density but no fat content of foods affected energy intake in lean and obese women. Am J Clin Nutr. 1999;69:863-71.

57. **Toubro S, Astrup A.** Randomised comparison of diets for maintaining obese subjects' weight after major weight loss: ad lib, low fat, high carbohydrate diet vs. fixed energy intake. BMJ. 1997;314:29-34.

58. **Harvey-Berino J.** The efficacy of dietary fat vs. total energy restriction for weight loss. Obes Res. 1998;6:202-7.

59. **Lichenstein AH, Van Horn L, for the AHA Nutrition Committee.** Science Advisory: very low fat diets. Circulation. 1998;98:935-8.

60. **Kris-Etherton PM, for the AHA Nutrition Committee.** Science Advisory: monounsaturated fatty acids and risk of cardiovascular disease. Circulation. 1998;100:1253-8.

61. **Krauss RM, Eckel RH, Howard Barbara, for the AHA Nutrition Committee.** Scientific Statement. Dietary Guidelines (revision 2000): a statement for health care professionals. Circulation. 2000;102:2296-311.

62. **Heilbronn LK, Noakes M, Clifton PM.** Effect of energy restriction, weight loss, and diet composition on plasma lipids and glucose in patients with type 2 diabetes. Diabetes Care. 1999;22:889-95.

63. **Gumbiner B.** Treating obesity in type 2 diabetes: calories, composition, and control. Diabetes Care. 1999;22:886-8.

64. **Van Horn L, for the AHA Nutrition Committee.** Fiber, lipids, and coronary heart disease: a statement for health care professionals. Circulation. 1997;95:2701-4.

65. **Ravussin E, Gautier J-F.** Metabolic predictors of weight gain. Int J Obes. 1999;23(suppl 1):37-41.

66. **Gibson SA.** Are high-fat, high-sugar foods and diets conducive to obesity? Int J Food Sci Nutr. 1996;47:405-15.

67. **Bolton-Smith C.** Intake of sugars in relation to fatness and micronutrient adequacy. Int J Obes. 1996;20(suppl 2):S31-3.

68. **Drewnowski A.** Sweetness and obesity. In: Sweetness. Dobbing J, ed. Berlin: Springer-Verlag; 1987:177-92.

69. **Leeds AR.** Dietary fibre: mechanisms of action. Int J Obes. 1987;11:3-7.

70. **Ludwig DS, Pereira MA, Kroenke CH, et al.** Dietary fiber, weight gain, and cardiovascular disease risk factor in young adults. JAMA. 1999;282:1539-46.

71. **American Dietetic Association.** Position Paper: Health implications of dietary fiber. J Am Diet Assoc. 1997;97:1157-9.

72. **Enns CW, Goldman JD, Cook A.** Trends in food and nutrient intakes by adults: NFCS 1977-78, CSFII 1989-91, and CSFII 1994-95. Family Economics and Nutrition Review. 1997;10:1-15.

73. **Hill AJ, Blundell JE.** Sensitivity of the appetite control system in obese subjects to nutritional and serotoninergic challenges. Int J Obes. 1991;14:219-33.

74. **Booth DA, Chase A, Campbell AT.** Relative effectiveness of protein in the late stages of appetite suppression in man. Physiol Behav. 1970;5:1299-302.

75. **de Jonge L, Bray GA.** The thermic effect of food and obesity: a critical review. Obes Res. 1997;5:622-31.

76. **Henry RH.** Protein content of the diabetic diet. Diabetes Care. 1994;17:1502-13.

77. **Skov AR, Toubro S, Ronn B, et al.** Randomized trial on protein vs. carbohydrate in ad libitum fat reduced diet for the treatment of obesity. Int J Obes. 1999;23:528-36.

78. **Rosenvinge JH, Skov A, Toubro S, et al.** Changes in renal function during weight loss induced by high vs. low-protein low-fat diets in overweight subjects. Int J Obes. 1999;23:1170-7.

79. **Tremblay A, St Pierre S.** The hyperphagic effect of a high-fat diet and alcohol intake persists after control for energy density. Am J Clin Nutr. 1996;63:479-82.

80. **American Dietetic Association.** Position Paper: Use of nutritive and nonnutritive sweeteners. J Am Diet Assoc. 1998;98:580-7.

81. **Council on Scientific Affairs.** Aspartame: review of safety issues. JAMA. 1985;254:400-2.

82. **Blundell JE, Hill AJ.** Paradoxical effects of an intense sweetner (aspartame) on appetite. Lancet. 1986;1:1092-3.

83. **Drewnowski A.** Intense sweetners and the control of appetite. Nutr Rev. 1995;53:1-7.

84. **Blackburn G, Kanders B, Lavin P, et al.** Aspartame facilitates weight loss and long term control of body weight. Int J Obes. 1993;17(suppl 1):46.

85. **Blackburn GL, Kanders BS, Lavin PT, et al.** The effect of aspartame as part of a multidisciplinary weight-control program on short- and long-term control of body weight. Am J Clin Nutr. 1997;65:409-18.

86. **Drewnowski A.** Fats and food acceptance: sensory, hedonic and attitudinal aspects. In: Food Acceptance and Nutrition. Solms J, Booth DA, Pangborn RM, Raunhardt O, eds. New York: Academic Press; 1988:189-204.

87. **American Dietetic Association.** Position Paper: Fat replacers. J Am Diet Assoc. 1998;98:463-8.

88. **Lawton CL.** Regulation of energy and fat intakes and body weight: the role of fat substitutes. Br J Nutr. 1998;80:3-4.

89. **Roberts SB, Pi-Sunyer FX, Dreher M, et al.** Physiology of fat replacement and fat reduction: effects of dietary fat and fat substitutes on energy regulation. Nutr Rev. 1998;56:S29-41.

90. **Miller DL, Castellanos VH, Shide DJ, et al.** Effect of fat-free potato chips with and without nutrition labels on fat and energy intakes. 1998;68:282-90.

91. **Miller GD, Groziak SM.** Impact of fat substitutes on fat intake. Lipids. 1996;31(suppl):S293-6.

92. **Lawson KD, Middleton SJ, Hassall CD.** Olestra, a nonabsorbed, noncaloric replacement for dietary fat: a review. Drug Metab Rev. 1997;29:651-703.

93. **Jacobson MF.** Olestra snacks compared with regular snacks. Ann Intern Med. 1999;131:866.

94. **Peters JC.** Fat substitutes and energy balance. Ann N Y Acad Sci. 1997;827:461-75.

95. **Thomson AB, Hunt RH, Zorich NL.** Review Article: Olestra and its gastrointestinal safety. Aliment Pharmacol Ther. 1998;12:1185-200.

96. **Jacobson MF, Brown MA, Whorton EB Jr.** Gastrointestinal symptoms following olestra consumption. JAMA. 1998;280:325-7.

97. **Kelly SM, Shorthouse M, Cotterell JC, et al.** A 3-month, double-blind, controlled trial of feeding with sucrose polyester in human volunteers. Br J Nutr. 1998;80:41-9.

98. **Lichtenstein AH, for the AHA Nutrition Committee.** *Trans*-fatty acids, plasma lipid levels, and risk of developing cardiovascular disease: a statement for health care professionals from the American Heart Association. Circulation. 1997;95: 2588-90.

99. **Ditschuneit H, Flechtner-Mors M, Johnson TD, Adler G.** Metabolic and weight loss effects of a long-term dietary intervention in obese patients. Am J Clin Nutr. 1999;69:198-204.

100. **Metz JA, Kris-Etherton PM, Morris CD, et al.** Dietary compliance and cardiovascular risk reduction with a prepared meal plan compared with a self-selected diet. Am J Clin Nutr. 1997;66:373-85.

101. **Wing RR.** Food provision in dietary intervention studies. Am J Clin Nutr. 1997;66:421-2.

102. Very low-calorie diets. National Task Force on the Prevention and Treatment of Obesity, National Institutes of Health. JAMA. 1993;270:967-74.

103. **Wadden TA, Frey DL.** A multicenter evaluation of a proprietary weight loss program for the treatment of marked obesity: a five-year follow-up. Int J Eat Disord. 1997;22:203-12.

104. **Drummond S, Crombie N, Kirk T.** A critique of the effects of snacking on body weight status. Eur J Clin Nutr. 1996;50:779-83.

105. **Bellisle F, McDevitt R, Prentice AM.** Meal frequency and energy balance. Br J Nutr. 1997;77(suppl 1):S57-70.

106. **Jenkins DJ, Wolever TM, Vuskan V, et al.** Nibbling versus gorging: metabolic advantages of increased meal frequency. N Engl J Med. 1989;321:929-34.

107. **Fabry P, Tepperman J.** Meal frequency: a possible factor in human pathology. Am J Clin Nutr. 1970;23:1059-68.

108. **Mann J.** Meal frequency and plasma lipids and lipoproteins. Br J Nutr. 1997;77(suppl 1):S83-90.

109. **Garrow JS, Durrant M, Blaza S, et al.** The effect of meal frequency and protein concentration on the composition of the weight lost by obese subjects. Br J Nutr. 1981;45:5-15.

110. **Schlundt DG, Hill JO, Sbrocco T, et al.** The role of breakfast in the treatment of obesity: a randomized clinical trial. Am J Clin Nutr. 1992;55:645-51.

111. **Morgan KJ, Zabik ME, Stampley GL.** The role of breakfast in diet adequacy of the US adult population. J Am Col Nutr. 1986;5:551-63.

112. **Klem ML, Wing RR, McGuire MT, et al.** A descriptive study of individuals successful at long-term maintenance of substantial weight loss. Am J Clin Nutr. 1997; 66:239-46.

7

■ ■ ■

Physical Activity and Exercise in the Treatment of Obesity

Jorge Calles-Escandon, MD

O besity, which can be characterized as the excessive storage of energy in the adipose tissue, is the end result of one of three general mechanisms: 1) increase in energy intake without proportionate increase in energy expenditure (EE), 2) decrease in EE without decrease in energy intake, and 3) a combination of 1 and 2. For physiologic purposes, energy intake is equivalent to food consumption because gastrointestinal absorption does not vary significantly in normal individuals over a wide range of dietary conditions. EE has been divided into three components (Fig. 7.1):

1. The *resting metabolic rate* (RMR) is defined as the energy expended by a person at rest under conditions of thermal neutrality. The basal metabolic rate (BMR) is more precisely defined as RMR measured soon after awakening in the morning, at least 12 h after the last meal. RMR differs from BMR by less than 10%, however, and therefore the terms are often used interchangeably. RMR is measured under defined conditions (after an overnight fast of 12 to 14 h, lying comfortably in a bed or sitting in a chair with no muscle movement and before ingestion of a meal). Approximately 60% of EE is RMR.

2. The *thermic effect of food*, which accounts for 10% to 15% of EE, is the energy used for the absorption and assimilation of food.

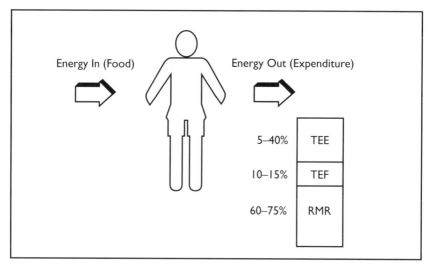

Figure 7.1   Energy balance equation. The components of energy expenditure in man are thermic effect of exercise (TEE), thermic effect of food (TEF), and resting metabolic rate (RMR).

Initially thought to be unique to proteins it is now recognized that there is also an increase in metabolic rate after ingestion of carbohydrate and fat.

3. The *thermic effect of physical activity or exercise* is the most variable component of EE; it ranges from nearly zero (total inactivity) to more than 50% (in elite athletes) of EE. This component can be further divided into *a)* spontaneous muscle movement ("fidgeting"), and *b)* voluntary, self-imposed increase in physical activity as it occurs during structure problems of exercise and/or sport participation.

The focus of this chapter is on EE associated with physical activity in the treatment of obesity. Recommendations are given for incorporating an exercise regimen and physical activity into a comprehensive treatment program for obese individuals. Other effects of exercise as they pertain to overall well-being are emphasized, and caveats are highlighted.

Exercise as a Thermogenic Effector

An increase in physical activity may induce negative energy balance through one or more of the following mechanisms:

1. Direct enhancement of EE (energy cost of the exercise *per se*)

2. Effects on the other two components of EE (RMR and food-induced thermogenesis [i.e., burning of calories])

3. Effects on energy intake

Energy Cost of Exercise

From a clinical and practical point of view, the energy cost of exercise has been oversold to individuals by a variety of nonmedical sources as well as from many physicians who glibly counsel obese patients to lose weight by simply exercising more (1). Some exercises do not significantly increase energy expenditure (Table 7.1). Moreover, although some of the activities (e.g., basketball, cross-country skiing, running) do increase EE substantially, this negative energy cost is achieved by a very intense and prolonged effort that is beyond that of most patients. Finally, after a certain level of fitness is attained, the body adapts and less energy is expended with further exercise bouts.

Table 7.1   Energy Costs of Exercise (in J/min)*

Walking	
Downstairs	1.2–2.4
Upstairs	3.4–7.2
Brisk walk (5 km/h)	1.2–2.4
Running	
8 km/h	2.2–4.3
11 km/h	2.4–6.0
21 km/h	3.6–7.2
Cycling	
8 km/h	1–2
21 km/h	2–4
Housework	0.8–1.5
Yard or garage work	0.8–2
Shoveling snow	1.5–3.0
Chopping wood	1.5–4.0
Lifting heavy things	4–8
Basketball	1.5–4.5
Cross-country skiing	2.4–5

* The energy cost of the activity is expressed in joules/minute (~0.24 cal/min); the lower limit applies to a person weighing ~57 kg, the upper limit to a person weighing ~115 kg. (Adapted from McArdle W, Katch F, Katch V. Exercise Physiology: Energy, Nutrition, and Human Performance. New York: Lea & Febiger; 1981.)

The mathematics of energy expenditure from exercise has also been oversimplified and has contributed to further misconceptions about energy expenditure and weight loss. From the energy cost of the exercise bout, one needs to subtract the ongoing RMR (which is independent of, but simultaneous to, the increase in EE of physical activity) from the energy cost of the exercise bout. When RMR is taken into account, the negative balance that can be achieved by a single bout of exercise is actually quite small compared with the total EE in a 24-h period. Thus the types and intensity of exercise that carry a high negative energy balance for a single bout are basically confined to those that can be undertaken by elite athletes or subjects with an excellent level of physical fitness.

Unfortunately, on a clinical basis and especially for the obese patient, it is unrealistic (even dangerous) to expect a level of exercise performance that in itself could be associated with a significant negative energy balance on the basis of a single bout per day. Nevertheless, this does not deter commercial enterprises from promoting their own agendas and thus spreading myths about the benefits of exercise for weight control.

Although from the quantitative and clinical point of view EE associated with exercise bouts is not thermodynamically important, it should be noted that when physical activity is undertaken on a regular basis, these repeated bouts of exercise may induce a significant cumulative energy loss. The critical point is that this loss may be important if, and only if, the negative energy balance is not accompanied by a compensatory increase in energy intake. Thus exercise cannot be used to substitute for or balance out dietary indiscretion. A widespread misconception is that energy (food) intake can be liberalized when participating in exercise activities. From a purely thermogenic perspective, the exercise-related energy loss *per se* cannot be considered as a single therapeutic tool for reducing body weight and, therefore, must be considered in conjunction with a comprehensive program that, again from a thermodynamic perspective, must include a defined limitation in energy intake.

Effect of Exercise on the Thermic Effect of Food

The effects of exercise on the thermic effect of food has been the subject of intense research in the last decades. Several investigators have documented a decrease in meal-induced thermogenesis in obese patients; this has led some to propose that this defect may explain and/or perpetuate the obese state. However, quantitatively, the thermic effect of food is a minor component of energy expenditure, accounting for no more than 10% to 15% of EE. As a consequence, a defect in this component would be associated with only a minimal difference in EE in obese versus lean individuals.

Example: A 70-kg subject with a 24-h EE of 600 kJ/day (143 cal/d) would have spent 60 to 72 kJ (14 to 17 cal/d) as that component of EE associated with food-induced thermogenesis. Because the defect in obese individuals is only ~25% (2), this would amount to only 16 to 17 kJ/day (3.8 to 4.0 cal/d). That could translate theoretically into a rate of weight gain of 3 kg/year, provided only fat tissue was gained and there was no change in food intake. However, the obese state is not only associated with an increase in fat mass but also with accretion of lean body mass. Thus the obese state is associated with a net increase in absolute EE via this gain in lean mass that accompanies the weight gain. In general, the ratio of gain of lean to fat tissue gain is 3:1. Lean body mass expends energy at a rate of around 7 kJ/d/kg (1.67 cal/d/lb). Therefore an increase in lean tissue of 2 or 3 kg would quickly offset the 25% defect in food-induced thermogenesis by adding an excess amount of EE to RMR. Effectively, this compensation would limit fat gain. Certainly, the clinically important increases in body weight (especially when body mass exceeds 35) cannot be explained by a reduction in food-induced thermogenesis.

From this example, it is reasonable to conclude that any intervention shown to increase or decrease the thermic effect of food will have a minimum impact on the overall regulation of EE and certainly will not be quantitatively important in the treatment of massive obesity. Still, exercise may change the thermic effect of food when 1) it acutely affects the thermogenesis associated with food ingestion, and 2) it is a chronic phenomenon associated with the training adaptation. The data available in the literature focus primarily on the acute interaction between exercise and food ingestion. Segal and colleagues (2-4) have compared lean and obese individuals. The evidence from these investigators supports an interaction between an acute bout of exercise and food ingestion in which the first enhances the thermic effect of the latter and vice versa. These authors have also demonstrated that the enhancement of food-induced thermogenesis by exercise is blunted in the obese patient. However, the energy to which this enhancement amounts is on the order of 5 to 12 kJ/d (1.2-2.9 cal/d). Thus, thermogenically, the potentiation of food-induced thermogenesis is negligible and the blunted response documented in obese individuals cannot explain their obese state. The latter is especially relevant within the context of the morbidly obese patient.

Data on the chronic effects of exercise and the thermic effect of food are scarce, but Leblanc et al (5) have shown that trained individuals have a decreased thermic effect of food. The investigators attribute the adaptation to lower concentrations of catecholamines in response to food ingestion and/or to the lower insulinemic response after meal ingestion that is typically observed in highly trained individuals. Studies have demonstrated a curvilinear relationship between maximum aerobic capacity (index of physical fitness) and the thermic effect of food (6). Moderate levels of training enhance the thermic effect of food, but high levels of training diminish it. Again, as pointed out previously, the amount of energy affected by exercise on thermogenesis is ~12 kJ/d (~2.9 cal/d). Energetically the cost is minimal and therefore therapeutically unimportant for obese patients.

Effect of Exercise on Resting Metabolic Rate

In theory, any effect of exercise on RMR could be extremely important because of the large percentage of total EE that RMR represents. Conceptually, the effects of exercise or physical activity could change the RMR either as an acute phenomenon and/or as part of the chronic adaptation to training. The acute effect of exercise on RMR is generally accepted. Most physiologists recognize the presence of the so-called "oxygen debt" after an acute bout of exercise. With respect to chronic effects, the magnitude and duration of this post-exercise increase in oxygen consumption during the basal state after an acute bout of exercise have been studied extensively, but no consensus has emerged.

Table 7.2 presents a compilation of studies (7-17) that have examined the effects of a bout of exercise on RMR It is evident that there are discrepant results. Different exercise prescriptions and different modes of exercise used for testing can explain some of the differences (e.g., duration, intensity, exercise performed, intermittent versus continuous protocols). The paradigms for the different studies cited in Table 7.2 also varied, and the control periods were not uniform. However, for purposes of critical analysis in this chapter, it is reasonable to assume that an acute bout of exercise can indeed increase EE. However, even accepting this effect of exer-

Table 7.2   Acute Effects of Exercise on Resting Metabolic Rate

Investigator	Increase in RMR?	Duration of Increase (h)
Bielinsky et al (7)	Yes	18
Maehlum et al (8)	Yes	3
Bahr and Machlum (9)	Yes	12
Tremblay et al (10)	Yes	16
Devlin and Horton (11)	Yes	16
Wolfe et al (12)	Yes	2
Sedlock et al (13)	No	
Blaza and Garrow (14)	No	
Freedman-Akabas et al (15)	No	
Pacy et al (16)	No	
Pivarnik and Wilkerson (17)	No	

cise on RMR, there is still no consensus among researchers on the magnitude and duration of this response.

Some investigators claim that the increase in RMR lasts for as long as 36 h after an acute bout of exercise, but most experts state that the increase is proportional to the intensity of the bout of exercise and lasts anywhere between 4 and 24 h. The magnitude of the increase (still a matter of debate) has been stated in several of these papers as between 2% and 15% of the RMR, with the most common observation being a 5% increase. This increase may seem trivial, but unlike the thermic effect of food and interaction with exercise as discussed above, it could be quantitatively very important if long-lived. Unfortunately, most of the studies have demonstrated that the effects of exercise are rather short-lived. Moreover, in practical terms, taking into consideration that a direct relationship exists between the intensity of the exercise bout and the increase in RMR, the impact of this phenomenon on weight regulation in clinically obese patients is not expected to be of great magnitude because of the incapacity of most of these patients to undertake exercise bouts of great intensity for prolonged periods of time. Therefore, from a purely thermodynamic perspective, the acute effect of exercise cannot be considered important in a program for weight loss, especially when one deals with massively obese individuals. Again, we encounter the common misperception about exercise serving as a substitute for indiscretions in dietary intake.

Studies on the effect of exercise on RMR as a chronic adaptation to training are mostly cross-sectional in design (Table 7.3) (5, 18-21) and have resulted in disparate results. Some studies have found an increase in RMR of between 7% and 10%; other studies did not confirm this increase. Therefore the available literature does not allow us to conclude that exercise has a chronic effect on RMR as part of the adaptation phenomenon to chronic exercise.

Of more interest and relevance are prospective studies yielding data that are more amenable to interpretation because the individuals who par-

Table 7.3   Cross-Sectional Studies on the Chronic Effects of Exercise on Resting Metabolic Rate

Investigator	Increase in RMR?	Magnitude (%)
Hill et al (18)	Yes	9
Poehlman et al (19)	Yes	7–11
Tremblay et al (20)	Yes	10
Leblanc et al (5)	No	
Hill et al (21)	No	

ticipated have been studied before and after the intervention. Several attempts have been made to study the effects of physical training on RMR. To establish a clinical perspective and as an attempt to reconcile some of the differences, the studies considered herein have been grouped as to whether weight loss was (or was not) a goal of the program (in general with dietary restrictions). The first cluster of studies (Table 7.4) (22, 23, 23a), in which no deliberate attempt was made to induce weight loss, suggests that exercise training *per se* does not change RMR or body composition significantly. The exception is a study conducted by Lawson et al (22) demonstrating a 5% increase in RMR. A second cluster of studies (Table 7.5) (20, 24, 25) comprised those in which moderate weight loss was an objective induced with a moderate restriction in dietary intake. Again, there are disparate conclusions. The bulk of evidence suggests that there is no change or even an increase in RMR when dietary restriction is combined with an exercise program. In general, it is accepted that dietary restriction should induce a decrease in RMR in conjunction with the decrease in excess lean body mass associated with obesity. Therefore the preservation of RMR documented in some of these studies or the increase in others can be considered as a very advantageous thermogenic effect of exercise. Rather unexpectedly, however, some of the studies in which severe dietary restriction and therefore substantial weight loss were attempted (Table 7.6) (21, 26-32) suggest that exercise training may actually reduce RMR. A possible explanation for this discrepancy may be the amount of energy restriction.

Table 7.4   Prospective Studies on the Effects of Exercise on Resting Metabolic Rate with No Dietary Restriction

Investigator	Increase in RMR?
Lawson et al (22)	Yes (5%)
Vallieres et al (23)	No
Bingham et al (23a)	No

Table 7.5   Prospective Studies on the Effects of Exercise on Resting Metabolic Rate and Moderate Weight Loss

Investigator	Increase in RMR?
Tremblay et al (20)	Yes
Nieman et al (24)	Yes
Belko et al (25)	No

Therefore it is conceivable that severe dietary restriction with its greater decrease in RMR than less severe dietary restriction may override the thermogenic effects of chronic exercise training to minimize excessive energy expenditure and preserve mass. This is one reason the NIH expert panel recommends slow progressive weight loss. Moreover, resistance exercise may help offset potential decreases in RMR by helping preserve some muscle mass that might normally be lost with caloric restriction.

Effects of Exercise on Total Energy Expenditure and Spontaneous Muscle Movement

A major breakthrough in the study of energy metabolism was achieved by the recent incorporation of the doubly-labeled water technique in human studies (33). With this method it is possible to measure the total EE in the free-living condition and the amount associated with physical activity by subtracting the RMR and the thermic effect of food. Thus, irrespective of

Table 7.6   Prospective Studies on the Effects of Exercise on Resting Metabolic Rate with Severe Dietary Restriction

Investigator	Study Conditions	Outcome
Hill et al (21)	10 women, 191 kJ/d with or without exercise	Exercise preserved lean body mass; RMR dropped in both groups
Saris and Van Dale (26, 27)	12 women, 12 weeks dietary restriction with or without exercise	Exercise induced more weight loss and blunted the decline in RMR
Tremblay et al (28)	6 women, 100 days 239 kJ deficit induced by exercise	6–11 kg loss; RMR and lean body mass preserved
Hammer et al (29)	26 women, 16 weeks, 191 kJ/d with exercise	No change in RMR; lean body mass preserved
Frey-Hewitt et al (30)	101 subjects, 3 groups (control, diet, exercise)	Diet decreased RMR (6–7 kg loss); exercise preserved RMR and lean body mass (4 kg weight loss)
Lemons et al (31)	40 women, 96 kJ with or without exercise	Exercise preserved RMR
Heymsfield et al (32)	191 kJ with or without exercise	Exercise induced a larger drop in RMR

the specific effect of exercise on any of the components of EE, if physical activity is useful in weight loss it must affect total EE. A provocative paper published by Roberts et al (34) measured total energy expenditure in infants born to lean and overweight mothers. An evaluation of the first year of life demonstrated that infants with a lower daily total EE gained more weight than other infants. Moreover, most of the excess body weight gained by these children could be correlated with a decrease in spontaneous physical activity. This research was supportive of a paper by Ravussin et al (35) who found that daily total EE (measured by indirect calorimetry in a respiratory chamber) was one of the most important contributors to body weight gain in adult Pima Indians. Of even more interest is a recent publication of Levine et al (36). These investigators found that spontaneous EE associated with spontaneous physical activity ("fidgeting") was a critical determinant of subsequent body weight gain, which confirmed and extended the results of Ravussin.

The results of these papers *in toto* suggest that actually physical activity associated with EE is a very important determinant of weight gain and strongly suggest an important role for an increase in physical activity in weight control programs. Most importantly, these studies point out a critical distinction about the role of exercise in overall weight management. Exercise and physical activity prevent weight gain rather than promote weight loss. This was eloquently demonstrated in an 18-month study in which those participants who combined caloric restriction and exercise for 8 weeks only lost 2 kg more than those who only restricted calorie intake (36a). However, over the next 16 months, those who continued to exercise were able to maintain weight loss, while those who discontinued exercise regained their weight. Thus, it is imperative that the patient understand the role of exercise in maintaining weight loss; the physician must reinforce the concept that exercise is not a substitute for controlling intake.

Effects of Exercise on Energy Intake

Data on this particular (but critical) area of research are rather scarce. Exercise may increase, decrease, or produce no change on energy intake. Cross-sectional observations on mill workers in West Bengal, India (37), suggest that individuals who sustain medium-to-very-heavy workloads have caloric intakes that increase in proportion to the energy expenditure associated with the intensity of the work produced. However, those individuals who did not have this level of activity and who were in comparison rather sedentary had no compensatory decrease in energy intake; therefore there was more obesity associated with sedentary work. This study was largely uncontrolled and as a consequence difficult to interpret. More careful and well-designed studies were those of Woo and colleagues (38-40). These investigators found that severely obese individuals did not compensate for food intake. Lean women increased food intake in proportion to EE associated with exercise training; however, obese individuals did not do so. Thus obese women seem to display a "dysregulation" of energy intake in relation to energy expenditure. The clinical applicability of this information remains to be determined.

Acute effects of exercise and appetite regulation have also been studied. King et al (41) found a reduction in energy intake only with very intense exercise (70% of the maximum aerobic capacity sustained for a full 60 min). Dempsey (42) measured estimated food intake after 18 weeks of a vigorous exercise program in obese and lean individuals. They did not find any measurable change in food intake. However, the data might be interpreted to suggest that exercise was able to blunt an increase in appetite, because there was no compensatory increase as could have been expected from the exercise program-related increase in EE. Thus the data (though scarce) suggest the possibility that exercise decreases energy intake. Such modulation seems to depend upon the intensity and duration of the exercise and to be related to body composition (at least in women (39, 40, 43)). The pathophysiologic and molecular bases of these putative effects of exercise on food intake deserve further research.

Summary

From the purely thermogenic point of view (i.e., ignoring the cardiovascular and psychologic benefits), the evidence shows that exercise may under some circumstances induce a modest negative energy balance both by the direct effect of energy cost of physical activity and more importantly by the effects of the exercise program on RMR. However, data also show that the magnitude of this energy deficit can easily be overcome with an increase in energy intake. Thus, from this perspective, exercise cannot be conceptualized as a sole agent for weight loss and must be considered as an adjunct to a comprehensive program aimed at weight control. The program by necessity must incorporate strategies to decrease energy intake. The overall assumption that a diet might be liberalized when someone is engaged upon an exercise program is a widespread misconception, and the health practitioner is in a unique situation to educate patients about this. More research is needed to determine the effects of exercise on dietary intake, because this might yield potentially more therapeutic gain for the obese patient than the thermogenic effect of exercise *per se*.

Exercise and the Prevention of Obesity

Farming experience has demonstrated in an empirical manner that animals kept physically inactive are fattened easier and better for sale. From these empirical observations a popular hypothesis has been that obesity development and maintenance are related to a decrease in physical activity and therefore that obesity might be prevented by maintaining or increasing levels of physical activity. Attempts to prove this popular belief have been undertaken by researchers. Obese girls and boys were compared with nonobese controls and matched for age, height, weight, and maturation (44, 45). The obese children were found to be much less active. A similar finding was observed in adult men and women when compared with normal weight controls (46).

It has been found that weight gain in obese children and adults occurs mainly during the winter months when physical inactivity is prevalent (47). Pacy et al (48) reviewed the studies that compare the activity of lean and obese individuals. Six of the ten studies reported that obese individuals displayed significantly reduced physical activity compared with lean controls. Williamson et al (49) noted that the low levels of recreational physical activity reported by the participants were strongly related to weight gain in both men and women. Unfortunately, from the data presented in all of these studies (as well those presented above), one cannot determine whether the reduced activity is the cause or consequence of obesity, because these were cross-sectional studies where the obese state was already defined. It is clinically self-evident that work tolerance is decreased in severely obese individuals. Theoretically this could create a vicious cycle in which obesity predisposes to physical inactivity and physical inactivity sustains the obese state.

Effects of Exercise on Weight Loss: Lessons from Clinical Trials

The underlying hypothesis that repeated bouts of exercise will increase EE in excess of energy intake and there will thus be a decrease in body weight has been tested in studies of relatively small numbers of individuals. Because of this, meta-analysis techniques have been used to evaluate the large amount of data that already exists in the literature. Meta-analysis has some caveats that limit its conclusions. Most of the studies have been performed in an outpatient setting, but some have been performed on inpatients. Meta-analysis studies cannot correct for these differences because by definition this technique uses a retrospective approach constrained to the original design of the specific studies analyzed. There is also a considerable variability in the length of the study periods. Moreover, variations in body composition, fat distribution, and background and family history have an impact on the outcome.

In spite of these caveats, the results of meta-analyses are noteworthy. Epstein and Wing (50) reported that exercise training consisting primarily of walking and/or running was very modest in its effects at reducing body weight. An average value of only 0.09 kg/wk can be attributed to exercise within the context of weight loss programs reported by these investigators. The exercise-associated weight loss seemed to be a function of the magnitude of the exercise as well as the frequency of the bouts. Ballor and Keesey (51) included a larger number of studies and both genders in their meta-analysis and a wide range of exercise modalities (walking, running, cycling). Most of the studies analyzed were at least 16 weeks long, with a frequency of least three bouts of exercise per week. Again, the conclusion of these investigators was that the effect of exercise was rather modest. Weight loss averaged 0.1 kg/wk, similar to the finding of Epstein and Wing. Ballor and Keesey, however, also found that incorporating exercise into a weight loss program was associated with an increase in lean body mass. A review of the literature published up to 1993 was undertaken by Garrow and Summerbell (52). Their analysis concluded that exercise induced a small amount of weight loss, about 0.1 kg/wk, a conclusion remarkably similar to those of the two studies just discussed. Thus, the overall conclusion of these studies is that exercise (when used for weight loss) results in very moderate losses in total body weight (0.1 kg/wk) and moderate losses of body fat but is associated with retention of lean body mass and sometimes even an increase.

In marked contrast, some other studies have reported large amounts of weight loss when using exercise as a modality for weight loss. These reports are not applicable to the general obese population because they were done under very special conditions. For example, reports (53, 54) on males in a 5-month training program under military conditions indicated an average weight loss of 12.5 kg, of which 12 kg were attributable to fat loss. The intensity of the exercise training program for these individuals was very high and included not only aerobic training but weapons training, field exercises, and drills. This type of exercise training is obviously not applicable to the general obese population but does demonstrate how much exercise is needed for it to be a primary modality for weight loss. Exercise of this nature may not be tolerated by very obese individuals because they are unable to exercise for very long periods of time and because they may be put at increased risk for joint injuries, orthopedic problems, and even cardiovascular events.

Because enhanced physical activity may promote EE (as reviewed above) many studies have used a combination of exercise and dietary restriction to elicit a greater weight loss than could be achieved with dietary restriction alone. It has also been hypothesized that exercise will prevent a decline in RMR that accompanies weight loss and may also preserve lean body mass. Using meta-analysis Ballor and Poehlman (55) concluded that exercise training reduced the amount of lean body mass loss during diet-induced weight loss. In a study by Hill et al (21) addition of an exercise program to energy restriction prevented the large drop in RMR associated with a deficit in energy intake. Of interest is that Kempen et al (56) found that specific fat loss in obese women was enhanced with incorporation of intense exercise in a program of weight loss (Fig. 7.2).

Data have been published that suggest exercise training may have the potential to change the proportion of fat and carbohydrate utilization at rest and during exercise and hence promote the preferential loss of fat depots. Intense exercise was associated with an increase in fat oxidation even when caloric intake was increased to match the energy deficit induced by the exercise. In this study (57), conducted under the controlled conditions of a metabolic research unit, it was demonstrated that exercise may shift the utilization of fuels and increase the oxidative use of fat, presumably in muscle, for energy generation. These data give support to the hypothesis that exercise training may be associated with an increase in fat oxidation and therefore with a loss of fat versus lean body mass.

Exercise and Weight Recidivism

It has been increasingly clear and might seem intuitively obvious that inclusion of exercise in weight reducing programs may help maintain the

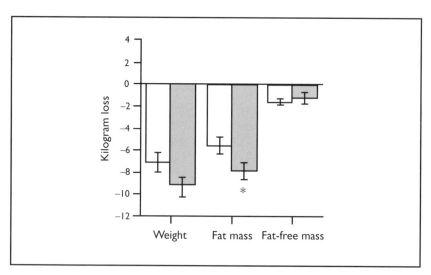

Figure 7.2   Total body weight loss, fat, and fat-free mass loss after 8 weeks of diet or diet with exercise treatment. Data are mean ± SE, and * indicates significantly different (*P* = 0.05) from diet. *White bar* = diet; *shaded bar* = diet and exercise. (From Kempen K, Saris W, Westerterp K. Energy balance during an 8 week energy-restricted diet with and without exercise in obese women. Am J Clin Nutr. 1995;62:722; with permission.)

weight loss. King et al (41) reported that weight loss after exercise alone, diet alone, or diet plus exercise was greatest in the last group, which suggests that the combination balance may be more effective for long-term maintenance of weight loss than either of the two alone. This overall conclusion was also reached by Pronk and Wing (58), who supported the idea that a combination of diet and exercise results in a better long-term maintenance of weight loss. It should be pointed out that most exercise programs incorporated into weight loss programs consist mainly of aerobic training.

Common sense and empirical knowledge suggest that the modality of exercise training may affect the amount of lean body mass loss as well as fat loss. Exercise physiologists have in general recognized that, although aerobic training is associated with fat loss, it is also associated with loss of lean body mass. In contrast, resistance (strength) training is associated with accretion of muscle mass, yet also possibly with fat mass gain. Formal testing of the effect of combination aerobic and strength training on inducing or maintaining weight loss has been rarely attempted. The few data available show that exercise training may affect body composition during weight loss programs (59). By including an exercise program after weight loss, aerobic training was associated preferentially with fat loss. In contrast, strength training was associated with an increase in lean body mass. Although it seems appealing from the clinical point of view to recommend that an exercise program for weight maintenance should include both modalities of exercise training, formal clinical trials using this mixed approach have not been published. We still need data to clarify whether fat mass also increases under such a regimen.

Two studies stand out as supporting the idea that long-term weight control is beneficially affected by regular exercise. A survey (60) showed that individuals who expended more than 1500 kcal/wk in self-reported physical activity regained only 24% of their initial weight, and those who expended more than 2000 kcal/wk of physical activity regained only 15% of their initial weight. The results are similar to those found by Pavlou et al (36a), who found that an EE of least 1500 kcal/wk was more successful in maintaining weight loss. Unfortunately, most patients have difficulty incorporating this level of activity into their lifestyle on a long-term on-going basis.

Metabolic Effects of Exercise

Muscle composition has also been related to body fatness. A higher content of type 1 skeletal muscle fiber is associated with a better metabolic profile (61). A change in the pattern of fiber composition in muscle induced by exercise has been proposed as a mechanism by which exercise could improve the metabolic profile of patients with obesity. Despite the fact that patients in one study maintained adiposity after 20 nights of exercise training, they improved their metabolic profile and showed reduced plasma glucose and insulin response in a standard oral glucose tolerance test, indirect evidence of amelioration of insulin resistance (Figs. 7.3 and 7.4) (62). Moreover, Despres et al (63) reported that 14 months of an exercise training program in obese women was able to elicit a greater loss of abdominal versus femoral adipose tissue. Because central distribution of obesity has been more highly correlated with metabolic abnormalities than has peripheral obesity, these data suggest that exercise might have a direct impact on metabolic characteristics of obese patients by inducing the preferential loss of the intra-abdominal content of fat rather than overall fat loss.

Nevertheless, overall fat mass and loss has an impact, and exercise may confer some protection against cardiovascular disease. This is illustrated by reports that individuals who had higher BMIs but were physically fit had lower mortality rates than sedentary individuals who were unfit and had low BMIs (64). A subsequent study (65) found that men who were overweight or obese (BMI > 27) but who also had a moderate-to-high level of physical fitness did not have elevated death rates compared with the general population. In fact, in that study, obese but physically fit individuals had death rates *lower* than normal weight men who were unfit. Therefore the hypothesis was advanced that it was exercise fitness that conferred cardiovascular protection independent of the degree of fatness. A much larger study was published in 1999 (66) with a more detailed investigation of body composition and cardiorespiratory fitness. In that study 21,925 men aged 30 to 83 were assessed (body composition and cardiorespiratory fitness). At follow-up there were 428 deaths. Although the percent of body fatness was directly associated with the risk of cardiovascular disease and mortality, this trend was attenuated to a significant degree by the cardiorespiratory fitness level. At all levels of fatness there was a decrease in the relative risk for cardiovascular disease and mortality for those individuals who were fit versus those who were unfit. Thus, independent of the effects of exercise training on the level of adiposity, these investigators have proposed that exercise should be recommended for all obese patients because it reduces cardiovascular disease and mortality.

Based on the foregoing data, interpreted with the caveat that there are not yet large long-term prospective intervention studies, it can be recommended that exercise training in conjunction with a weight loss program is beneficial for the obese patient. This benefit may not be directly related to the energetic cost of exercise bouts or to the thermogenic effects of exercise training. The important information (derived from trials) is that exercise has beneficial overall effects on cardiovascular status and metabolic profile that may be important in decreasing the effects of obesity on morbidity and mortality.

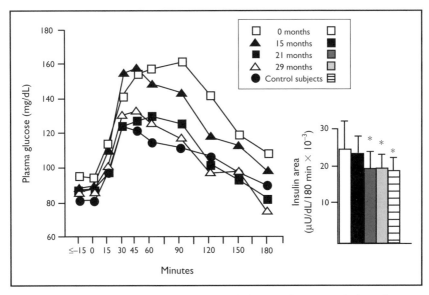

Figure 7.3   Plasma glucose levels during an oral glucose tolerance test in four obese women before and after 15, 21, and 29 months of aerobic exercise. Their values are compared with 22 nonobese female control subjects. Body fat was not completely normalized by the exercise training. * indicates significant differences. (From Tremblay A, Després J, Maheux J, et al. Normalization of the metabolic profile in obese women by exercise and a low fat diet. Med Sci Sports Exerc. 1991;23:1326; with permission.)

Exercise as a Change in Behavior

An excellent review of this specific topic has been recently published (67), and the reader is referred to that report for further information. The challenge for practitioners is the specific implementation of several changes to facilitate increased physical activity. For patients, the challenge is making exercise a part of daily life activities, not just as a temporary remedy for control of body weight. For these purposes, models of behavioral change can be useful when designing feasible plans and monitoring progress. Individual progress can then be viewed as a series of five stages of readiness: precontemplation, contemplation, preparation, action, and maintenance (see Chapter 6, Table 6.3 and discussion thereof).

Recommendations

Most clinical studies on exercise have focused on cardiorespiratory issues. It is still not known which is the optimal prescription for exercise: 1) to maintain or achieve significant weight loss, or 2) to induce a betterment of

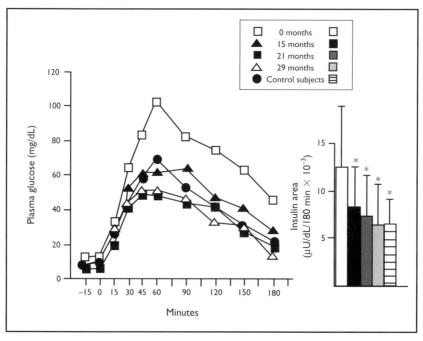

Figure 7.4   Plasma insulin levels during an oral glucose tolerance test in four obese women before and after 15, 21, and 29 months of aerobic exercise. Their values are compared with 22 nonobese female control subjects. Body fat was not completely normalized by the exercise training. * indicates significant differences. (From Tremblay A, Després J, Maheux J, et al. Normalization of the metabolic profile in obese women by exercise and a low fat diet. Med Sci Sports Exerc. 1991;23:1326; with permission.)

the metabolic profile. This has created a number of misconceptions about the role of exercise in weight loss, some of which have been discussed above. In the context of an exercise prescription, the major misunderstanding is that what is needed for cardiorespiratory fitness is not adequate for weight control. Specifically, the public health education program promoting at least 20 min of exercise at least 3 times weekly has been very effective for cardiovascular fitness but cannot be extrapolated as adequate for weight control. In fact, as concluded by the NIH expert panel, essentially 30 min of daily moderate-intensity activity is needed. Moreover, because the *combined* effects of intensity and duration are important, a balance between the two is essential. Low-intensity, long-duration exercise may be the most effective way to achieve and maintain body fat loss (68, 69).

A critical component is the role of the physician in motivating patients to change behavior, particularly in encouraging physical activity. Patients who received very brief (5 min) counseling from their physician promoting increased physical activity, followed by a brief "booster" telephone call 2 weeks later, did better than control patients who received no physician counseling (70). Thus even a brief talk exerts powerful effects on behavior if the words come from a physician. The initial discussion when counseling patients on an increase in physical activity should focus on

1. Current physical activity

2. Previous attempts to become engaged in an exercise or physical activity program

3. Barriers that the patient cites to becoming engaged in an exercise program

4. Benefits that the patient identifies that could be positive for the patient and the patient's family

The responses can then be integrated into the patient's stage of readiness to determine what type of counseling is appropriate and tailoring it the individual's particular situation. For example, if the patient is at an early phase (precontemplation or contemplation), the physician should provide information about the health and weight loss benefits of physical activity in order to motivate the patient to move into the next phase. The physician may want to discuss the barriers as well as the benefits of physical activity that would follow the patient's behavioral change. At this stage the physician may recommend that the patient become engaged in small but definitive changes in physical activities. An opportunity should be given to the patient to incorporate these changes into his or her lifestyle. At follow-up, any increase in physical activity should be viewed as a success and communicated as such. Patients in the preparation or action stage should be given more specifics about exercise and advice on how to overcome the barriers impeding full behavioral change.

No systematic studies have definitively determined at what time during a weight management treatment plan exercise is most effectively implemented from behavioral, metabolic, and physiologic perspectives. Intuitively, one may consider that an exercise program would be beneficial after weight loss in moderately overweight to obese individuals when it is more likely these patients are physically capable of undertaking exercise at the level needed to achieve sufficient deficit in energy balance to sustain weight loss. Anecdotally, it seems at least some weight loss needs to occur before patients are capable of increasing physical activity in general, let alone undertaking structured exercise. Thus it is more pragmatic to recommend exercise as a strategy after a certain amount of weight loss has been achieved and when cardiovascular function has improved to the extent that the patient is in a better position to become engaged in a rigorous program of physical activity.

Practical recommendations for patients include

1. Eventually exercise on a daily basis because the metabolic effects of exercise are evanescent in nature.

2. Divide 30 min of exercise into either two or three mini-bouts of 15 or 10 min to be undertaken before breakfast, before lunch, and before dinner. There is a growing body of evidence (e.g., 51, 67, 68, 71, 72) that multiple short bouts of exercise are at least as effective as a single long bout and that they have obvious logistical advantages.

3. Self-monitoring the heart rate can be used to make sure that exercise is undertaken at adequate intensity as well as to provide immediate positive feedback. A number of formulas can be used, usually based on the percent of maximum predicted heart rate; most result in a recommendation of 140 to 150 beats/min. It is important for patients to understand that this value refers to sustained heart rate.

4. Most patients need to begin slowly and progress in incremental steps. In some cases, exercise may require "mini-bouts" of as little as 1 min of intensive exercise (i.e., peak heart rate of 140 to 150 beats/min) followed by 8 to 9 min of relaxed activity. The duration of the intense period is then to be slowly increased on a weekly basis, adding 1 min at a time until the full 10 to 15 min bout is reached.

5. Incorporate self-monitoring of activity and exercise into the food diary.

6. For patients who do not become engaged in physical activity, behavioral interventions focused on problem solving are needed. Try to determine the nature of the patient's problem with exercising, times and locations at which the barrier or problem occurs, and if others are involved in this barrier.

After the patient is given the weight treatment plan, follow-up and reinforcement are of paramount importance. The patient should be contacted by staff on the telephone almost on a weekly basis to encourage and maintain his or her enthusiasm for participation. If the clinic budget and structure allows, postcards can be effective as well.

Summary

Obesity is a chronic condition that requires life-long management. Exercise has benefits beyond the energetic effects that include improvement in insulin sensitivity and cardiovascular fitness. Physicians must incorporate a few minutes into their interviews to discuss physical activity with patients. The patient's current and past levels of physical activity should be assessed; barriers must be identified and benefits of weight loss discussed. By spending as little as 3 to 5 min in counseling, physicians can play a critical role in promoting health. Specific goals should be set and follow-up implemented. Collaborating with an exercise physiologist and other health care professionals is often useful and should be considered for cases that are particularly challenging.

■   ■   ■

Key Points

- Exercise alone is not an effective weight loss therapy. Regular exercise may help achieve a significant cumulative energy loss, but this energy loss will not result in significant weight loss unless energy intake is limited as well.

- Exercise and physical activity are critical determinants in preventing weight gain rather than in inducing weight loss.

- Aerobic training is associated with both fat loss and loss of lean body mass, whereas resistance training accentuates loss of muscle mass. However, few studies exist that compare training modalities with weight loss.

- Before embarking on an exercise regimen, obese patients should first achieve some weight loss so that they are physically able to sustain the increase in activity.

- Exercise has been shown to confer cardiovascular protection and beneficial metabolic effects independent of weight loss.

- The physician has a key role in motivating patients to change physical activity behavior; follow-up and reinforcement are crucial to the maintenance of the program.

ACKNOWLEDGMENTS
This work was completed in part with funds from NIH Grant RO1 AG14784-01A1.

■   ■   ■

REFERENCES

1. **McArdle W, Katch F, Katch V.** Exercise Physiology: Energy, Nutrition and Human Performance. New York: Lea & Febiger; 1981.
2. **Segal KR, Pi-Sunyer FX.** Exercise, resting metabolic rate and thermogenesis. Diab Met Rev. 1986;2:19-34.

3. **Kissileff H, Pi-Sunyer F, Segal K, et al.** Acute effects of exercise on food intake in obese and nonobese women. Am J Clin Nutr. 1990;52:240

4. **Segal KR, Gutin B, Nyman AM, Pi-Sunyer FX.** Thermic effect of food at rest, during exercise and after exercise in lean and obese men of similar body weight. J Clin Inv. 1985;76:1107-12.

5. **Leblanc J, Diamond P, Cote J, Labrie A.** Hormonal factors in reduced post-prandial heat production of exercise-trained subjects. J Appl Physiol. 1984;56:772-6.

6. **Poehlman ET, Malby CL, Badylak SF, Calles J.** Aerobic fitness and resting energy expenditure in young adult males. Metabolism. 1989;38:85-90.

7. **Bielinsky R, Schutz Y, Jequier E.** Energy metabolism during the postexercise recovery in man. Am J Clin Nutr. 1985;42:69-82.

8. **Maehlum S, Grandmontagne M, Newsholme E, Sejersted OM.** Magnitude and duration of post-exercise oxygen consumption in healthy young subjects. Metabolism. 1986;35:425-9.

9. **Bahr R, Maehlum S.** Excess post-exercise oxygen consumption: a short review. Acta Physiol Scand. 1986;123:99-104.

10. **Tremblay A, Nadeau A, Fournier G, Bouchard C.** Effect of a three day interruption of exercise training on resting metabolic rate and glucose induced thermogenesis in trained individuals. Int J Obes. 1988;12:163-8.

11. **Devlin J, Horton ES.** Potentiation of the thermic effect of insulin by exercise: differences between lean, obese and non-insulin dependent diabetic men. Am J Clin Nutr. 1986;43:884-90.

12. **Wolfe RR, Klein S, Carraro F, Weber JM.** Role of triglyceride-fatty acid cycle in controlling fat metabolism in humans during and after exercise. Am J Physiol. 1990;258:E382-E389.

13. **Sedlock DA, Fissinger JA, Melby CL.** Effect of exercise intensity and duration on post-exercise energy expenditure. Med Sci Sports Exerc. 1989;21:626-36.

14. **Blaza S, Garrow JS.** Thermogenic response to temperature, exercise and food stimuli in lean and obese women, studied by 24 hour direct calorimetry. Br J Nutr. 1983;49:171-80.

15. **Freedman-Akabas S, Colt E, Kissileff HR, Pi-Sunyer FX.** Lack of sustained increase in Vo_2 following exercise in fit and unfit subjects. Am J Clin Nutr. 1985;41:545-9.

16. **Pacy PJ, Barton N, Webster JD, Garrow JS.** The energy cost of aerobic exercise in fed and fasted normal subjects. Am J Clin Nutr. 1985;42:764-8.

17. **Pivarnik JM, Wilkerson JE.** Recovery metabolism and thermoregulation of endurance trained and heat acclimatized men. J Sports Med Phys Fit. 1988;28:375-80.

18. **Hill JO, Heymsfield SB, McMannus C, DiGirolamo M.** Meal size and thermic response to food in male subjects as a function of maximum aerobic capactiy. Metabolism. 1984;33:743-9.

19. **Poehlman E, McAuliffe TL, Van Houten D, Danforth E Jr.** Influence of age and endurance training on metabolic rate and hormones in healthy men. Am J Physiol. 1990;259:E66-E72

20. **Tremblay A, Fontaine E, Poehlman ET, et al.** The effect of exercise training on resting metabolic rate in lean and moderately obese individuals. Int J Obes. 1986;10:511-7.

21. **Hill JO, Sparling PB, Shield TW, et al.** Effects of exercise and food restriction on body composition and metabolic rate in obese women. Am J Clin Nutr. 1987; 46:622-30.

22. **Lawson S, Webster JD, Pacy PJ, Garrow J.** Effect of a 10 week aerobic exercise programme on metabolic rate, body composition and fitness in lean sedentary females. Br J Clin Pract. 1987;41:684-8.

23. **Vallieres F, Tremblay A, St.-Jean L.** Study of the energy balance and the nutritional status of highly trained female swimmers. Nutr Res. 1989;9:708.

23a. **Bingham SA, Goldberg GR, Coward WA, et al.** The effect of exercise and improved physical fitness on basal metabolic rate. Br J Nutr. 1989;61:155-73.

24. **Nieman DC, Haigh JL, De Guia ED, Register UD.** Reducing diet and exercise training effects on resting metabolic rates in mildly obese women. J Sports Med Phys Fit. 1988;28:79-88.

25. **Belko Z, Van Loan M, Barbieri TF, Mayclin P.** Diet, exercise, weight loss, and energy expenditure in moderately obese women. Int J Obes. 1987;11:93-104.

26. **Saris W, Van Dale D.** Effects of exercise during VLCD diet on metabolic rate, body composition and aerobic power: pooled data of four studies. Int J Obes. 1989;13:169.

27. **Van Dale D, Saris WH, Schoffelen PFM, Ten Hoor F.** Does exercise give an additional effect in weight reduction regimes? Int J Obes. 1987;11:367-75.

28. **Tremblay A, Nadeau A, Despres JP, et al.** Long-term exercise training with constant energy intake: effect on glucose metabolism and resting energy expenditure. Int J Obes. 1990;14:75-84.

29. **Hammer R, Barrier C, Roundy E, et al.** Calorie-restricted low-fat diet and exercise in obese women. Am J Clin Nutr. 1989;49:77.

30. **Frey-Hewitt B, Vranizan KM, Dreon DM, Wood PD.** The effect of weight loss by dieting or exercise on resting metabolic rate in overweight men. Int J Obes. 1990;14:327-34.

31. **Lemons AD, Kreitzman N, Coxon A, Howard A.** Selection of appropriate exercise regimens for weight reduction during VLCD and maintenance. Int J Obes. 1989;13(Suppl 2):119-23.

32. **Heymsfield SB, Casper K, Hearn J, Guy D.** Rate of weight loss during underfeeding; relation to physical activity. Metabolism. 1989;38:215-23.

33. **Schoeller D, Ravussin E, Schutz Y, et al.** Energy expenditure by doubly labeled water: validation and proposed calculation. Am J Physiol. 1986;250:R823.

34. **Roberts SB, Savage J, Coward WA, et al.** Energy expenditure and intake in infants born to lean and overweight mothers. N Engl J Med. 1988;318:461-6.

35. **Ravussin E, Lillioja S, Knowler W, et al.** Reduced rate of energy expenditure as a risk factor for body weight gain. N Engl J Med. 1988;318:467.

36. **Levine JA, Eberhardt NL, Jensen MD.** Role of nonexercise activity thermogenesis in resistance to fat gain in humans [see Comments]. Science. 1999;283:212-4.

36a. **Pavlou K, Krey S, Steffee W.** Exercise as an adjunct to weight loss and maintenance in moderately obese subjects. Am J Clin Nutr. 1989;49:1115-23

37. **Mayer J, Roy P, Mirta K.** Relation between caloric intake, body weight, and physical work: studies in an industrial male population in West Bengal. Am J Clin Nutr. 1956;4:169

38. **Pi-Sunyer X, Woo R.** Effect of exercise on food intake in human subjects. Am J Clin Nutr. 1985;42:983-90.

39. **Woo R, Garrow J, Pi-Sunyer F.** Effect of exercise on spontaneous calorie intake in obesity. Am J Clin Nutr. 1982;36:470.

40. **Woo R, Garrow J, Pi-Sunyer F.** Voluntary food intake during prolonged exercise in obese women. Am J Clin Nutr. 1982;36:478.

41. **King N, Burley V, Blundell J.** Exercise-induced suppression of appetite: effects on food intake and implications for energy balance. Eur J Clin Nutr. 1994;48:715.

42. **Dempsey J.** Anthropometrical observations on obese and nonobese young men undergoing a program of vigorous physical exercise. Res Q. 1964;35:275.

43. **Woo R, Pi-Sunyer F.** Effect of increased physical activity on voluntary intake in lean women. Metabolism. 1985;34:836.

44. **Johnson M, Burke B, Mayer J.** Relative importance of inactivity and overeating in the energy balance of obese high school girls. Am J Clin Nutr. 1956;4:37.

45. **Stefanki P, Heald F, Mayer J.** Caloric intake in relation to energy output of obese and nonobese adolescent boys. Am J Clin Nutr. 1959;7:55.

46. **Chirico A, Stunkard A.** Physical activity and human obesity. N Engl J Med. 1960;263:935.

47. **Porter W.** Season variation in the growth of Boston school children. Am J Physiol. 1920;52:121.

48. **Pacy P, Webster J, Garrow J.** Exercise and obesity. Sports Med. 1986;3:89.

49. **Williamson D, Madans J, Anda R, et al.** Recreational physical activity and ten-year weight change in a US national cohort. Int J Obes. 1993;17:279.

50. **Epstein L, Wing R.** Aerobic exercise and weight. Addict Behav. 1980;5:371.

51. **Ballor D, Keesey R.** A meta-analysis of the factors affecting exercise-induced changes in body mass, fat mass and fat-free mass in males and females. Int J Obes. 1991;15:717-26.

52. **Garrow J, Summerbell C.** Meta-analysis: effect of exercise, with or without dieting, on the body composition of overweight subjects. Eur J Clin Nutr. 1995;49:1.

53. **Lee L, Kumar S, Leong L.** The impact of five-month basic military training on the body weight and body fat of 197 moderately to severely obese Singaporean males aged 17-19 years. Int J Obes. 1994;18:105.

54. **Sum C, Wang K, Choo C, et al.** The effect of a 5 month supervised program of physical activity on athropometric indices, fat free mass, and resting energy expenditure in obese male military recruits. Metabolism. 1994;43:1148.

55. **Ballor D, Poehlman E.** Exercise-training enhances fat-free mass preservation during diet-induced weight loss: a meta-analytical finding. Int J Obes. 1994;18:35.

56. **Kempen K, Saris W, Westerterp K.** Energy balance during an 8 week energy-restricted diet with and without exercise in obese women. Am J Clin Nutr. 1995;62:722.

57. **Calles-Escandon J, Goran MI, O'Connell M, et al.** Exercise increases fat oxidation at rest unrelated to changes in energy balance or lipolysis. Am J Physiol. 1996;270:E1009-E1014.

58. **Pronk N, Wing R.** Physical activity and long-term maintenance of weight loss. Obes Res. 1994;2:587.

59. **Ballor DL, Harvey-Berino JR, Ades PA, et al.** Contrasting effects of resistance and aerobic training on body composition and metabolism after diet-induced weight loss. Metabolism. 1996;45:179-83.

60. **Ewbank P, Darga L, Lucas C.** Physical activity as a predictor of weight maintenance in previously obese subjects. Obes Res. 1995;3:257.

61. **Wade A, Marbut M, Round J.** Muscle fiber type and aetiology of obesity. Lancet. 1990;335:805.

62. **Tremblay A, Despres J, Maheux J et al.** Normalization of the metabolic profile in obese women by exercise and a low fat diet. Med Sci Sports Exerc. 1991;23: 1326.

63. **Despres J, Pouliot M, Moorjani S, et al.** Loss of abdominal fat and metabolic response to exercise training in obese women. Am J Physiol. 1991;261:E159

64. **Blair SN, Kohl HW III, Paffenbarger RS Jr, et al.** Physical fitness and all-cause mortality: a prospective study of healthy men and women. JAMA. 1989;262:2395-401.

65. **Barlow CE, Kohl HW III, Gibbons LW, et al.** Physical fitness, mortality and obesity. Int J Obes Relat Metab Disord. 1995;19:S41-S44.

66. **Lee CD, Blair SN, Jackson AS.** Cardiorespiratory fitness, body composition, and all cause and cardiovascular disease mortality in men. Am J Clin Nutr. 1999;69: 373-80.

67. **Leermakers EA, Dunn AL, Blair SN.** Exercise management of obesity. Med Clin North Am. 2000;84:419-40.

68. **Donnelly JE, Jacobsen DJ, Synder Heelan K, et al.** The effects of 18 months of intermittent versus continuous exercise on aerobic capacity, body weight and composition, and metabolic fitness in previously sedentary, moderately obese females. Int J Obes. 2000;24:566-72.

69. **Lee I-M, Sesso HD, Paffenbarger RS.** Physical activity and coronary heart disease risk in men: does the duration of exercise episodes predict risk? Circulation. 2000;102:981-6.

70. **Calfas KJ, Long BJ, Sallis JF, et al.** A controlled trial of physician counseling to promote the adoption of physical activity. Prev Med. 1996;25:225-33.

71. **DeBusk RF, Stenestrand U, Sheehan M, Haskell WL.** Training effects of long versus short bouts of exercise in healthy subjects. Am J Cardiol. 1990;65:1010-3.

72. **Pratt M.** Benefits of lifestyle activity versus structured exercise. JAMA. 1999; 281:375-6.

8

■ ■ ■

Behavioral Treatment of Obesity in the Primary Care Setting

David B. Sarwer, PhD

Leslie G. Womble, MD

Robert I. Berkowitz, MD

The 1998 NIH Expert Panel Report on the Identification, Evaluation, and Treatment of Overweight and Obesity in Adults (1) stressed that the management and treatment of obesity require a life-long, reciprocal effort between the patient and practitioner. The patient's readiness to change must be taken into account to achieve the two primary goals outlined in the report: 1) attain 10% loss of initial body weight over a period of 6 months, and 2) prevent weight regain. To help the patient accomplish these goals, primary care physicians have several treatment options. Behavioral interventions include a combination of diet modification, increased physical activity, and behavioral skills training. In addition, physicians have the option of pharmacologic agents, which can and, it is the contention of this chapter, should be used in combination with behavioral modification.

Behavioral Assessment of the Obese Patient

A comprehensive assessment of the obese patient is necessary before selecting a treatment option (2). Ideally, the treating physician will complete the assessment; however, given the multifactorial nature of obesity as well as the prevalence of the condition, physician-assistants, nurses, or dietitians may also play major roles. In conjunction with the initial assessment, there should be access to a psychologist or psychiatrist for consultation on related mental health issues. This initial assessment has been described in detail in Chapter 5 and elsewhere (2, 3). Specifically, the practitioner needs to evaluate factors that contribute to the patient's obesity, the psychosocial status of the patient, the goals and expectations of treatment, and the timing of the weight loss efforts. These four assessment areas are summarized by the acronym *BEST*, which represents the *B*iological (see Chapter 5), *E*nvironmental, *S*ocial-psychological, and *T*emporal factors associated with weight loss (Table 8.1).

Table 8.1   BEST Assessment of Obesity

Biological Factors	**Environmental Factors**
Onset of obesity	Binge eating
Family history	Eating habits
Contributing illnesses	Exercise and activity levels
Prader-Willi syndrome	
Hypothalamic tumors	**Social-Psychological Factors**
Pituitary tumors	Social relationships
Hypothyroidism	Job satisfaction
Polycystic ovary syndrome	Life goals
Atypical depression	Coping strategies
Medications	Co-morbid psychological factors
Antidepressants	Depression
Tricyclics	Psychiatric conditions
Monamine oxidase inhibitors	Bulimia nervosa
Antipsychotics	Psychosis
Clozapine	Severe anxiety
Chlorpromazine	
Perphenazine	**Temporal Factors**
Clopenthixol	Motivation
Thiothixene	Readiness
Olanzapine	
Lithium	
Anticonvulsants	
Valproic acid	
Carbamazepine	
Steroids	
Corticosteroids	
Ovarian steroids	
Antidiabetics	
Insulin	
Sulfonylureas	
Thiazolidinediones	
Antineoplastics	

Environmental Factors

The practitioner should assess the presence of eating disorders, binge eating being the most significant associated with obesity. Binge eating is defined as consumption of a large amount of food (i.e., an amount that would be considered large by others) in a brief period of time, and the eating is accompanied by a feeling of loss of control (4). Binge eating occurs in approximately 15% to 20% of obese persons treated in specialty clinics but in only about 2% of the population (5). Obese binge eaters may require psychotherapeutic treatment before or in addition to weight reduction.

To assess the possibility of binge eating, the practitioner can begin by determining the general eating habits of the patients by reviewing food records. This may require the assistance of a registered dietitian (see Chapter 6). These records typically include all food and beverage consumption over the course of several days. The general composition of the patient's diet, approximate daily calorie intake, and specific eating patterns can be gleaned from the records. In the absence of food records, ask the patient to describe food and beverage intake over the past 24 h as well as food and beverage intake on a typical weekend. It is important for the practitioner to be aware that overweight patients often consume large amounts of high-caloric beverages, including regular sodas, sweetened iced tea, and fruit juice. By failing to ask about beverage intake, the practitioner may miss a large number of calories consumed by the patient.

Practitioners should also assess the patient's exercise and activity level. Ask patients about their participation in more traditional forms of recreation and exercise, such as aerobics, tennis, jogging, or walking, and about their daily lifestyle activity, such as stair use and daily walking (6). Not surprisingly, many overweight and obese individuals are quite often sedentary, frequently due to the physical discomfort associated with activity.

Social/Psychological Factors

Practitioners frequently initiate weight loss treatment knowing very little about the persons they are treating. Although obesity is the focus of treatment, practitioners should spend some time learning about other dimensions of the patient's life because they almost always have a bearing on the obese condition. These areas include intimate and social relationships, job satisfaction, life goals, and coping strategies. The physician should attempt to understand how weight affects and is affected by these factors, and what life changes the patient anticipates with weight loss.

Practitioners should evaluate for the presence of co-morbid psychological factors, particularly depression and increased stress. Approximately 25% to 35% of obese patients treated in university and hospital clinics present with co-morbid psychopathology such as depression (7). A recent national survey suggests that obese women, compared with individuals of a normal body weight, are more likely to suffer from depression, contemplate suicide, and report previous suicide attempts (8). Obesity was associated with a 37% increased risk of depression for women. In contrast, for men obesity was associated with a 25% decreased risk of depression. It appears that it is the severely obese patients who account for the higher prevalence of depression; the prevalence of depression in moderately obese patients is no higher than that for the general population (9). These findings underscore the importance of physicians evaluating both the medical conditions and psychological functioning of their obese patients. Practitioners can screen for depression by asking about mood, changes in sleep and appetite, feelings of guilt or worthlessness, and lack of enjoyment in daily activities. There are a number of standard instruments available to assist the practitioner, such as the Beck Depression Inventory (BDI). If depression is suspected, practitioners should also evaluate the presence of suicidal ideation, a condition that takes immediate precedence over weight management and that must be treated before embarking on a weight loss program.

Body shape and size may affect the self-esteem and body image of overweight and obese patients. Many obese persons avoid social situations due to embarrassment or, if they do attend such events, they are frequently a source of frustration and upset (9a). The practitioner should ask all patients if their weight and shape affects how they feel about themselves.

Several behavioral and psychiatric conditions may contraindicate behavioral treatment of obesity. The presence of bulimia nervosa—binge eating with loss of control, which is accompanied by compensatory behaviors including vomiting, laxative abuse, or excessive exercise—warrants further psychiatric evaluation and treatment. Persons with an active substance abuse disorder are inappropriate for weight loss treatment. Patients experiencing an acute psychiatric disorder, including active psychosis or extreme anxiety, also require psychiatric care. Although obesity is often associated with an increase in depressive symptoms (8, 9), it is the occurrence of a major depressive episode that contraindicates behavioral obesity treatment. Mild or situational depression may be treated simultaneously with weight management; this should be determined on a case-by-case basis.

Timing Factors

The practitioner also should determine the patient's interest and motivation for weight loss at the particular time of visit (6). A distressing event such as the onset of a weight-related illness, failure to fit into yet another size of clothing, or urging by friends or family members are examples of events that often prompt patients to seek treatment. However, it is the evaluation of the patient's motivation to lose weight independently of the events that triggered the interest in weight reduction that is the critical component of the assessment process. The provider should also evaluate the level of stress in the life of the patient at the time of the assessment. Heightened stress levels are associated with attrition from weight reduction treatment (1). Thus the patient should be relatively free of major stressors for the months of treatment. When there are high levels of stress, weight maintenance and weight gain prevention rather than weight loss should be the focus of treatment efforts. An understanding of the patient's motivation and stress level will help the patient and practitioner determine the patient's readiness to change at the time the patient presents in the office.

Treatment Goals

The assessment should conclude with a discussion of the patient's goals. Patients typically enter treatment desiring to obtain a specific weight, often one that is 25% to 35% less than their starting body weight (10). Recent studies have found that patients expected to lose 25% of starting body weight at the end of one year, and that they expected to lose this weight even though they were told during initial assessment that they would only lose 5% to 15% of starting weight during the program (11, 12). Clearly, obese individuals desire greater weight losses than the present generation of treatments is able to deliver.

One of the greatest challenges for practitioners treating obesity is helping patients adopt more realistic weight loss goals, typically 5% to 15% of initial weight (2). While patients may initially bristle at such modest losses, studies suggest that a 10% weight loss will improve many of the health complications of obesity (e.g., hypertension, abnormal glucose tolerance, abnormal lipid concentrations) (13). Thus qualitative and behavioral outcomes of weight loss should be emphasized: the health benefits as well as the improvements in mobility, appearance, body image, and self-esteem associated with a weight loss as low as 10%. However, a 10% weight loss may often not improve psychosocial functioning of some patients to the desired extent. If further improvements in body image and self-esteem are desired, a referral for psychotherapy may be appropriate. Once the patient has accepted the benefits and limitations of these losses, the patient and practitioner can select a treatment approach.

Treatment Recommendations

The 1998 NIH guidelines specified treatment recommendations for the obese patient based upon the patient's body mass index (BMI), fat distribution, level of fitness, and the presence of co-morbid medical conditions or other risk factors (see Chapter 5) (1). These guidelines can provide a useful template for determining appropriate treatment options. In 1991, Brownell and Wadden published a conceptual scheme of a three-stage process for selecting a weight loss treatment approach (14). Similar to the NIH guidelines, this approach provides treatment recommendations based on BMI. It also provides suggestions for treatment options of different intensity.

Figure 8.1 shows a three-stage process for selecting a weight loss treatment using the aforementioned conceptual scheme of Brownell and Wadden.* Behavior-modification strategies, which are discussed below, should be used with all patients. For patients with a BMI < 30 kg/m^2, behavior modification in a variety of forms (self-directed programs, commercial weight loss programs, self-help programs, physician-based counseling) is the primary treatment recommended. Pharmacotherapy can be used for those patients who do not experience success with a behavioral program after 6 months. For patients with a BMI of 30 to 40 kg/m^2, behavior modification can be used in combination with pharmacotherapy. Behavior modification is also necessary for long-term treatment of persons with a BMI > 40 kg/m^2 who undergo gastric surgery.

Co-morbid conditions are a factor in treatment. For example, many patients with a BMI of 27 to 29 kg/m^2 do not have health complications and, as previously mentioned, for these patients behavior modification is the primary recommendation. In contrast, the practitioner may wish to consider pharmacotherapy for an individual with a BMI of 29 kg/m^2 who also has type 2 diabetes. Patients with significant psychiatric problems, or who want more support in changing diet and exercise habits, can be referred for adjunct care.

Integrating Behavioral Treatment with Nutrition Therapy and Physical Activity

The primary goal of the behavioral treatment of obesity is to help obese individuals identify and modify inappropriate eating, exercise, and thinking habits that contribute to their weight problem (6). Although not all obese persons have inappropriate eating and exercise habits (15), behavioral treatment can provide obese persons with a set of skills with which to control their obesity, regardless of its etiology. This therapeutic approach acknowledges the role of genetic, metabolic, and hormonal influences on body weight (6), but the focus of treatment is on changing behavior.

Most successful diet and exercise programs use behavioral modification strategies. These programs typically emphasize principles of behavioral treatment, including self-monitoring, problem solving, stimulus control, and nutrition education. These programs often include the use of

---

*The treatment scheme shown in Figure 8.1 is the recommendation of the authors and therefore not identical to the model and recommendations proposed in the NIH report. —EDITOR

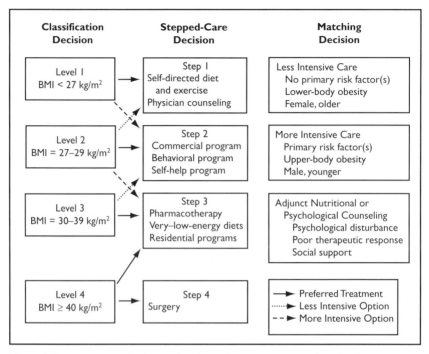

Figure 8.1   A conceptual scheme showing a three-stage process for selecting a treatment approach. The first step (Classification Decision) divides patients into four levels based on BMI. This level dictates which of the four steps would be appropriate in the second stage (Stepped-Care Decision). This ensures that the least intensive, costly, and risky approach will be used. The *solid arrow* between the two boxes identifies the treatment most likely to be appropriate. The *dotted arrow* indicates a less intensive option, where there is a reduced need for weight reduction because of the absence of risk factors. The *dashed arrow* indicates a more intensive option, one appropriate for patients with a significant co-morbid condition. The third stage (Matching Decision) is used to make the final treatment selection, based on the assessment of the patient's need for weight reduction, as judged by the actual presence of co-morbid conditions or other risk factors. See text for discussion. (Courtesy of Thomas A. Wadden, PhD, and Kelly Brownell, PhD.)

treatment manuals, such as the LEARN Program for Weight Control (16). Such programs typically emphasize, in a step-by-step, weekly format, principles of behavioral treatment. Programs of this format may be particularly useful in the primary care setting, because they provide patients with materials to work with between office visits. Three of the key components of behavioral treatment—self-monitoring, nutrition counseling, and exercise—are focused on below. (Those interested in reading more about the behavioral treatment of obesity are referred to reviews specifically on this topic (3, 17, 18)).

Self-Monitoring

Self-monitoring is considered the cornerstone of behavioral treatment for obesity (2, 3). It is useful during both weight loss and weight maintenance because it provides the patient and provider with a detailed record of food and beverage intake. Patients frequently report that self-monitoring makes them more aware of what they consume, which often leads them to decrease intake. Patients often remark that recording keeps them from eating certain things "because I don't want to write it down." Patients will frequently show weight reduction soon after they start recording their food and beverage intake. In addition to recording what and how much they eat and drink each day, patients indicate the time, place, activity, and emotions experienced while eating. This more-detailed monitoring allows the patient to identify maladaptive eating patterns. Problem solving and stimulus control techniques can be taught to interrupt these patterns. Stimulus control is used to modify the precursors of eating to create a more restricted set of environmental events that trigger eating. For example, monitoring forms may reveal that an individual eats snack foods while talking on the telephone even after just eating a meal. The corresponding intervention may involve avoiding food intake while talking on the telephone or limiting consumption to one carefully selected snack.

Because the meeting between the patient and provider in the primary care setting is brief, completion of monitoring and similar homework exercises is thought to be critical to long-term behavior change (15). A more intensive cognitive-behavioral intervention by a mental health professional may be required for those patients who resist keeping food records, or for those patients who demonstrate more complex eating patterns triggered by frequent, strong emotional experiences. These strategies involve identifying thoughts that are irrational (e.g., "I am a failure when it comes to losing weight") and then cognitively restructuring those irrational thoughts with counterstatements.

Nutrition Education

Early behavioral treatment programs for obesity did not include formal nutrition education; however, as summarized in the NIH report, due to evidence that a portion-controlled, low-fat, high-carbohydrate diet promotes both good cardiovascular health and lower body weight, all good behavioral treatment programs now include a nutrition education component. Many behavioral programs provide patients with general nutrition education rather than prescribe a rigid diet (16).

Most nutritionists recommend a diet composed of no more than 30% calories from fat, 12% from protein, and the remainder from carbohydrate (19). The Food Guide Pyramid (see Chapter 6, Fig. 6.1) (20) can be used as a guide to making food choices; the food groups are shown in proportion to the recommended daily servings. The Food Guide Pyramid encourages individuals to consume 6 to 11 servings of bread, cereal, rice, and pasta; 3 to 5 servings of vegetables; 2 to 4 servings of fruit; 2 to 3 servings of milk, yogurt, and cheese; and 2 to 3 servings of meat, poultry, fish, and eggs each day. Using these serving guidelines, dieting women and men usually limit their calories to 1200 and 1500 kcal, respectively, whereas nondieting women and men typically consume 1800 and 2500 kcal/day, respectively. To meet the caloric intake range of 1200 to 1500 calories, patients often need to eat at the low end of the recommended number of bread servings (6 to 8 servings).

Dieters are encouraged to consume foods that they enjoy without avoiding "forbidden foods". These foods, typically high in fat and sugar content, include chocolate, cookies, ice cream and other high-calorie items such as fried chicken and fast-food meals. It is acceptable for patients to eat these foods but in moderation. They are asked to reduce the portion size of these foods when possible. Examples of behavior modification techniques are encouraging patients to eat ice cream out of a smaller bowl and to order the small-serving size of foods like French fries in fast-food restaurants. As a result, the patients do not feel deprived, and they may be less likely to overindulge when they eventually eat a "forbidden food".

In clinics focused on behavioral approaches to weight loss, general nutritional education is provided and patients are encouraged to eat a healthy well-balanced diet based on the principles of the Food Guide Pyramid. Patients are seldom provided with a day-to-day diet or eating plan that details specific foods and portion sizes. Instead, the patient ultimately determines the specific content of the diet, based on individual food preferences. This approach is thought to be the most successful for long-term weight control (3).

Exercise

The health benefits of regular exercise are unarguable; however, exercise may only modestly contribute to weight loss. The addition of regular exercise to a 1200 kcal/d diet may increase weight loss by only 2 to 3 kg during a typical 16 to 20 week behavioral program (21, 22). Thus the practitioner should avoid overstating the weight-reducing effects of exercise. It should be emphasized that the role of regular exercise appears to be important for long-term weight maintenance rather than as an effective means of weight loss *per se*. Numerous studies show that those patients who lose weight and keep it off exercise regularly. In contrast, weight regainers do not appear to exercise regularly (see Chapter 7) (23-25).

Programmed activity and lifestyle activity are two broad categories of exercise (16). Regularly planned periods (e.g., 20 to 40 min) of physical exertion at a high intensity level (e.g., 60% to 80% of maximum heart rate) such as running, swimming, cycling, and aerobic workouts are examples of programmed activity. Many obese patients do not like participating in programmed activity because of the physical discomfort (joint and muscle pain, excessive sweating) and the potential psychological upset (concerns about finding appropriate clothing or social stigmatization). Moreover, many are not capable of such a regimen, at least initially, and it may be medically contraindicated. Encouraging patients to increase lifestyle activity is more amenable to these patients. Thus, from a behavioral perspective, increasing activity levels by, for example, taking the stairs, parking far from building entrances, and discarding remote controls are examples of lifestyle activity that can be incorporated into day-to-day patterns of living (26). The main goal of this form of activity is to increase energy expenditure without worrying about level of intensity.

Behavioral programs typically encourage patients to increase both forms of activity (27). Walking can be considered both a programmed and lifestyle activity and may be an ideal form of exercise for obese individuals (28). For most participants, programmed activity begins with walking two or three times a week for about 15 to 20 min at a time. A recent study found that a program of diet and increased lifestyle activity (30 min/day) may be just as beneficial to one's health as a program consisting of diet plus vigorous activity (3 step-aerobic classes per week). Both groups expressed similar significant improvements in weight, systolic blood pressure, and serum lipid and lipoprotein levels (28).

Although the effects of exercise on weight loss in the short term appears to be modest, a recent study suggests that high levels of exercise may improve weight loss in the long-term. Researchers showed that 150 min/wk of exercise equivalent to a brisk walk improved weight loss over an 18-month period (29). This same study also showed that those patients who exercised at least 200 min/wk lost significantly more weight than those exercising between 100 to 150 min/wk and those exercising less than 100 min/wk. It is unclear whether such an amount of exercise is realistic outside of a controlled clinical trial. Therefore patients should be encouraged to exercise at least 150 min/wk. This exercise could be done in one long continuous session or in several short intermittent sessions, whichever is more convenient. Patients should also be reminded that any amount of exercise is better than none at all.

Physicians must work with patients to identify specific goals for increasing physical activity along with strategies for attaining them. When setting an exercise goal, patients need to specify what, where, when, and for how long they are going to do the activity of choice. Patients should be encouraged to keep track of their activity level by recording it on their food monitoring forms. The physician should follow up on the specific exercise plan at each scheduled visit. In general, health care providers should follow up with their patients on all of their treatment recommendations at the next patient contact. Failing to follow up with patients indirectly conveys the message that the recommendation was not important.

Results of Behavioral Therapy

Short-Term Behavioral Treatment

A review of the behavioral treatment studies published from 1991 to 1995 suggests that behavioral approaches produce weight losses consistent with the current weight loss recommendations. On average, women lost 9% of their starting body weight in a 22-week treatment period (3). Attrition rates in these studies were less than 20%, which suggests that most people who actually entered treatment completed treatment. Whether these low attrition rates outside the realm of controlled research trials are attainable remains to be determined. These weight losses from behavioral therapy also are consistent with the weight losses achieved by the majority of the antiobesity drugs available over the past decade (30-32). The similarity of weight losses for behavioral and pharmacologic treatments for obesity is often surprising to patients and practitioners alike, because weight loss medications are often mischaracterized, particularly by the popular press, as the "magic bullet" of weight control.

Patients who received 20 weeks of behavior therapy for weight loss typically regain about 30% to 35% of the weight loss in the year following treatment (33). Even with weight regain, most patients still meet the criteria of success proposed by the Institute of Medicine: "Successful long-term weight control by our definition means losing at least 5% of body weight...and keeping below our definition of successful weight loss for at least 1 year" (34). Furthermore, several studies (35, 36) but not all (37) have shown that losses of this magnitude are associated with long-term (>1 year) improvement in lipid, lipoprotein, and glucose levels.

Until recently, study results indicated that weight regain generally increased over time and that patients frequently regained 100% of their weight loss within 5 years (33). Although discouraging, this finding is not surprising if we think about obesity as a chronic disorder such as hypertension. For example, if a patient discontinued antihypertensive medication after 20 weeks, few practitioners would expect the patient to have adequate blood pressure control following termination of the medication. Continuous, long-term care is expected and needed for hypertension; and this type of care is increasingly thought to be necessary for the treatment of obesity. This perspective is reinforced by more recent data indicating that 5-year outcomes using lifestyle interventions in the context of a comprehensive weight management program are much better than they were 10 years ago (33). Approximately 30% of patients are able to sustain the 10% weight loss goal set forth by the recent NIH report. Thus practitioners are strongly advised to encourage patients to think of behavioral change as a lifestyle approach that they will incorporate for the rest of their lives rather than to think of behavioral change as short-term.

Long-Term Behavioral Treatment

Due to the problem of weight regain following the cessation of active treatment, several studies have extended the duration of treatment and have demonstrated the benefits of long-term behavioral treatment (38-41). One study found that patients who attended group maintenance sessions every-other-week for 1 year following weight reduction maintained 13.0 kg of their 13.2 kg end-of-treatment weight loss. Those who did not receive such therapy maintained only 5.7 kg of a 10.8 kg loss (38). Maintenance sessions appear to provide patients the support and motivation needed to continue to practice weight control skills, such as keeping food records, exercising regularly, and weighing themselves at least weekly (42). In addition, although social support is often hard to quantify in an empirical sense, many patients report that continued contact with their treatment group is beneficial. Thus physicians with an active obesity practice may want to consider adding a social support component, such as a newsletter or electronic mail contacts, to facilitate long-term adherence.

Three caveats to long-term behavioral treatment can be noted. First, increasing treatment duration is not associated with substantially larger weight losses than those found in short-term treatment (40). Therefore the goal of long-term treatment should be the maintenance of weight loss rather than striving for additional losses. Second, it appears, from somewhat limited data, that follow-up visits need to occur at least every-other-week to sustain a 10% weight loss (43). Infrequent contact is not likely to be sufficient to sustain patients' attention to and motivation for behavior change. Thus physicians should consider including other medical staff, such as nurses and physician assistants, to meet with patients on a regular basis. Third, it appears that long-term behavioral treatment delays, rather than prevents, weight regain. When maintenance sessions are discontinued, patients regain weight (38, 41). These results suggest the need for even longer-term care (i.e., beyond 1 year) (42). Such therapy, however, is difficult to provide, even when resources are available. The addition of pharmacotherapy may provide assistance with the long-term maintenance of weight loss.

Nevertheless, as noted above, outcomes using lifestyle intervention are improving. More evidence is available from the recently established National Weight Control Registry (NWRC) in which researchers are examining the characteristics of individuals who are successful at the long-term maintenance of weight loss (23). Persons in the registry (629 women and 155 men) have lost an average of 30 kg and maintained a minimum of 13.6 kg weight loss at the end of 5 years; 70% reported early onset (prepubescent) of obesity, and 73% had at least one parent who was overweight. Therefore, despite the familial and probable genetic predisposition to being overweight, these patients were able to lose and maintain a significant amount of weight. Approximately half of the group reported losing weight through a formal program, whereas the other half lost weight on their own, which suggests that at least some individuals are acting on public health education campaigns. To help maintain weight loss, the members of the registry reported restricting food intake in many different ways, such as restricting certain kinds of foods, eating all foods in limited quantities, counting calories, and counting fat grams. Members also engaged in high levels of physical activity such as walking and stair climbing. In addition, regular self-monitoring (e.g., food records and weekly weighing) also appears to be an important strategy for long-term weight control. Clearly, this information suggests that there are different methods for maintaining weight loss. Therefore it may be particularly important to help the patient identify specific maintenance techniques that best fit the lifestyle of the patient.

A Combined Behavioral/Pharmacologic Approach

Behavioral and pharmacologic treatments as single therapies for obesity both result in a reduction in weight of about 10%. Pharmacological treatments, however, appear to be more effective in the long-term management of obesity. A number of studies have demonstrated that patients who remain on medication can maintain weight loss of 7% to 8% of initial weight for greater than a 1-year period (30-32). This kind of weight maintenance is also possible for patients receiving behavioral care, although it seems to take much more time and effort for both patient and practitioner to sustain these losses.

As discussed above, behavioral modification induces weight loss by helping patients control their *external* environment. Food records help patients identify patterns in their eating. The desire to eat is controlled by taking steps to prevent situations in which the triggers are especially salient. For example, patients might take a different route home to avoid passing a favorite fast-food restaurant, remove high fat foods from the home, or avoid eating while watching television. In contrast, traditional and current phamacologic agents induce weight loss by modifying *internal* signals associated with eating. Sibutramine, which is a serotonin and norepinephrine reuptake inhibitor, operates by giving patients feelings of satiety or fullness, which ultimately results in a decrease in appetite (44). Orlistat, a gastrointestinal lipase inhibitor, prevents absorption of fat (32). Because behavioral modification and pharmacologic treatment differ in their mechanisms of action, it follows that they may serve to augment one another in a treatment setting.

A study by Craighead and colleagues 20 years ago supports this idea of the additive effects of behavioral modification and pharmacologic treatment (45). The combination of medication (fenfluramine, which is no longer available) with weekly group behavioral modification resulted in a 15.3 kg (approximately 16%) weight loss in 26 weeks. This loss was significantly greater than that achieved by either group behavioral modification without medication (10.9 kg; approximately 11%) or pharmacotherapy alone (6.0 kg; about 7%). Although this study is limited by the use of a medication no longer available, the results do suggest the potential beneficial effects of a combined treatment approach.

A recent study using sibutramine provides further evidence for the efficacy of this approach (12). In this study, 53 women were treated with sibutramine and randomized to one of three treatment conditions. Patients in the first group (Drug-Alone) received sibutramine alone for the 1-year treatment period. They met briefly with a physician ten times over the course of this year to evaluate potential side effects. The second group (Drug-Plus-Lifestyle) received the medication and attended group lifestyle modification sessions lasting 90-min and ate a 1200 kcal/d diet. These groups met weekly for the first 20 weeks and monthly thereafter. The third group (Combined Treatment) also received the medication and attended 90-min group meetings like the participants in the second group. This group was also prescribed a 1000 kcal/d portion-controlled diet using a nutritional supplement for the first 16 weeks. Following those 16-weeks, these patients gradually decreased their consumption of the supplement until they were eating a 1200 to 1500 kcal/d diet as prescribed for the first two groups.

The Drug-Plus-Lifestyle group and the Combined Treatment group lost significantly more weight (10.8 ± 10.2% and 16.5 ± 8.0%, respectively) than the Drug Alone group (4.1 ± 6.3%). The women in the two groups with behavior modification also reported significantly more satisfaction with their weight change, health, appearance, and self-esteem (12). These data support the contention that pharmacologic interventions in combination with lifestyle modification results in a more optimal outcome.

Behavioral Treatment in the Primary Care Setting

Despite the apparent benefits of combining behavioral and pharmacologic therapies in efficacy studies, there are several obstacles to the approach in "real world" clinical practice. Few primary care practices are equipped to provide intensive behavioral treatment and, additionally, they face many obstacles to providing treatment in our current health care delivery system.

To address some of these issues, the effectiveness of combining the two treatment approaches was investigated by one of the authors (RIB) and others (46). In this study, 26 women were randomized to one of two treatment groups. One group (n = 13) of women took medication (fenfluramine and phentermine) and participated in 90-min group behavior modification meetings. These classes met weekly for the first 18 weeks, biweekly from weeks 19 to 40, and monthly from weeks 41 to 52. The second group (n = 13) also received medication but instead of attending group meetings they met with a physician for 15 to 20 min ten times over the course of 1 year. During the physician visits, they received behavioral modification for weight loss. Weight loss for the two groups was equal. Therefore this study demonstrated that a primary care physician-directed behavioral program can substitute for a traditional group behavior therapy approach.

The study had a number of limitations, however. First, the patients took 60 mg of fenfluramine and 15 mg of phentermine (the popular Fen-Phen), and the former has since been removed from the market. Second, the sample size ($n = 26$) was small. Third, the physician (RIB) who administered the lifestyle modification is a psychiatrist who specializes in obesity, making it questionable whether these findings would generalize to internal medicine physicians. To address these limitations, the study is currently being replicated on a larger scale with the use of an approved medication (sibutramine) and with internal medicine physicians administering the brief behavior modification for weight management.

Successful Long-Term Weight Control

To maximize the likelihood of successful long-term weight management and patient satisfaction, it is important for the patient to accept modest weight loss and to adhere to a long-term treatment. It is also important that the collaborative relationship between the patient and provider be recognized.

Acceptance of Modest Weight Losses

A number of experts (1, 19, 34, 47), though not all (48), believe that patients should seek weight losses that are 5% to 15% of their initial body weight. Patients can achieve and maintain this weight loss with long-term behavior therapy and/or long-term pharmacotherapy (see Chapter 12). The question remains, however, whether patients are accepting of this modest weight loss. Foster et al (11) showed that there is a large gap between the weight loss that patients desire and the weight loss they can attain. At the end of a 48-week treatment program, patients achieved a mean weight loss of 16.3 kg (16.4% reduction in initial body weight), only half of the loss they wanted to achieve (32% reduction in initial body weight). In addition, 20% of the patients achieved a weight loss that was disappointing to them and 47% did not even achieve a disappointing weight loss.

The results of this study highlight the importance of reviewing with patients their weight loss expectations. The practitioner needs to clearly relate to the patient what he or she can expect to lose during a weight loss program and what improvements he or she can expect to see in mood, body image, and health complications. The practitioner also needs to reiterate the positive health outcomes of a 5% to 15% weight loss to help the patient become more accepting of these modest weight losses. The principal goal of obesity therapy is to improve health. While patients typically desire to improve their appearance through weight loss, this is a secondary goal of treatment. By failing to highlight these important points, the patient may hold on to unattainable goals, which will likely lead to frustration and disappointment and ultimately may be related to weight gain.

A Long-Term Collaborative Relationship

The use of behavioral modification (or behavioral modification and pharmacotherapy) in primary care practice has the potential to improve the treatment of obese persons. This success may be strongly related to the collaborative relationship that can be established between patient and practitioner. Despite frustrations with weight loss and weight regain, long-term weight control can be achieved. In addition to accepting modest weight losses of 5% to 15% of initial body weight, patients must also believe that obesity is a chronic disorder that, like essential hypertension or diabetes, requires long-term care (42). Maintaining weight loss requires just as much effort as losing the weight. Unfortunately, patients (and often physicians) rarely find weight maintenance as exciting as weight loss. Patients need to recognize that they need to make long-tem behavioral changes and may need to take medications long-term to maintain weight loss (45). Health care professionals need to acknowledge to patients that they recognize how challenging and frustrating weight control can be. Apathetic physicians who are uninterested in helping patients with weight control can contribute to the helpless feeling that many obese persons experience. This is particularly important, because obese patients are often the objects of prejudice and discrimination. By working together in a collaborative, respectful manner, physicians and patients increase the likelihood of successful long-term weight control.

■　■　■

Key Points

- Behavioral therapy uses learning principles to develop and implement strategies to change lifestyle habits.
- Evaluation of the patient with obesity should focus on the biological and environmental causes of the obesity, the psychosocial status of the patient, and the patient's level of motivation.
- Patients should be counseled to accept realistic weight loss goals, generally 5% to 15% of their initial weight. It should be stressed that health benefits as well as improvements in appearance can be accomplished even with what patients may consider only modest weight losses.

- Behavioral treatment integrates nutrition therapy with exercise programs while focusing on changes to the eating, activity, and mental habits that contribute to obesity.

- Self-monitoring helps the patient identify maladaptive eating patterns that are then corrected through the use of problem-solving stimulus control techniques.

- Pharmacologic treatment yields best results when combined with behavioral modification.

■   ■   ■

REFERENCES

1. **NIH Obesity Education Initiative Expert Panel.** Clinical guidelines on the identification, evaluation, and treatment of overweight and obesity in adults: the evidence report. Obes Res. 1998;6:51S-209S.

2. **Wadden TA, Sarwer DB.** Behavioral treatment of obesity: new approaches to an old disorder. In: Goldstein D, ed. The Management of Eating Disorders. Totowa, NJ: Humana Press; 1999:173-99.

3. **Sarwer DB, Wadden TA.** The treatment of obesity: what's new, what's recommended. J Womens Health. 1999;8:483-92.

4. **Spitzer RL, Devlin M, Walsh TB, et al.** Binge eating disorder: a multisite field trial of the diagnostic criteria. Int J Eat Disord. 1992;11:191-203.

5. **Yanovski SZ.** Binge eating disorder: current knowledge and future directions. Obes Res. 1993;1:306-24.

6. **Wadden TA, Foster GD.** Behavioral assessment and treatment of markedly obese patients. In: Wadden TA, VanItallie TB, eds. Treatment of the Seriously Obese Patient. New York: Guilford Press; 1992:290-330.

7. **Fitzgibbon ML, Stolley MR, Kirschenbaum DS.** Obese people who seek treatment have different characteristics than those who do not seek treatment. Health Psychol. 1993;12:342-5.

8. **Carpenter KM, Hasin D, Allison DB, Faith MS.** Relationships between obesity and DSM-IV major depressive disorder, suicide ideation, and suicide attempts: results from a general population study. Am J Public Health. 2000;90:251-7.

9. **Hsu GLK, Benotti PN, Dwyer SB, et al.** Nonsurgical factors that influence the outcome of bariatric surgery: a review. Psychosom Med. 1998;60:338-46.

9a. **Sarwer DB, Wadden TA, Foster GD.** Assessment of body image dissatisfaction in obese women: specificity, severity, and clinical significance. J Consult Clin Psychol. 1998;66:651-4.

10. **Foster GD, Wadden TA, Vogt RA.** Body image before, during and after weight loss treatment. Health Psychol. 1997;16:226-9.

11. **Foster GD, Wadden TA, Vogt RA.** What is a reasonable weight loss?: Patients' expectations and evaluations of obesity treatment outcomes. J Consult Clin Psychol. 1997;65:79-85.

12. **Wadden TA, Berkowitz RI, Sarwer DB, et al.** Benefits of lifestyle modification in the pharmacologic treatment of obesity: a randomized trial. Arch Intern Med. 2001;161:218-27.

13. **Blackburn GL.** Effect of degree of weight loss on health benefits. Obes Res. 1995;3:211s-216s.

14. **Brownell KD, Wadden TA.** The heterogeneity of obesity: fitting treatments to individuals. Behav Ther. 1991;22:153-77.

15. **Wadden TA, Bell ST.** Obesity. In: Kazdin AE, Hersen M, Bellack AS, eds. International Handbook of Behavior Modification and Therapy. 2nd ed. New York: Plenum Publishing; 1990:449-73.

16. **Brownell KD.** The LEARN Program for Weight Control. Dallas: American Health Publishing; 1991.

17. **Wadden TA, Steen SN.** Improving the maintenance of weight loss: the ten percent solution. In: Angel A, Anderson H, Bouchard C, et al, eds. Progress in Obesity Research; VII. London: John Libbey; 1996:745-50.

18. **Wing RR.** Behavioral approaches to the treatment of obesity. In: Bray GA, Bouchard C, James WPT, eds. Handbook of Obesity. New York: Marcel Dekker; 1998:855-73.

19. **Agricultural Research Service.** Report of the Dietary Guidelines Advisory Committee on the Dietary Guidelines for Americans; 1995.

20. **National Livestock and Meat Board.** Food Guide Pyramid. Chicago; 1993.

21. **Perri MG, McAdoo WG, McAllister DA, et al.** Enhancing the efficacy of behavior therapy for obesity: effects of aerobic exercise and a multicomponent maintenance program. J Consult Clin Psychol. 1986;54:670-5.

22. **Wadden TA, Vogt RA, Anderson RE, et al.** Exercise in the treatment of obesity: effects of four interventions on body composition, resting energy expenditure, appetite, and mood. J Consult Clin Psychol. 1997;65:269-77.

23. **Klem ML, Wing RR, McGuire MT, et al.** A descriptive study of individuals successful at long-term maintenance of substantial weight loss. Am J Clin Nutr. 1997;66:239-46.

24. **Ballor DL, Poehlman ET.** Exercise training enhances fat-free mass preservation during diet-induced weight loss: a meta-analytical finding. Int J Eat Disord. 1994;18:35-40.

25. **Saris WHM.** Fit, fat, and fat-free: the metabolic aspects of weight control. Int J Obes. 1998;22:S15-S21.

26. **Brownell KD, Stunkard AJ.** Physical activity in the development and control of obesity. In: Stunkard AJ, ed. Obesity. Philadelphia: WB Saunders; 1980:300-24.

27. **Fox KR.** A clinical approach to exercise in the markedly obese. In: Wadden TA, VanItallie TB, eds. Treatment of the Seriously Obese Patient. New York: Guilford Press; 1992:354-82.

28. **Andersen RE, Wadden TA, Bartlett SJ, et al.** Effects of lifestyle activity vs. structured aerobic exercise in obese women: a randomized trial. JAMA. 1999;281:335-40.

29. **Jakicic JM, Winters C, Lang W, Wing RR.** Effects of intermittent exercise and use of home exercise equipment on adherence, weight loss, and fitness in overweight women: a randomized trial. JAMA. 1999;282:1554-60.

30. **Davidson MH, Hauptman J, DiGirolamo M, et al.** Weight control and risk fac-

tor reduction in obese subjects treated for 2 years with orlistat: a randomized controlled trial. JAMA 1999;281:235-42.

31. **Jones SP, Smith IG, Kelly F, Gray JA.** Long-term weight loss with sibutramine. Int J Obes. 1995;19(Suppl):41.

32. **Sjostrom L, Rissanen A, Andersen T, et al.** Randomized placebo-controlled trial of orlistat for weight loss and prevention of weight regain in obese patients. Lancet. 1998;352:167-72.

33. **Wadden TA, Sternberg JA, Letizia KA, et al.** Treatment of obesity by very-low-calorie diet, behavior therapy and their combination: a five-year perspective. Int J Obes. 1990;51:167-72.

34. **Institute of Medicine.** Weighing the Options: Criteria for Evaluating Weight Management Programs. Washington, DC: Government Printing Office, 1995.

35. **Pi-Sunyer FX.** A review of long-term studies evaluating the efficacy of weight loss in ameliorating disorders associated with obesity. Clin Ther. 1996;18:1006-35.

36. **Wing RR.** Effect of modest weight loss on changes in cardiovascular risk factors: are there differences between men and women or between weight loss and maintenance? Int J Obes. 1995;19:67-73.

37. **Wadden TA, Anderson DA, Foster GD.** Two-year changes in lipids and lipoproteins associated with the maintenance of a 5% to 10% reduction in initial weight: some findings and some questions. Obes Res. 1999;7:170-1.

38. **Perri MG, McAllister DA, Gange JJ, et al.** Effects of four maintenance programs on the long-term management of obesity. J Consult Clin Psychol. 1988;56:529-34.

39. **Viegener BJ, Perri MG, Nezu AM, et al.** Effect of an intermittent, low-fat, low-calorie diet in the behavioral treatment of obesity. Behavior Ther. 1990;21:499-509.

40. **Wadden TA, Foster GD, Letizia KA.** One-year behavioral treatment of obesity: comparison of moderate and severe caloric restriction and the effects of weight maintenance therapy. J Consult Clin Psychol. 1994;62:165-71.

41. **Wing RR, Blair EH, Marcus MD, et al.** Year-long weight loss treatment for obese patients with type 2 diabetes: does including an intermittent very-low-calorie diet improve outcome? Am J Med. 1994;97:354-62.

42. **Wadden TA, Sarwer DB, Berkowitz RI.** Behavioral treatment of the overweight patient. Bailliere's Clin Endocrin Metab. 1999;13:93-107.

43. **Jeffery RW, Thorson C, Burton LR, et al.** Strengthening behavioral interventions for weight loss: a randomized trial of food provision and monetary incentives. J Consult Clin Psychol. 1993;61:1038-45.

44. **Lean MEJ.** Sibutramine: a review of clinical efficacy. Int J Obes. 1997;21:30S-36S.

45. **Craighead LW, Stunkard AJ, O'Brien RM.** Behavior therapy and pharmacotherapy for obesity. Arch Gen Psychiatry. 1981;38:763-8.

46. **Wadden TA, Berkowitz RI, Vogt RA, et al.** Lifestyle modification in the pharmacologic treatment of obesity: a pilot investigation of a potential primary care approach. Obes Res. 1997;6:278-84.

47. **World Health Organization.** Obesity: Preventing and Managing the Global Epidemic. Geneva: World Health Organization; 1998.

48. **Jeffery RW, Wing RR, Mayer RR.** Are smaller weight losses or more achievable weight loss goals better in the long term for obese patients? J Consult Clin Psychol. 1998;66:641-5.

9

Pharmacologic Therapy for Obesity

Mehmood A. Khan, MD

John V. St. Peter, PharmD

For some patients with obesity, weight loss treatment that combines diet modification, an exercise program, and behavioral changes is effective. However, because the success rate of such a regimen is often poor, pharmacotherapy may be indicated for certain patients. Pharmacologic therapy must be used in conjunction with behavioral (diet and exercise) strategies and therefore still requires a high level of patient motivation and involvement. Because several factors, such as appetite and energy expenditure, regulate body weight, the pharmacotherapy of obesity requires an understanding of that subject.

Regulation of Body Weight

Central Receptor Systems

Multiple receptor systems, including those of the biogenic amines, are known to either stimulate or decrease food intake in both animals and humans. Serotonin, also known as 5-hydroxytryptamine (5-HT), and cells known to respond to 5-HT are found throughout the central nervous system (CNS) and its periphery. At least seven distinct subfamilies of 5-HT receptors have been cloned, each with one or more subtypes (1). Currently two major noradrenergic receptor subtypes are recognized (α and β), each with multiple subtypes (2). Histamine and dopamine also demonstrate multiple-receptor subtypes; however, their role in the regulation of eating behavior and food intake is less well documented. Direct stimulation of 5-HT_{1A} and noradrenergic α-2 receptors increases food intake, whereas the opposite occurs with 5-HT_{2C} and noradrenergic α-1 or β-2 receptor activation. In animal models, stimulating histamine receptor subtypes 1 or 3 and dopamine receptor subtypes 1 or 2 results in lowering of food intake. Table 9.1 summarizes the major effects of direct receptor stimulation, inhibition, or changes in synaptic cleft amine concentrations on food intake.

Peptides

Since the 1950s it had been conjectured that weight was controlled via hormone interaction at the level of the hypothalamus (3). The protein product of the mouse obese gene (*ob*) described in 1994 appears to be the signaling mechanism between peripheral energy storage and hypothalamic feeding centers (3, 4). This protein was called *leptin* (after "leptos", the Greek for "thin"). The *ob/ob* genetically obese mouse does not produce leptin,

Table 9.1   Effects of Various Neurotransmitters, Receptors, and Peptides on Food Intake

Neurotransmitter/Receptor/Peptide	Action	Food Intake
Norepinephrine	Increase concentration	Decrease
α^{-1}	Stimulate receptor	Decrease
α^{-2}	Stimulate receptor	Increase
β^{-2}	Stimulate receptor	Decrease
Serotonin	Increase concentration	Decrease
5-HT_{1A}	Stimulate receptor	Increase
5-HT_{1B}	Stimulate receptor	Decrease
5-HT_{1C}	Stimulate receptor	Decrease
Histamine		
H-1	Stimulate receptor	Decrease
H-3	Stimulate receptor	Decrease
Dopamine		
D-1	Stimulate receptor	Decrease
D-2	Stimulate receptor	Decrease
Leptin	Increase concentration	Decrease
Neuropeptide Y	Increase concentration	Increase
Galanin	Increase concentration	Increase

and this animal's marked hyperphagia subsides with leptin supplementation. The human leptin homologue has been cloned, and various animal studies have demonstrated that leptin is produced in the periphery by white and possibly brown adipocytes (5). Additionally, it appears that the sympathetic nervous system (SNS), via β-3 adrenoceptors, inhibits leptin expression (5). Unlike the leptin-deficient *ob/ob* mouse, obese human serum leptin levels increase as fat cell mass increases. There is a direct relationship between serum leptin concentrations and various markers of obesity such as percent body fat, body mass index (BMI), and serum insulin concentrations (6). Thus humans appear to be resistant to the satiety effects of leptin, and it is unknown whether leptin supplementation in humans will decrease obesity. Leptin appears to provide a peripheral link that is signaling the CNS about the status of fat cell mass. A second peptide, neuropeptide Y (NPY), is being intensely studied for its effects on feeding. NPY elicits many effects both peripherally and centrally including appetite stimulation. Most recently, messenger RNA for two new appetite-stimulating proteins called *orexins* has been observed to be concentrated in the lateral hypothalamus (7). The relationships between the sympathetic nervous system, leptin, NPY, orexins, and other hormones such as insulin and glucocorticoids are still evolving (8). Exogenous manipulation of these proteins may provide future pharmacotherapeutic approaches to obesity management.

Energy Balance

The net balance of energy ingested relative to energy expended by an individual over time determines the degree of obesity. Energy stores will increase if there is imbalance between intake and expenditure. An individual's metabolic rate at rest is the single largest determinant of energy expenditure. It is important to determine metabolic rate under standardized conditions, which has given rise to terms such as *resting metabolic rate* (RMR) and *basal metabolic rate* (BMR). RMR is defined as the energy expended by a person at rest under conditions of thermal neutrality. BMR is more precisely defined as the RMR measured soon after awakening in the morning, at least 12 h after the last meal. Metabolic rate increases after eating, based upon the size and composition of the meal. It reaches a maximum approximately 1 h after the meal is consumed and essentially returns to basal levels 4 h after the meal. This increase in metabolic rate is known as the *thermogenic effect* of food (9). RMR may include the residual thermic effect of a previous meal and may be lower than BMR during quiet sleep. BMR and RMR differ by less than 10%, and the terms are frequently used interchangeably. An obvious approach to obesity therapy is to increase BMR or RMR. In practice this has been difficult to achieve long term in a safe and effective manner.

Peripheral Storage and Thermogenesis

Adipose tissue is generally divided into two major types, white and brown (10). The primary function of white adipose tissue is lipid manufacture, storage, and release. Lipid storage occurs in response to insulin and lipid release occurs during periods of calorie restriction, when insulin levels are suppressed. Brown type is notable for its ability to dissipate energy via a process of uncoupled mitochondrial respiration (10). The exact roles of each of these tissue subtypes are better defined in animal models than in humans. Adipose tissue is highly innervated by the sympathetic nervous system and adrenergic stimulation is known to activate lipolysis in fat cells as well as increase energy expenditure in adipose tissue and skeletal muscle. These properties provide a potential pharmacologic avenue for altering energy balance and changing weight status.

A major focus of research in obesity pharmacotherapy has centered on the activity of adrenergic receptors and their effect on adipose tissue with respect to energy storage and expenditure or thermogenesis (10, 11). All three subtypes of β-adrenergic receptors (β-1, β-2, and β-3) appear to be active in fat cell function. The β-3 receptor appears to be less responsive than β-1 and β-2 with respect to activation via norepinephrine. This has led to the development of specific β-3 adrenoceptor agonists. However, apparent differences in selectivity and responsiveness between animal and human β-3 receptors have complicated the drug development process. *In vivo* studies in humans suggest that the β-3 receptor may be largely responsible for adipose tissue adrenergic-mediated increases in thermogenesis (12). Genetic polymorphisms have been identified in the β-2 and β-3 receptor systems that are associated with obesity or excess weight gain (13, 14). Thus genetic susceptibility for excess weight status may, in part, be related to adrenergic dysfunction. The development of effective pharmacotherapies involving these receptor systems may be delayed pending definitive identification of receptor subtype contributions.

General Pharmacologic Approach to Therapy

The success of obesity therapy has most often been measured as weight loss over study periods of up to 12 months. Successful obesity treatment plans have incorporated diet, exercise, behavior modification (with or without pharmacologic therapy), and/or surgical intervention. Strategies for the pharmacologic management of obesity have centered on the CNS and/or peripheral (non-CNS) sites that regulate human energy balance. Table 9.2 lists the most common obesity pharmacotherapeutic agents.

Numerous studies of the effects of central appetite suppressant agents on weight status have been completed since the 1970s (15, 16). Questions

Table 9.2   Obesity Pharmacotherapeutic Agents

Class	Availability	Dosages, mg
Noradrenergic agents		
Methamphetamine HCl (desoxyephedrine HCl)	R_x*	5–15
Amphetamine sulfate	R_x*	5–30
Dextroamphetamine sulfate (Dexedrine)	R_x*	5–30
Amphetamine/dextroamphetamine mixtures (Adderall)	R_x*	5–30
Benzphetamine (Didrex)	R_x*	25–150
Phendimetrazine (Prelu-2, Bontril, Plegine, X-Trazine)	R_x	70–105
Phentermine (Fastin, Oby-trim, Adipex-P, Ionamin)	R_x	15–37.5
Diethylpropion (Tenuate, Tenuate Dospan)	R_x	75†
Mazindol (Mazanor, Sanorex)	R_x	1–3
Phenylpropanolamine (Accutrim, Dexatrim, others)	OTC	75
Ephedrine (various)	OTC/unlabeled use	20–60
Serotonergic agents		
Fenfluramine (Pondamin)	Removed from market	60–120
Dexfenfluramine (Redux)	Removed from market	15–30
Fluoxetine (Prozac)	R_x/unlabeled use**	60
Sertraline	R_x/unlabeled use**	200
Noradrenergic/serotonergic Sibutramine (Meridia)	R_x	5–15
Gastroinestinal lipase inhibitor Orlistat (Ro 18-0647)	R_x	150–360

*High abuse potential; not indicated for treatment of obesity.
†25 mg tid or 75 mg qd if using extended-release formulation.
**Efficacy unproven.

have been raised regarding the quality and interpretability of some of these data (17). The National Task Force on the Prevention and Treatment of Obesity concluded that short-term anorexic agent use may be unjustified because of the predictable weight regain that occurs upon discontinuation of therapy. However, long-term pharmacotherapy may have a place in the treatment of obesity for patients who have no obvious contraindications to available drug therapy (18). Guidance for a multidisciplinary obesity team approach to therapy has been given in a joint statement by the American Association of Clinical Endocrinologists (AACE) and the American College of Endocrinology (ACE) (19).

The recent discovery of cardiac valve disease related to serotonergic appetite suppressant use, however, affirms the Task Force's warning for further study of available therapies before widespread implementation of routine obesity pharmacotherapy (20-22). The following sections outline the current status of pharmacologic agents for obesity therapy, focusing on proposed mechanisms, dosing recommendations, potential side effects, and monitoring parameters.

Noradrenergic Agents

Amphetamines

The appetite-suppressant effects of amphetamines were well recognized by the 1930s. Amphetamines activate central noradrenergic receptor systems as well as dopaminergic pathways, at higher doses, by stimulating neurotransmitter release. Increases in blood pressure and mild bronchodilation are attributed to peripheral α- and β-receptor activation. The powerful stimulant and addictive potential of the amphetamines relative to other available agents has resulted in their general avoidance for the treatment of obesity (19, 23). Based on safety concerns and their addictive potential, amphetamines have no place in the treatment of obesity.

Phentermine

Phentermine, structurally similar to amphetamine, has less severe CNS stimulation and a lower abuse potential. It appears to enhance norepinephrine and dopamine neurotransmission. Phentermine is available in immediate-release and sustained-release formulations; however, the value of sustained-release formulations can be questioned based upon the reported phentermine plasma half-life of 12 to 24 h (15). A single dose once daily in the morning provides effective appetite suppression throughout the day. Divided doses immediately before meals are common, however. Doses above the maximum given on the label do not improve effectiveness (24). Evening or bed-time dosing should be avoided because of possible insomnia.

Significant increases in blood pressure, palpitations, and arrhythmias can occur with phentermine administration. Use is not advisable in hypertensive patients and those with unstable cardiovascular function. The potential for hypertensive crisis with coadministration of phentermine and monoamine oxidase (MAO) inhibitors is noted in product labeling because of the documented cases of this syndrome seen with coadministration of amphetamine or noradrenergic derivatives and MAO inhibitors (25). Similar warnings have been noted regarding concomitant use of tricyclic antidepressants; this is less well documented, however (26). With MAO inhibitors, a minimum washout time of 14 days before the use of any adrenergic agent is suggested to avoid excessive adrenergic stimulation syndromes. Phentermine use is contraindicated in patients who abuse substances such as cocaine, phencyclidine, and methamphetamine, again, because of the potential for excessive adrenergic stimulation syndromes and abuse potential. Mydriasis from adrenergic stimulation can worsen glaucoma, and thus patients with glaucoma should not receive phentermine. Diabetic patients may experience altered insulin or oral hypoglycemic dosage requirements soon after beginning therapy and before seeing any substantial weight loss.

Phentermine is an effective adjunct to diet, exercise, and behavior modification for producing weight loss in excess of that seen with placebo (15, 27). Intermittent and continuous phentermine therapy appear to elicit comparable weight loss (28). However, most individuals experience weight regains during therapy and generally after discontinuing use (15). Despite its recent extensive off-label use in combination with the fenfluramine derivatives and the occurrence of cardiac valvulopathy, phentermine monotherapy when prescribed to carefully selected patients is relatively safe if monitored properly and thus remains a short-term pharmacotherapy for obesity.

Mazindol

Mazindol is chemically distinct from amphetamines and phentermine. Its tricyclic structure results in amphetamine-like appetite suppression. Direct stimulation of hypothalamic activity and norepinephrine reuptake inhibition are potential mazindol mechanisms (29). Mazindol undergoes extensive hepatic metabolism and approximately 50% of an administered dose is recovered in urine, mostly as conjugated metabolites. The pharmacokinetics of mazindol has not been extensively described; however, dosing is based upon an elimination half-life of 10 h (15). Clinically, the drug is given once daily, 1 to 3 mg, before the morning or noon meal. However, some clinicians employ multiple small doses, 1 mg, given just before meals. Efficacy trials of single versus multiple daily doses are not available.

Dry mouth commonly occurs with mazindol use, and difficulty with urination is possible. Fewer patients complain of CNS stimulation with manzindol than with either phentermine or the amphetamines. Additionally, fewer cardiovascular adverse effects have been reported. Thus, obese patients with mild-to-moderate hypertension may be treated with mazindol.

Contraindications for use, similar to those for phentermine, include concurrent MAO inhibitors, glaucoma, symptomatic cardiovascular disease, and stimulant substance abuse. Mazindol has been noted to cause lithium toxicity with concurrent use (30). Early studies in type 2 diabetic patients treated with mazindol demonstrated no need for changes in oral hypoglycemic therapy (31). More recently, improved insulin sensitivity with mazindol treatment was documented using euglycemic clamp studies (32). Caution and close monitoring of insulin or oral hypoglycemic dosage are advisable when treating obese diabetic patients with this therapy. Several placebo-controlled trials have demonstrated the effectiveness of mazindol as a short-term therapy for weight reduction (15).

Diethylpropion

Diethylpropion stimulates norepinephrine release from presynaptic storage granules. Increased adrenergic neurotransmitter concentrations activate hypothalamic centers that result in decreased appetite and food intake. This drug undergoes extensive first-pass hepatic metabolism. Active metabolites are renally eliminated and account for approximately 70% of administered dose. The elimination half-life of these metabolites is approximately 8 h (24). Less than 10% of the parent compound is recovered in urine. No specific dosing recommendations exist for use in patients with renal or hepatic insufficiency. Diethylpropion can be taken in divided daily doses, generally 25 mg three times daily before meals. An extended-release formulation is also employed by some clinicians, usually as 75 mg taken once daily in the morning or midmorning. Both dosing regimens are effective in achieving short-term weight loss in excess of placebo (15). Complaints of insomnia increase if late afternoon dosing is used. Diethylpropion causes less CNS stimulation than mazindol and generally causes less insomnia than phentermine. Patients with severe hypertension or significant cardiovascular disease should not receive diethylpropion. However, it is one of the safest noradrenergic appetite suppressants, and its use has been recommended in patients with mild-to-moderate hypertension or angina pectoris (33). Diabetic patients may experience decreased insulin or oral hypoglycemic dosage requirements soon after beginning therapy and before any substantial weight loss. More frequent blood glucose self-monitoring and medical follow-up are warranted when treating diabetic patients with diethylpropion.

Phenylpropanolamine

Although commonly classified as a noradrenergic anorexic, phenylpropanolamine (PPA) is atypical with regard to its mechanism and site of action. PPA racemates, D- and L-norephedrine, have chemical structures similar to amphetamine (34). The levoenantiomer has more potent anorexic effects. Centrally, PPA appears to stimulate α-adrenergic receptors without additionally activating the dopaminergic or β-adrenergic systems as seen with amphetamine (34). PPA appears to preferentially activate medial as opposed to lateral hypothalamic regions (34). Although PPA-induced increases in brown adipose tissue thermogenesis have been seen in animals, this is less evident in humans (35). PPA exhibits an elimination half-life of 4 to 6 h in humans with approximately 90% of an administered dose recovered unchanged in urine (36). Both immediate- and extended-release formulations are available in the United States over-the-counter. The extended release formulations are generally used in weight management products and commonly employ a daily dose of 75 mg.

PPA use can result in nervousness, insomnia, headache, nausea, and dizziness. Most adverse effects are self-limited; however, case reports of severe side-effects such as hypertensive crisis, intracranial hemorrhage, and seizure exist (37). A meta-analysis of PPA clinical trials has indicated that PPA use results in weight loss in excess of placebo but somewhat less than that seen with prescription anorectics (38). Differences in weight loss were most apparent in studies lasting longer than 4 weeks. The adrenergic action of PPA can elevate blood glucose in patients with impaired glucose tolerance, including overt diabetes, by increasing gluconeogenesis and glycogen breakdown.

Patients with diabetes mellitus, hypertension, or heart disease should be intensely monitored when PPA therapy is started. Some products contain combinations of caffeine and PPA. Concurrent use of caffeine and PPA results in elevations of caffeine plasma levels and potentially excess adrenergic stimulation (39). As with the other adrenergic agents, concurrent use of PPA and MAO inhibitors should be avoided because of accelerated hypertension (25). A case-control study is underway to help determine whether PPA use is related to serious adverse events, specifically hemorrhagic stroke. Available information implicates PPA as a cause of hemorrhagic stroke (40), and the FDA has announced its intention to reclassify PPA from category I (safe and effective) to category III (needs more data to prove safety) (41, 41a, 41b, 41c).

Ephedrine

Chemically related to PPA (± norephedrine), ephedrine may be a viable obesity pharmacotherapy. It appears to suppress appetite and increase energy expenditure via release of presynaptic norepinephrine and direct stimulation of thermogenic β-adrenergic receptors (42). The efficiency of ephedrine stimulation is somewhat blunted by physiologic feedback systems involving adenosine and various prostaglandins (43). This notion has stimulated research to characterize the effect of ephedrine in the presence of adenosine and prostaglandin antagonists such as caffeine and aspirin (44, 45). Ephedrine in combination with caffeine has enhanced appetite suppression and thermogenesis compared with placebo and other anorectics over time periods of up to 6 months (16, 42, 46). Oral doses of 20 mg ephedrine and 200 mg caffeine up to three times daily have been studied (47, 48).

The spectrum of side effects with ephedrine and ephedrine/caffeine combinations is similar to that seen with other noradrenergic agents. Side effects are more notable at higher doses and most commonly include tremor, agitation, nervousness, increased sweating, and insomnia; palpitations and tachycardia have also been reported. Patients with diabetes, hypertension, or cardiovascular disease (including arrhythmic conditions) should not self-medicate with ephedrine-containing products without evaluation by a physician. Ephedrine is available both with and without a prescription; neither form is approved by the FDA for use as an obesity therapy (49, 50).

Serotonergic Agents

Serotonin is an important neurotransmitter involved in many human physiologic systems. Sleep-wake cycles, sensitivity to pain, blood pressure, and mood and eating behaviors have links to serotonin activity. Increasing central serotonin levels decreases the amount of food consumed and prolongs the time between food intake (23). Some serotonergic agents increase central serotonin concentrations via stimulating release of pre-synaptic stores and/or inhibition of reuptake into storage granules. Additionally, either the parent compound or metabolites of these agents may also directly stimulate post-synaptic 5-HT receptors (51). Peripheral serotonin effects on appetite, such as slowing gastric motility, have also been described (23). A major distinction between serotonergic and noradrenergic agents is that the former lack the central stimulant effects and abuse potential observed with the latter (15, 52); conversely, decreased wakefulness, altered sleep patterns, and changes in affect can be seen.

Fenfluramine
This orally active, racemic mixture (D-, L-fenfluramine) was used extensively as monotherapy for appetite suppression for many years. Fenfluramine increases synaptic serotonin concentration via reuptake inhibition and possibly by increasing serotonin release. An early, double-blind, placebo-controlled trial in obese patients demonstrated that fenfluramine 20 mg three times daily had similar efficacy as daily phentermine 30 mg (53). Average weight loss after 20 weeks of therapy ranged from 7.5 to 10 kg. Both medications were more effective than placebo, which attained 4.4 kg average loss (53). Additionally, this trial was one of the first to include a treatment arm employing the combination of fenfluramine (30 mg before the evening meal) and phentermine (15 mg in the morning). Combination dosages were half that used in the monotherapy arms and achieved average weight loss of 8.5 kg with fewer reported side effects.

Subsequently, Weintraub et al completed classic placebo-controlled studies in a small cohort of obese patients that stimulated widespread interest in and use of the combination of fenfluramine and phentermine (Fen/Phen) for weight management (54-62). This combination provided, in most cases, enhanced anorexia with weight loss in excess of placebo (15, 63). Additionally, it appears that phentermine coadministration decreased some of the anxiety and confusion sometimes associated with fenfluramine (52). Weight loss with this combination was associated with improvements in blood pressure, lipid profile, and glucose tolerance (60, 61, 64). The long-term effectiveness of this combination was never clearly documented, however, and weight regain, while less than that lost, occured during the second year of use in many patients (64, 65). Fenfluramine was withdrawn from world-wide markets in 1997 because of its relation to cardiac valvular insufficiency and valvular structural abnormalities (see Serious Adverse Effects below) (20-22, 66).

Dexfenfluramine

The D-isomer of fenfluramine was used extensively in Europe before its release in the United States in 1996. Dexfenfluramine increased synaptic serotonin concentrations via reuptake inhibition. Additionally, *in vitro* observations demonstrated that its metabolite, dexnorfenfluramine, directly stimulated 5-HT_{2C} receptors (51). This compound was the first in the United States to receive approval for chronic use. Dexfenfluramine was more effective than placebo in promoting weight loss as part of a program in conjunction with diet and exercise (15, 16). Additional effectiveness with the addition of phentermine was also noted with this agent (67). As a derivative of fenfluramine, it was also removed from the world-wide markets because of potential cardiac valve problems (see Serious Adverse Effects below) (22, 66).

Selective Serotonin Reuptake Inhibitors and Antidepressants

It is interesting that some of the serotonergic appetite-suppressing agents were first studied as antidepressants and then noted to have effects on weight. However, one of the popular misconceptions about these agents is they facilitate weight loss. As a class, selective serotonin reuptake inhibitors (SSRIs) are generally weight-neutral, but this is nevertheless advantageous for psychiatric therapy because so many of the antidepressants, such as the tricyclic antidepressants, are associated with weight gain (2, 68). The National Task Force on the Prevention and Treatment of Obesity has reviewed many randomized, double-blind, placebo-controlled weight loss clinical trials using fluoxetine and one with sertraline (18, 69). Patients receiving fluoxetine (60 mg per day) demonstrate initial weight loss of 2 to 4 kg on average, but weight regain occurs in spite of continued medication use such that no difference is noted between fluoxetine and placebo over periods of up to 1 year (70). Similar findings are noted using sertraline (200 mg per day) as an adjunct to help maintain weight loss with very-low-calorie diet (VLCD) (69). A direct relation exists between the amount of weight loss and the sum of fluoxetine and norfluoxetine plasma concentrations. Higher plasma concentrations are associated with greater weight loss (71). Despite the potential benefits, clinical trials indicate that it is unlikely fluoxetine will be useful for long-term weight loss and weight maintenance.

Antidepressant serotonin reuptake inhibitors are not approved by the FDA as weight management agents, and they are not currently recommended for routine treatment of obesity (18, 19). Nevertheless, some practitioners continue to prescribe these agents "off-label" for the treatment of obesity, either alone or in combination with phentermine (72). The safety and efficacy of phentermine-SSRI combinations are unclear. A recent case report of adverse experiences (impaired mentation, tremor, hyperreflexia, and gastrointestinal symptoms) with unintentional concurrent use of phentermine and fluoxetine reinforces the need for caution by prescribers of unlabeled combination therapy (73). Serious adverse effects such as primary pulmonary hypertension and cardiac valve abnormalities (see Serious Adverse Effects below) in excess of background prevalence have not been reported in relation to SSRI use for obesity therapy. Consistent with this, a recent case study in patients with aortic valve insufficiency confirmed by cardiac ultrasound demonstrated no difference in the rate of SSRI use in patients with or without aortic valve insufficiency (74).

Noradrenergic/Serotonergic

Sibutramine

The noradrenergic/serotonergic compound is an orally active racemic mixture that became available in the United States in early 1998. The parent compound and two active metabolites appear to increase synaptic concentrations of serotonin (5-HT), norepinephrine (NE), and dopamine via reuptake inhibition. The active metabolites (M_1 and M_2) are more potent than the parent sibutramine. Reuptake inhibition appears to be greatest for norepinephrine, followed by serotonin, with dopamine the least inhibited. Sibutramine, M_1 and M_2 do not directly stimulate serotonergic (5-HT_1 or 5-HT_2), noradrenergic (α-1, α-2, β-1, β-2, β-3) or dopamine receptors (75). It is thought that sibutramine induces weight loss by both decreasing appetite and maintaining or increasing thermogenesis via the combined effects on 5-HT and NE reuptake inhibition, with recent data suggesting its appetite-suppressing effects predominate (75, 76). In humans, the degree to which these effects can be attributed to central versus peripheral activity is unknown. Sibutramine is subject to hepatic first-pass metabolism via $CYP3A_4$ (77). Moderate changes in sibutramine and/or metabolite disposition have been seen with ketoconazole coadminstration (77). M_1 and M_2 area-under-the-curve increased by 58% and 20% respectively, with concurrent ketoconazole (200 mg twice daily for 7 days). Smaller changes have been noted with concurrent erythromycin and cimetidine. The active metabolites M_1 and M_2 exhibit elimination half-lives of 14 and 16 h respectively (77, 78). Further metabolism of the active metabolites results in conjugates that are renally eliminated. The pharmacokinetics of sibutramine allows for a single daily oral dosing.

Sibutramine has been studied in clinical trials in doses from 1 to 30 mg daily and demonstrates a relatively clear dose-response relationship. Weight loss from daily doses of 1 mg is, on average, no different than from placebo. The recommended starting dose is 10 mg daily, with a recommended dose range of 5 to 15 mg daily.

Dry mouth, anorexia, insomnia, constipation, appetite increase, dizziness, and nausea were noted two to three times more frequently in sibutramine-treated subjects than in placebo-treated subjects (77, 78). Significant increases in systolic and diastolic blood pressure as well as pulse rate have been noted with sibutramine use (77). Baseline blood pressure should be established before beginning therapy, and close monitoring is required when using this agent.

Sibutramine product labeling indicates that among the most serious contraindications are coronary artery disease, stroke, congestive heart failure, and arrhythmias (78). Like other centrally acting appetite suppressants, sibutramine should not be used in patients receiving MAO inhibitor therapies. Sibutramine is listed as a Schedule IV prescription substance in spite of being noted as having no street value by recreational substance users (78). Primary pulmonary hypertension has not been reported with sibutramine use (see Serious Adverse Effects below). Echocardiographic assessments of a small cohort of patients from clinical trials, with approximately 6 months exposure, do not demonstrate the cardiac valve problems seen with the fenfluramine derivatives (77).

Based upon 12-month clinical trials, weight loss with sibutramine therapy appears to be most significant during the first 6 months of therapy. Twenty-nine percent of placebo-treated patients in these trials attained a 5% reduction in total body weight after 12 months (78). Using sibutramine at 10 and 15 mg per day resulted in 56% and 65% of patients respectively achieving at least a 5% reduction in total body weight (78). A 10% reduction in body weight was achieved by 8% of placebo-treated patients, whereas 30% and 39% of sibutramine 10 and 15 mg per day respectively obtained this level of weight reduction. There is, on average, a tendency for weight regain after 6 months of treatment. However, in the context of a closely supervised weight management program (i.e., patients treated with a VLCD for 4 weeks who lost at least 6 kg, then treated with a conventional diet and sibutramine), all patients (100% response) continued to lose weight and then maintain weight loss for 1 year compared with only 42% on placebo who were able to sustain weight loss (79). Thus, in selected patients, this agent can be very effective.

As with other centrally active appetite suppressants, weight regain occurs with cessation of therapy (80). Safety and efficacy beyond 1 year of exposure to sibutramine are uncertain.

Lipase Inhibitor (Orlistat)

The percentage of dietary intake as fat has been implicated as a contributing factor in the development of obesity. Fat represents an extremely dense energy source, one that provides 9 kcal/g compared with approximately 4 kcal/g from protein or carbohydrate. In humans, most of accumulated body fat excess is derived from dietary sources because of a limited capacity to synthesize fat directly from carbohydrate. Gastrointestinal (gastric, pancreatic, and carboxylester) lipases are essential in the absorption of the long-chain triglycerides commonly found in Western diets. Additionally, lipase is known to play a role in facilitating gastric emptying and secretion of other pancreaticobiliary substances (81).

Orlistat (Xenical, RO 18-0647) is a synthetic derivative of lipstatin, a natural lipase inhibitor produced by *Streptomyces toxyticini*. Orlistat is minimally absorbed and selectively inhibits gastrointestinal lipases (82). Lipase inhibition results in decreased formation of free fatty acids from dietary triglyceride. Additionally, lower luminal free fatty acid concentrations result in malabsorption of cholesterol (17).

Orlistat induces weight loss by a persistent lowering of dietary fat absorption. Clinical studies employing orlistat as an adjunct to diet therapy demonstrated dose-dependent reductions in fat absorption. Pharmacodymanic modeling using early clinical trial data demonstrated half-maximal inhibition of fat absorption from orlistat doses of 98 mg/d, with maximal effects at around 400 mg/d (83). Clinically, as much as a 30% reduction in fat absorption occurs with daily doses of 360 mg (83, 84). No additional decrease in fat absorption occurs with doses above 400 mg/d (83). Therefore the approved dosing is 120 mg with meals (typically 3 doses/d). Orlistat must be taken with foods that contain fat in order to exert its effect. However, varying either meal content with regard to fat/fiber ratio or the timing of drug ingestion relative to meals demonstrated little effect on the inhibition of fat absorption (85, 86).

Orlistat treatment in conjunction with a low-calorie diet over 1 year in a small cohort of obese subjects resulted in a maintained 7% to 9% decrease in body weight as opposed to placebo-treated subjects who experienced weight regain at 6 to 7 months of therapy (87). A 2-year study demonstrated weight loss of 10% (~10 kg) during the first year compared with 6% (~6 kg) in the placebo (88). Some weight regain occurred during year 2, but 57% who continued on orlistat maintained at least 5% weight loss versus 37% in the placebo group. Similar results have been demonstrated in a more recent large clinical trial (89) and in a trial in the primary care setting (90), and improvements in risk factors have been demonstrated as well (91).

Orlistat may also have a role in treating patients suffering from co-morbidities. A 1-year, randomized, double-blind, placebo-controlled trial of orlistat in obese patients with type 2 diabetes has been completed (92).

This trial demonstrated that prolonged use of orlistat results in significant sustainable weight loss with improvements in glycemic control and lipid profile. Additionally, a significant number of orlistat-treated diabetic patients either decreased or discontinued oral sulfonylurea therapy during and throughout the trial. Thus, with continued lifestyle intervention, this agent may prove to be an acceptable long-term medication supplement in medically supervised weight loss programs.

While unanimously recommended for approval by an FDA advisory committee in 1997, the FDA subsequently requested further information regarding the occurrence of breast cancer during clinical trials. An overall breast cancer incidence of 0.6% (9 cases, all female) was noted in the orlistat treatment versus 0.1% (1 case, female) with placebo. In retrospect, evidence of malignancy, before study participation, was apparent in 8 of the 9 orlistat-treated patients. Clarification of this issue resulted in orlistat approval by the FDA in 1998.

At least one gastrointestinal complaint (e.g., soft stools, abdominal pain/colic, flatulence, fecal urgency or incontinence) is initially reported in up to 80% of individuals using orlistat (93, 94). These complaints are most common in the first 1 to 2 months of therapy, are mild-to-moderate in severity, and tend to improve with continued orlistat use. Orlistat-induced malabsorption of fat-soluble vitamins has been documented (87, 95). Therefore a multivitamin supplement is recommended during therapy with this agent. Despite its definite effects on fat absorption and gastrointestinal motility, orlistat does not appear to change the pharmacokinetic or dynamic profiles of numerous other agents. Controlled studies of concurrent administration of contraceptives, digoxin, glyburide, phenytoin, pravastatin, warfarin, extended-release nifedipine, captopril, atenolol, furosemide, and ethanol have documented minimal effects (82).

Peptides

Many different endogenous peptides, which play various roles in the regulation of food intake, have been identified in animals and humans. Leptin originates in the adipocyte and is proposed to function as a peripheral feedback messenger with respect to fat storage (see Regulation of Body Weight above). NPY and galanin are two CNS peptides that appear to similarly stimulate food consumption but have differing effects on preference to carbohydrate or fat as well as substrate metabolism (96). NPY and galanin are thought to exert minimal effects on protein intake; however, a third, less well described, CNS peptide growth hormone-releasing factor stimulates protein ingestion. Carbohydrate ingestion and utilization is related to NPY hypothalamic activity, specifically in the arcuate and medial paraventricular nucleus. Galanin activity, centering in the lateral paraventricular nucleus and medial preoptic areas, increases both carbohydrate and fat intake, with preferential effects on fat consumption and utilization (96). NPY enhances fat synthesis via an increased respiratory quotient and utilization of carbohydrate. Galanin appears to slow energy expenditure (96). NPY and galanin modulate the release of insulin, corticosterone, and vasopressin, further affecting nutrient intake behaviors and substrate metabolism. NPY is associated with increased levels of insulin, corticosterone, and vasopressin, whereas decreases are seen with galanin (96). The macronutrient intake, energy utilization, and endocrine effects of NPY are most consistent with those seen in chronic obesity. Future pharmacotherapies may develop based upon knowledge of the effects of these endogenous peptides.

Recombinant leptin has been administered subcutaneously to humans (97). A Phase 1 tolerability and dose-ranging study demonstrated some initial prospects for exogenous leptin administration. Participants were randomly assigned to receive either leptin or placebo and were given exercise and nutrition counseling. The placebo-controlled study was not designed to demonstrate efficacy, but preliminary data analysis of 165 male and female participants showed that 19% of placebo-treated patients versus 30% to 45% of leptin-treated subjects lost at least 2 kg over 28 days of study. Thirty obese participants remained in the study through 90 days of therapy. Not all of the leptin doses studied elicited weight loss. Placebo-treated individuals lost an average of 1.5 kg, and subjects exposed to some of the leptin doses lost 2 to 4 kg. These potentially effective doses are being used in Phase 2 trials involving obese patients with and without type 2 diabetes. Some study participants suffered local injection site reactions, and systemic antibodies were detected at higher leptin doses in some patients. Second-generation leptin molecules are being developed to reduce injection site reactions that will potentially improve tolerance for higher doses.

Herbal, Natural, and Food Supplement Weight Loss Therapies

Many individuals, whether or not clinically overweight or obese, choose to undertake weight loss regimens without medical monitoring and incorporate the ingestion of herbal, natural, or food supplement products. It is important to remember that the FDA does not strictly regulate the manufacture and labeling of these products. Thus quality control of these products is highly variable (e.g., potency varies widely from label), and their safety and efficacy are not required to be established before marketing, unlike prescription medications. Table 9.3 lists some of the common constituents found in many of these products.

Chromium
The effectiveness of chromium as an agent for weight loss is unclear. The hexavalent form of this trace element is thought to be carcinogenic,

Table 9.3   Weight Loss Agents in Herbal, Natural, and Food Supplements*

Herbal/Natural/Food Supplements	Active Moiety	Proposed Effect
Chromium picolinate	Chromium	?
Ma huang	Ephedrine derivatives	Noradrenergic
St. John's wort	Hypericin	Serotonergic/MAO inhibition
White willow bark	Salicylate	Inhibits norepinephrine breakdown
Calcium pyruvate	Pyruvate	?
Guarana extract	Caffeine	Noradrenergic
Various tea extracts	Caffeine	Noradrenergic
Garcinia cambogia extract (citrin)	Hydroxycitric acid	?

*Safety and efficacy not documented.
? Proposed mechanism unclear.

whereas the trivalent form found in human food sources is essentially non-toxic (98). Chromium is considered an essential micronutrient and, experimentally in animals, is an insulin cofactor active in carbohydrate, protein, and lipid metabolism (98). In humans, insulin resistance has been reported in a few cases of apparent severe chromium deficiency during long-term total parenteral nutrition. There is no reliable means of assessing total body chromium status, so to establish the diagnosis of deficiency is difficult.

The tryptophan metabolite, picolinic acid, forms a complex with trivalent chromium, which improves bioavailability. Food sources with highly available chromium include brewer's yeast, calf liver, American cheese, and wheat germ (98). A recent double-blind, placebo-controlled study of chromium picolinate as a supplement to aerobic exercise in the treatment of obesity failed to demonstrate any effectiveness (99).

Ma huang

Ma huang is a traditional Chinese medicine manufactured from various parts of the *Ephedra* species. This species is known to produce L-ephedrine, D-pseudoephedrine, L-norephedrine, D-norpseudoephedrine, l-*N*-methylephedrine, and D-*N*-methylpseudoephedrine (100). The FDA Center for Food Safety and Applied Nutrition has completed an analysis of several products labeled as containing ma huang; ephedrine-type alkaloids were detected in concentrations ranging from 0 to 56 mg/g (100). Although it is difficult to determine actual exposure to active entities when using ma huang, side effects and cautions are similar to those for ephedrine (see Ephedrine above). The

FDA has proposed constraints on allowable ephedrine alkaloid concentrations and combinations with other stimulants such as caffeine in dietary supplements (101). From 1994 to mid-1997, the FDA received over 800 reports of serious adverse events, including seizures, stroke, and death, coincident with ephedrine-containing dietary supplement use. Those dangers were reinforced by a recent update of the FDA database (101a). These preparations should be avoided in patients with diabetes, hypertension, and other cardiovascular disease. One problem with many ma huang products is the lack of consistency in labeling versus actual product content.

St. John's Wort
St. John's wort, a perennial flowering plant (*Hypericum perforatum*), has been employed as a medicinal herb for thousands of years. Its use in weight loss and herbal supplements is probably based upon the proposed effects of its constituent naphthodianthrones (hypericin and pseudohypericin). These are thought to be inhibitors of monoamine oxidase and would be expected to increase synaptic concentrations of monoamines such as serotonin and norepinephrine. Consistent with these assumptions, *Hypericum* extracts appear to be more effective than placebo in the treatment of depression (102). However, *in vitro* studies have not been able to substantiate direct monoamine oxidase inhibition at physiologic hypericin concentrations, and recognized antidepressant effects may be due to other constituents (103, 104). The risks of concurrent use of *Hypericum* derivatives and other adrenergic and serotonergic compounds have not been characterized. St. John's wort has not been studied with respect to its role in obesity management, and its safety and efficacy as a treatment modality in the self-management of obesity are unclear.

White Willow Bark
White willow bark is a natural source of salicylate, a prostaglandin inhibitor. Prostaglandin inhibition may enhance adrenergic stimulation via inhibition of norepinephrine breakdown (see Ephedrine above).

Guarana Extract and Various Tea Extracts
Guarana and various tea extracts are sources of caffeine that have inherent adrenergic properties as well as increase the effects of stimulant substances such as ephedrine or ephedra alkaloids (see Ephedrine above). There may also be additional properties related to catechin polyphenols that promote thermogenesis above and beyond the effects of their caffeine content (105, 105a).

Garcinia cambogia
Garcinia cambogia, a popular extract containing hydroxycitric acid, which inhibits citrtate lyase *in vitro* and interferes with the TCA cycle to ultimately

promote fat oxidation, purports to be a thermogenic agent (marketed as a "fat burner"). However, its efficacy has yet to be proven. Recent clinical trials have demonstrated that despite its *in vitro* effects, it does not result in any changes in fat oxidation in either the resting or exercise state nor does it promote overall weight loss (106, 107).

Chitosan

Chitosan is derived from mollusk shells and marketed as a fat chelating agent. However, there is no evidence that fat excretion increases with chitosan (108).

Severe Adverse Effects

Severe adverse effects have been reported with almost all of the appetite-suppressant agents discussed in this chapter. Because of combination or multiple use patterns by many patients, it is often difficult to identify direct causal relationships. Therefore all practitioners treating patients who are current users of, or have been exposed to, anorectic agents should maintain a high index of suspicion for the occurrence of severe adverse effects. Primary pulmonary hypertension and cardiac valvulopathy, as discussed below, appear to occur most frequently with the use of fenfluramine derivatives.

Primary Pulmonary Hypertension

Primary pulmonary hypertension (PPH) is a condition in which high pressures of unknown etiology in the pulmonary vasculature result in increased right ventricular afterload. Various causal relationships have been suggested including recent pregnancy, cocaine use, cirrhosis, genetic susceptibility, oral contraceptive use, and infection with the human immunodeficiency virus. Afflicted individuals have an impaired ability to increase cardiac output in response to exertion and can present with vague complaints of dyspnea, chest pains, and sometimes syncope. Progression of this disorder causes right-sided heart failure and death. About 50% of cases may spontaneously remit. In the unremitting cases, the condition responds poorly to medical management; patients have a median survival from diagnosis of about 2.5 to 3 years. The estimated annual incidence of this condition is one or two cases per million population.

In Europe, during the 1960s, an increase in the incidence of PPH was noted during the same time period that an adrenergically active appetite suppressant, aminorex fumarate, was marketed. A return to the baseline incidence of PPH was observed after aminorex was removed from use. Overall, an increased risk of developing PPH appears possible with use of some of the noradrenergic and serotonergic appetite suppressants, either alone or in combination (109-112). Specifically, the estimated odds ratio for occurrence of PPH with use of fenfluramine derivatives is stated as about 6 and possibly greater than 20 with use over 3 months duration (111, 112). The 20-fold increased PPH prevalence is similar to the rate of fatality from penicillin anaphylaxis (10-20/million exposures) (113). To date, PPH has not been identified as a problem with PPA, sibutramine, or the SSRI compounds.

Cardiac Valvulopathy

Cardiac valve disease is known to occur coincidentally with serotonergic compounds (methysergide and ergotamine) and disease states (carcinoid disease) that result in systemic elevations of serotonin (114, 115). A form of cardiac valvular disease has been recognized coincidentally with the use of serotonergic appetite suppressants. Clinical investigators initially described 24 cases of symptomatic valvular heart disease in women, mean age 44 years, with no previous history of cardiac disease and a common association with exposure to the combination of fenfluramine-phentermine (Fen/Phen) (20). Cardiac ultrasonography demonstrated multivalvular regurgitation and abnormal valve morphology. Eight of the 24 cases demonstrated newly documented pulmonary hypertension, with right ventricular systolic pressures ranging from 52 to 93 mm Hg. Mitral valve replacement was required in 5 of the 24 cases. Three of these five were concurrently exposed to SSRI or TCA compounds. Average exposure to Fen/Phen was 11 months (range, 1 to 28 months).

Subsequently, a prevalence study using echocardiography was performed in 233 appetite-suppressant-exposed patients and 233 age-, gender- and BMI-matched control subjects (22). A significantly increased prevalence of mostly aortic insufficiency was described in the exposed patients who had been treated with dexfenfluramine alone, dexfenfluramine/phentermine, or Fen/Phen for an average of 20.5 months. The investigators found that 1.3% of control subjects versus 22.7% of exposed patients demonstrated mild or greater aortic insufficiency. This study demonstrated a highly significant risk for cardiac valve insufficiency with appetite suppressant use (odds ratio, 22.6; $P < 0.001$; 95% confidence interval, 7.1 to 114.2). Fewer individuals demonstrated mitral or tricuspid insufficiency than the original case reports. A subsequent report confirmed the association with aortic insufficiency but not mitral regurgitation (115a) and demonstrated that the background prevalence of mild or greater aortic insufficiency in unexposed obese patients is similar to that of the general population under 50 years of age.

In the months preceding fenfluramine derivative removal from worldwide markets, a randomized, double-blind, placebo-controlled trial of two formulations of dexfenfluramine was begun. At the time of market withdrawal, 1212 obese patients had been randomized to one of two dexfenfluramine formulations or placebo. Patients were exposed to either dexfenfluramine alone or placebo for a median of 75 to 77 days. Echocardiograms, within 30 days of stopping medication, were completed in 1072 study subjects, with relatively equal distribution between the treatment groups. Approximately 80% were women. Preliminary findings were reported via a press release at the 1998 American College of Cardiology meeting and subsequently published (116). The investigators noted that significant aortic insufficiency (mild or greater) was detected in 5.0% and 5.8% of dexfenfluramine-treated patients (immediate-release and sustained-release groups, respectively) and 3.6% of placebo-treated patients. In their analysis, no difference in valve disease was noted between drug- and placebo-treated groups ($P = 0.43$), which suggests that relatively short exposure to dexfenfluramine alone carries minimal risk for valve problems. The background prevalence of mild or greater aortic insufficiency reported in the placebo group is twofold to threefold higher than in previous reports (22, 117-121).

Valvular insufficiency is not readily appreciated on physical exam in many patients with appetite-suppressant-related valvular disease but is detectable via cardiac ultrasonography. An understanding of risk factors, etiology, progression, and natural history of this drug-related valve disease is evolving. The Department of Health and Human Services has issued interim recommendations for health care providers for dealing with this valvulopathy. These include antibiotic prophylaxis for some dental and surgical procedures depending upon the degree of valve incompetence (66). Most of the current research regarding this valvulopathy has centered on serotonergic pharmaceuticals. Interestingly, significant aortic insufficiency has been reported in women who have consumed "Chinese herbs" as part of a weight loss routine; a direct causal relationship with the herbal preparations, however, is unclear because these weight loss routines also included fenfluramine and diethylpropion (122).

Serotonin Syndrome

Concern regarding the potential occurrence of serotonin syndrome has been heightened with the increasing number of serotonergic agents being employed in the treatment of obesity, depression, and migraine. The serotonin syndrome is defined by a spectrum of symptoms that develop coincidentally with the administration of multiple serotonergic agents (123). Excess peripheral and central serotonergic stimulation may be involved, leading to a constellation of symptoms (124). Specific diagnostic criteria include the presence of at least three of the following symptoms: fever, shivering, confusion, agitation, tremor, ataxia, hyperreflexia, sweating, or diarrhea. Although the syndrome is generally mild, severe episodes can include seizures, dyspnea, hypotension, hypertension, arrhythmias, renal failure, disseminated intravascular coagulation, and death.

Serotonin syndrome occurs most commonly in patients consuming combinations of serotonergic agents. The largest number of reported cases center around MAO inhibitors taken concurrently with SSRIs, dextromethorphan, meperidine, and tricyclic antidepressants (123). Case reports also include combinations of SSRIs with tryptophan, lithium, pentazocine, and dextromethorphan. Sumatriptan, a popular therapy for migraine, has been linked to syndrome development in a small number of patients who were also receiving an SSRI (125). Interestingly, this review compiled a number of cases of SSRI-sumatriptan and MAO inhibitor-sumatriptan use without problems. No information regarding the safety of sumatriptan and noradrenergic or serotonergic obesity therapies was given. The apparent unpredictable nature of combination serotonergic therapy dictates extreme caution in these polypharmacy situations.

Evaluation of Therapeutic Outcomes

Figure 9.1 depicts an approach to determining appropriate types of treatment for the overweight/obese individual based on the guidelines outlined in the NIH report (126).* The decision to treat any overweight/obese patient is dependent upon the degree and distribution of obesity present, the motivation of the patient to lose weight, and the potential benefits and risks of weight loss. Pharmacotherapy should only be considered after at least 6 months of lifestyle intervention have been attempted without meeting goals. Under these circumstances, pharmacotherapy may be appropriate for carefully selected overweight individuals with BMI $\geq$ 27 kg/m^2 and those with BMI $\geq$ 30 kg/m^2 with or without weight-related, immediate life-threatening medical conditions. From the health care professional perspective, drug therapy for obesity should always be considered as a supplement to an integrated program of diet, exercise, and behavior modification (including group support). A complete medical and medication history is essential in determining appropriate obesity drug therapy. Consideration must be given to alcohol, nicotine, caffeine, and herbal or food supplement use as well as prescription and nonprescription drugs.

Specific weight goals should be established that are consistent with medical needs and patient personal desire. For most obese patients, a weight-loss goal of 5% to 10% to no more than 30% of initial weight is reasonable. An average rate of weight loss after the first month of therapy is around 1 lb/wk. Patients should not be allowed to attain weight less than their estimated ideal weight. Assessment of patient progress should be documented in a health care setting once or twice monthly for 1 or 2 months, then monthly thereafter (19). Each encounter should document weight, waist circumference, BMI, blood pressure, medical history, and patient assessment of obesity medication tolerability (19). Chronic use of obesity medications should be consistent

---

*Though based on the NIH guidelines, Figure 9.1 incorporates recommendations of the authors. Figure 9.1 itself was not created by the NIH and is therefore not necessarily identical to its proposed guidelines.—EDITOR

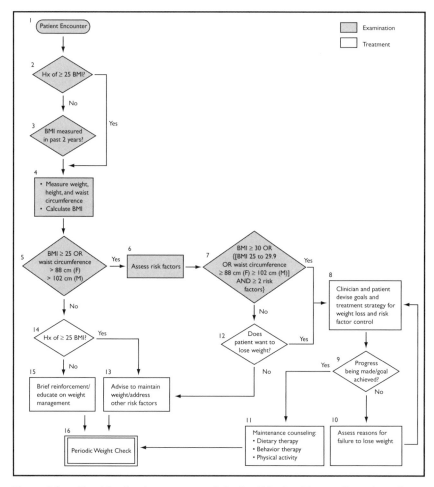

Figure 9.1   Algorithm for the treatment of obesity. This algorithm applies only to the assessment of obesity and subsequent decisions based on that assessment. It does not reflect any initial overall assessment for other conditions and diseases that the physician may wish to make.

with approved product labeling. Medication therapy should be discontinued after 3 to 4 months if the patient has failed to demonstrate weight loss or maintenance of prior weight. In fact, most labeling instructions indicate that re-evaluation should occur if the patient does not achieve an average weight loss of 1 lb/wk in the first month of therapy. Per the NIH report, recommended follow-up is within the first 2 weeks, monthly for 3 months, then quarterly for the first year. However, as always, clinical judgement on a case-by-case basis should be invoked, particularly in patients with co-morbidities.

Even in lower risk patients, regular follow-up is crucial to assist the patient in sustaining weight loss.

The recent AACE/ACE statement on obesity provides a patient evaluation checklist, a validated survey of general well-being, and sample informed consent forms that can be used in the screening and follow-up of patients receiving obesity pharmacotherapy as part of a weight loss program (19). The Short Form 36 (SF-36) has also been used as a quality-of-life evaluation tool for obese patients undergoing programmatic weight loss. Quarterly assessments of well-being and quality of life using validated assessment tools can be helpful in objectively quantifying the effectiveness of therapy as well as potential drug-induced side effects (e.g., depression) (19).

Patients with diabetes who are receiving weight loss medication require more intensive medical monitoring, and self-monitoring of blood glucose that also involves an endocrinologist, a registered dietician, and/or diabetes educator should be considered. Some centrally acting weight loss agents, such as the serotonergic agents, have direct effects that immediately improve glucose tolerance, even before significant weight loss. Insulin therapy may therefore need to be adjusted with the start of obesity medication therapy. Peripherally active agents, such as orlistat, have also been shown to decrease oral hypoglycemic agent requirements in type 2 diabetic patients (92). However, this effect was noted later on in therapy and more directly correlated with weight loss. Some diabetic patients may require daily telephone contact with a health-care provider to assist in adjusting their hypoglycemic therapy. Weekly patient visits to a health care setting may be necessary for 1 or 2 months until the effects of diet, exercise, and weight loss medication become more predictable. Assessment of hemoglobin A_{1c} as frequently as every 3 months may be appropriate in weight-losing patients with type 2 diabetes to aid in adjustment of hypoglycemic therapy. Lipid profiles can normalize or improve with weight loss. Lipid status should be assessed semi-annually or annually in patients with hyperlipidemia to determine the need for continued hyperlipidemia therapies. Weight loss can also result in normalization of blood pressure in hypertensive obese patients. Assessment of appropriateness of antihypertensive therapy should occur with each follow-up visit. (See Chapter 4 for contraindications to weight loss in patients with type 2 diabetes mellitus.)

Pharmacoeconomic Considerations

There are few data regarding economic consequences of treating obesity. One study evaluated the savings in prescription costs following a 12-week weight reduction program in 40 type 2 diabetic patients (127). Patients lost an average of 33.7 lb over the study period. A cost analysis was completed on 32 of 40 patients who were taking antihypertensive and/or antidiabetic medications using the out-of-pocket costs for these medications at the beginning of the study and after one year. The patients sustained a mean weight loss of 19.8 lb over the next year. The average cost of these prescriptions at the beginning compared with the 1-year follow-up was $63.30 versus $32.50 per month. The estimated annual average saving in prescription costs per patient was $443. A recent study confirmed these findings and extended them to demonstrate significant savings for obese patients with hyperlipidemia and cost-neutral for hypertension (128).

Money magazine caught consumer eyes with a 1997 article entitled, "Shrink Your Weight While Keeping Your Wallet Plump" (129). This analysis evaluated out-of-pocket expenses per pound lost for several different diet options including Weight Watchers, Ultra Slim Fast, Redux (dexfenfluramine), Jenny Craig, and Optifast. Jenny Craig costs included purchase of food products, and Redux and Optifast costs included physician monitoring. Weight Watchers and Ultra Slim fast were lowest at $8 to $9 per pound lost, whereas Jenny Craig and Optifast came in high at $59 and $84, respectively, per pound lost. Redux fell in the middle at $28 per pound lost. Cost of side effects, quality-of-life parameters, and probability of long-term weight loss with the various products/services were not included in this analysis.

Martin and colleagues compared the costs associated with medical and surgical treatment of obesity (130). Medical therapy groups received diet therapy only (no medications), and cost included weekly clinic visits for behavioral modification. A successful outcome was defined as loss of at least one third of excess body weight above ideal body weight. Patients were monitored for 2 years, some for as long as 7 years, so long-term weight control could be addressed. As expected, the costs of surgery were much higher than medical therapy over the first two years ($24,000 versus $3000). However, when costs were extrapolated to 6 years, the cost per pound lost for medical therapy exceeded surgical therapy (about $313 versus $261 per pound lost).

It is clear from these data that weight loss can be expensive for the consumer. Prospectively designed cost-benefit or cost-effectiveness analyses are needed to determine if costs of weight loss therapy or surgery are balanced by lower costs of hospitalizations for other medical problems associated with obesity or the additional life-years gained. Quality-of-life measures also need to be taken into consideration when evaluating this type of data.

Conclusion

It is clear that obesity is a lifelong condition. Currently, orlistat is the only pharmacotherapy available in the United States that has been demonstrated to be effective, for up to 2 years in selected patients. Longer-term results will require further research. Weight regain occurs in most individuals regardless of the therapeutic modalities used. Nevertheless, in recent years increasingly effective treatments have been developed. Pharmacotherapy can augment the role of lifestyle changes and diet and therefore serve a useful role in weight treatment therapy.

■ ■ ■

Key Points

- The agents most commonly used in the pharmacologic treatment of obesity include noradrenergic agents, serotonergic agents, noradrenergic/serotonergic agents, lipase inhibitors, and peptides.
- Serotonergic agents reduce appetitie and/or increase satiety without the central stimulant effects and abuse potential associated with noradrenergic agents.
- Lipase inhibitors cause weight loss by lowering dietary fat absorption.
- Herbal therapies are not held to the same FDA efficacy and safety standards as prescription medication. Therefore the quality and potency of such products are highly variable and do not necessarily reflect the content shown on the label. Herbal preparations should generally be avoided in patients with diabetes, hypertension, and cardiovascular disease.
- Severe adverse effects have occurred with the use of some appetite suppressants, with the most serious including primary pulmonary hypertension, cardiac valvulopathy, and serotonin syndrome.
- Pharmacologic therapy for obesity should always be used in conjunction with nutritional intervention, an exercise program, and behavioral treatment. Drug therapy should be considered only after the patient has not met weight loss goals after 6 months of lifestyle intervention strategies.

■ ■ ■

REFERENCES

1. **Baez M, Kursar JD, Helton LA, et al.** Molecular biology of serotonin receptors. Obes Res. 1995;3(Suppl 4):441S-447S.
2. **Bloom FE.** Neurotransmission and the central nervous system. In: Goodman and Gilman's The Pharmacologic Basis of Therapeutics. Hardman JG, Gilman AG, Limbird LE, eds. New York: McGraw-Hill; 1996:267-93.

3. **Caro JF, Sinha MK, Kolaczynski JW, et al.** Leptin: the tale of an obesity gene. Diabetes. 1996;45:1455-62.

4. **Misra A, Garg A.** Leptin: its receptor and obesity. J Investig Med. 1996;44:540-8.

5. **Giacobino JP.** Role of the beta-3 adrenoceptor in the control of leptin expression. Horm Metab Res. 1996;28:633-7.

6. **Considine RV, Sinha MK, Heiman ML, et al.** Serum immunoreactive-leptin concentrations in normal-weight and obese humans. N Engl J Med. 1996;334:292-5.

7. **Barinaga M.** New appetite-boosting peptides found. Science. 1998;279:1134.

8. **Woods SC, Seeley RJ, Porte DJ, Schwartz MW.** Signals that regulate food intake and energy homeostasis. Science. 1998;280:1378-83.

9. **Garrow JS.** Energy Balance and Obesity in Man. New York: Elsevier/North Holland Biomedical Press; 1978.

10. **Lowell BB, Flier JS.** Brown adipose tissue, beta-3 adrenergic receptors, and obesity. Annu Rev Med. 1997;48:307-16.

11. **Vidal-Puig A, Solanes G, Grujic D, et al.** UCP3: an uncoupling protein homologue expressed preferentially and abundantly in skeletal muscle and brown adipose tissue. Biochem Biophys Res Commun. 1997;235:79-82.

12. **Liu YL, Toubro S, Astrup A, Stock MJ.** Contribution of beta-3 adrenoceptor activation to ephedrine-induced thermogenesis in humans. Int J Obes Relat Metab Disord. 1995;19:678-85.

13. **Large V, Hellstrom L, Reynisdottir S, et al..** Human beta-2 adrenoceptor gene polymorphisms are highly frequent in obesity and associate with altered adipocyte beta-2 adrenoceptor function. J Clin Invest. 1997;100:3005-13.

14. **Clement K, Vaisse C, Manning BS, et al.** Genetic variation in the beta-3 adrenergic receptor and an increased capacity to gain weight in patients with morbid obesity. N Engl J Med. 1995;333:352-4.

15. **Bray GA.** Use and abuse of appetite-suppressant drugs in the treatment of obesity. Ann Intern Med. 1993;119:707-13.

16. **Cerulli J, Lomaestro BM, Malone M.** Update on the pharmacotherapy of obesity. Ann Pharmacother. 1998;32:88-102.

17. **Drent ML, van der Veen EA.** Lipase inhibition: a novel concept in the treatment of obesity. Int J Obes Relat Metab Disord. 1993;17:241-4.

18. **National Task Force on the Prevention and Treatment of Obesity.** Long-term pharmacotherapy in the management of obesity. JAMA. 1996;276:1907-15.

19. **Bray GA.** AACE/ACE Obesity Statement. Endocr Pract. 1997;3:163-208.

20. **Connolly HM, Crary JL, McGoon MD, et al.** Valvular heart disease associated with fenfluramine-phentermine. N Engl J Med. 1997;337:581-8.

21. **Graham DJ, Green L.** Further cases of valvular heart disease associated with fenfluramine-phentermine. N Engl J Med. 1997;337:635.

22. **Khan MA, Herzog CA, St Peter JV, et al.** The prevalence of cardiac valvular insufficiency assessed by transthoracic echocardiography in obese patients treated with appetite-suppressant drugs. N Engl J Med. 1998;339:713-8.

23. **Noach EL.** Appetite regulation by serotoninergic mechanisms and effects of D-fenfluramine. Neth J Med. 1994;45:123-33.

24. **Silverstone T.** Appetite suppressants: a review. Drugs. 1992;43:820-36.

25. **Dawson JK, Earnshaw SM, Graham CS.** Dangerous monoamine oxidase inhibitor interactions are still occurring in the 1990s. J Accid Emerg Med. 1995;12:49-51.

26. **Lasagna L.** Safety. In: Phenylpropanolamine: A Review. Lasagna L, ed. New York: John Wiley & Sons; 1988;191-300.

27. **Valle-Jones JC, Brodie NH, O'Hara H, et al.** A comparative study of phentermine and diethylpropion in the treatment of obese patients in general practice. Pharmatherapeutica. 1983;3:300-4.

28. **Truant AP, Olon LP, Cobb S.** Phentermine resin as an adjunct in medical weight reduction: a controlled, randomized, double-blind prospective study. Curr Ther Res Clin Exp. 1972;14:726-38.

29. **Angel I.** Central receptors and recognition sites mediating the effects of monoamines and anorectic drugs on feeding behavior. Clin Neuropharmacol. 1990;13:361-91.

30. **Amdisen A.** Lithium and drug interactions. Drugs. 1982;24:133-9.

31. **Sanders M, Breidahl H.** The effect of an anorectic agent (mazindol) on control of obese diabetics. Med J Aust. 1976;2:576-7.

32. **Nishikawa T, Iizuka T, Omura M, et al.** Effect of mazindol on body weight and insulin sensitivity in severely obese patients after a very-low-calorie diet therapy. Endocr J. 1996;43:671-7.

33. **American Medical Association.** Drugs Used in Obesity. 1995;2439.

34. **Wellman PJ.** Overview of adrenergic anorectic agents. Am J Clin Nutr. 1992;55: 193S-198S.

35. **Alger S, Larson K, Boyce VL, et al.** Effect of phenylpropanolamine on energy expenditure and weight loss in overweight women. Am J Clin Nutr. 1993;57:120-6.

36. **Lasagna L.** Basic pharmacology. In: Phenylpropanolamine: A Review. Lasagna L, ed. New York: John Wiley; 1988;84-190.

37. **Lake CR, Gallant S, Masson E, Miller P.** Adverse drug effects attributed to phenylpropanolamine: a review of 142 case reports. Am J Med. 1990;89:195-208.

38. **Greenway FL.** Clinical studies with phenylpropanolamine: a meta-analysis. Am J Clin Nutr. 1992;55:203S-205S.

39. **Lake CR, Rosenberg DB, Gallant S, et al.** Phenylpropanolamine increases plasma caffeine levels. Clin Pharmacol Ther. 1990;47:675-85.

40. **Kernan WN, Viscoli CM, Brass LM, et al.** Phenylpropanolamine and the risk of hemorrhagic stroke. N Engl J Med;.2000;343:1826-32.

41. **United States Food and Drug Administration, DoODP.** March 9, 1993. Docket #81N-0022; OTC Weight Control Drug Products for Human Use; Comment #LET86. Docket #81N-0022; OTC Weight Control Drug Products for Human Use; Comment #LET86.

41a. FDA Paper on Phenylpropanolamine (PPA); 11/6/00.

41b. Public Health Advisory. Subject: Safety of Phenylpropanolamine (PPA); 11/6/00.

41c. Science Background Statement on Safety of Phenylpropanolamine (PPA); 11/6/00.

42. **Astrup A, Breum L, Toubro S.** Pharmacological and clinical studies of ephedrine and other thermogenic agonists. Obes Res. 1995;3(Suppl 4):537S-540S.

43. **Dulloo AG.** Ephedrine, xanthines and prostaglandin-inhibitors: actions and interactions in the stimulation of thermogenesis. Int J Obes Relat Metab Disord. 1993;17(Suppl 1):S35-S40.

44. **Dulloo AG, Seydoux J, Girardier L.** Paraxanthine (metabolite of caffeine) mimics caffeine's interaction with sympathetic control of thermogenesis. Am J Physiol. 1994;267:E801-4.

45. **Dulloo AG, Seydoux J, Girardier L.** Potentiation of the thermogenic antiobesity effects of ephedrine by dietary methylxanthines: adenosine antagonism or phosphodiesterase inhibition? Metabolism. 1992;41:1233-41.

46. **Breum L, Pedersen LK, Ahlstrom F, Frimodt-Moller J.** Comparison of an ephedrine/caffeine combination and dexfenfluramine in the treatment of obesity: a double-blind multi-centre trial in general practice. Int J Obes Relat Metab Disord. 1994;18:99-103.

47. **Astrup A, Breum L, Toubro S, et al.** The effect and safety of an ephedrine/caffeine compound compared to ephedrine, caffeine and placebo in obese subjects on an energy restricted diet: a double-blind trial. Int J Obes Relat Metab Disord. 1992;16:269-77.

48. **Astrup A, Toubro S, Cannon S, et al.** Thermogenic synergism between ephedrine and caffeine in healthy volunteers: a double-blind, placebo-controlled study. Metabolism. 1991;40:323-9.

49. **Williams DM, Self TH.** Asthma products. In: Handbook of Nonprescription Drugs. Covington TR, Berardi RR, Young LL, eds. Washington, DC: American Pharmaceutical Association; 1996;157-77.

50. **Tietze KJ.** Cold, cough, and allergy products. In: Handbook of Nonprescription Drugs. Covington TR, Berardi RR, Young LL, eds. Washington, DC: American Pharmaceutical Association; 1996;133-56.

51. **Curzon G, Gibson EL, Oluyomi AO.** Appetite suppression by commonly used drugs depends on 5-HT receptors but not on 5-HT availability. Trends Pharmacol Sci. 1997;18:21-5.

52. **Brauer LH, Johanson CE, Schuster CR, et al.** Evaluation of phentermine and fenfluramine, alone and in combination, in normal, healthy volunteers. Neuropsychopharmacology. 1996;14:233-41.

53. **Weintraub M, Hasday JD, Mushlin AI, Lockwood DH.** A double-blind clinical trial in weight control: use of fenfluramine and phentermine alone and in combination. Arch Intern Med. 1984;144:1143-8.

54. **Weintraub M.** Long-term weight control: the National Heart, Lung, and Blood Institute funded multimodal intervention study [erratum appears in Clin Pharmacol Ther. 1992;52:323]. Clin Pharmacol Ther. 1992;51:581-5.

55. **Weintraub M, Sundaresan PR, Madan M, et al.** Long-term weight control study. I (weeks 0 to 34). The enhancement of behavior modification, caloric restriction, and exercise by fenfluramine plus phentermine versus placebo. Clin Pharmacol Ther. 1992;51:586-94.

56. **Weintraub M, Sundaresan PR, Schuster B, et al.** Long-term weight control study. II (weeks 34 to 104). An open-label study of continuous fenfluramine plus phentermine versus targeted intermittent medication as adjuncts to behavior modification, caloric restriction, and exercise. Clin Pharmacol Ther. 1992;51:595-601.

57. **Weintraub M, Sundaresan PR, Schuster B, et al.** Long-term weight control study. III (weeks 104 to 156). An open-label study of dose adjustment of fenfluramine and phentermine. Clin Pharmacol Ther. 1992;51:602-7.

58. **Weintraub M, Sundaresan PR, Schuster B, et al.** Long-term weight control study. IV (weeks 156 to 190). The second double-blind phase. Clin Pharmacol Ther. 1992;51:608-14.

59. **Weintraub M, Sundaresan PR, Schuster B, et al.** Long-term weight control study. V (weeks 190 to 210). Follow-up of participants after cessation of medication. Clin Pharmacol Ther. 1992;51:615-8.

60. **Weintraub M, Sundaresan PR, Cox C.** Long-term weight control study. VI. Individual participant response patterns. Clin Pharmacol Ther. 1992;51:619-33.

61. **Weintraub M, Sundaresan PR, Schuster B.** Long-term weight control study. VII (weeks 0 to 210). Serum lipid changes. Clin Pharmacol Ther. 1992;51:634-41.

62. **Weintraub M.** Long-term weight control study: conclusions. Clin Pharmacol Ther. 1992;51:642-6.

63. **Tuominen S, Hietola M, Kuusankoski M.** Double-blind trial comparing fenfluramine, phentermine and dietary advice on treatment of obesity. Int J Obes. 1980; 14:138.

64. **Hartley GG, Nicol S, Halstenson C, et al.** Long-term results from phentermine, fenfluramine, diet, behavior modification, and exercise for treatment of obesity [Abstract]. Obes Res. 1997;5:58S.

65. **Spitz AF, Schumacher D, Blank RC, et al.** Long-term pharmacologic treatment of morbid obesity in a community practice. Endocr Pract. 1997;3:269-75.

66. Cardiac valvulopathy associated with exposure to fenfluramine or dexfenfluramine: U.S. Department of Health and Human Services interim public health recommendations, November 1997. MMWR   Morb Mortal Wkly Rep. 1997;46:1061-6.

67. **Khan MA, St.Peter JV, Hartley GG, et al.** The effect of adding phentermine to weight management therapy in patients with declining response to dexfenfluramine alone [Abstract]. Obes Res. 1997;5:22S.

68. Fluoxetine (Prozac®) and other drugs for treatment of obesity. Med Lett Drugs Ther. 1994;36:107-8.

69. **Wadden TA, Bartlett SJ, Foster GD, et al.** Sertraline and relapse prevention training following treatment by very-low-calorie diet: a controlled clinical trial. Obes Res. 1995;3:549-57.

70. **Goldstein DJ, Rampey AHJ, Enas GG, et al.** Fluoxetine: a randomized clinical trial in the treatment of obesity. Int J Obes Relat Metab Disord. 1994;18:129-35.

71. **Goldstein DJ, Rampey AHJ, Roback PHJ, et al.** Efficacy and safety of long-term fluoxetine treatment of obesity: maximizing success. Obes Res. 1995;3(Suppl 4):481S-490S.

72. **Anchors M.** Fluoxetine is a safer alternative to fenfluramine in the medical treatment of obesity. Arch Intern Med. 1997;157:1270.

73. **Bostwick JM, Brown TM.** A toxic reaction from combining fluoxetine and phentermine. J Clin Psychopharmacol. 1996;16:189-90.

74. **St Peter JV, Khan MA, Singh AH, et al.** Case study of aortic valve insufficiency and selective serotonin reuptake inhibitor use [Abstract]. Circulation. 1999;100:I-519.

75. **Stock MJ** Sibutramine: a review of the pharmacology of a novel anti-obesity agent. Int J Obes Relat Metab Disord. 1997;21(Suppl 1):S25-S29.

76. **Danforth E Jr.** Sibutramine and thermogenesis in humans. Int J Obes. 1999;23:1007-8.

77. Sibutramine hydrochloride monohydrate (Meridia®). Product information. Knoll Pharmaceutical Company; 1997.

78. **Lean ME** Sibutramine: a review of clinical efficacy. Int J Obes Relat Metab Disord. 1997;21(Suppl 1):S30-S36.

79. **Apfelbaum M, Vague P, Ziegler O, et al.** Long-term maintenance of weight loss after very-low-calorie diet: a randomized blinded trial of the efficacy and tolerability of sibutramine. Am J Med. 1999;106:179-84.

80. **Bray GA, Ryan DH, Gordon D, et al.** A double-blind randomized placebo-controlled trial of sibutramine. Obes Res. 1996;4:263-70.

81. **Schwizer W, Asal K, Kreiss C, et al.** Role of lipase in the regulation of upper gastrointestinal function in humans. Am J Physiol. 1997;273:G612-20.

82. **Guerciolini R.** Mode of action of orlistat. Int J Obes Relat Metab Disord. 1997;21(Suppl 3):S12-23.

83. **Zhi J, Melia AT, Guerciolini R, et al.** Retrospective population-based analysis of the dose-response (fecal fat excretion) relationship of orlistat in normal and obese volunteers. Clin Pharmacol Ther. 1994;56:82-5.

84. **Hauptman JB, Jeunet FS, Hartmann D.** Initial studies in humans with the novel gastrointestinal lipase inhibitor Ro 18-0647 (tetrahydrolipstatin). Am J Clin Nutr. 1992;55:309S-313S.

85. **Guzelhan C, Odink J, Niestijl Jansen-Zuidema JJ, Hartmann D.** Influence of dietary composition on the inhibition of fat absorption by orlistat. J Int Med Res. 1994;22:255-65.

86. **Hussain Y, Guzelhan C, Odink J, et al.** Comparison of the inhibition of dietary fat absorption by full versus divided doses of orlistat. J Clin Pharmacol. 1994;34:1121-5.

87. **James WP, Avenell A, Broom J, Whitehead J.** A one-year trial to assess the value of orlistat in the management of obesity. Int J Obes Relat Metab Disord. 1997;21(Suppl 3):S24-30.

88. **Sjostrom L, Rissanen A, Andersen T, et al, for the European Multicentre Orlistat Study Group.** Randomised placebo-controlled trial of orlistat for weight loss and prevention of weight regain in obese patients. Lancet. 1998;352:167-72.

89. **Davidson MH, Hauptman J, Digirolamo M, et al.** Weight control and risk factor reduction obese subjects treated for 2 years with orlistat: a randomized controlled trial. JAMA. 1999;281:235-42.

90. **Hauptman J, Lucas C, Boldrin M, et al, for the Orlistat Primary Care Study Group.** Orlistat in the long-term treatment of obesity in primary care settings. Arch Fam Med. 2000;9:160-7.

91. **Rossner S, Sjostrom L, Noack R, et al, for the European Orlistat Obesity Study Group.** Weight loss, weight maintenance, and improved cardiovascular risk factors after 2 years treatment with orlistat for obesity. Obes Res. 2000;8:49-61.

92. **Hollander PA, Elbein SC, Hirsch IB, et al.** Role of orlistat in the treatment of obese patients with type 2 diabetes: a 1-year randomized double-blind study. Diabetes Care. 1998;21:1288-94.

93. **Tonstad S, Pometta D, Erkelens DW, et al.** The effect of the gastrointestinal lipase inhibitor, orlistat, on serum lipids and lipoproteins in patients with primary hyperlipidaemia. Eur J Clin Pharmacol. 1994;46:405-10.

94. **Drent ML, Larsson I, William-Olsson T, et al.** Orlistat (Ro 18-0647), a lipase inhibitor, in the treatment of human obesity: a multiple dose study. Int J Obes Relat Metab Disord. 1995;19:221-6.

95. **Melia AT, Koss-Twardy SG, Zhi J.** The effect of orlistat, an inhibitor of dietary fat absorption, on the absorption of vitamins A and E in healthy volunteers. J Clin Pharmacol. 1996;36:647-53.

96. **Leibowitz SF.** Brain peptides and obesity: pharmacologic treatment. Obes Res. 1995;3(Suppl 4):573S-589S.

97. Amgen announces leptin causes weight loss in humans and plans for two phase 2 trials. http://www.Amgen.com. 1997.

98. **National Research Council.** Trace elements. In: Recommended Dietary Allowances. Washington, DC: National Academy Press; 1998:195-246.

99. **Trent LK, Thieding-Cancel D.** Effects of chromium picolinate on body composition. J Sports Med Phys Fitness. 1995;35:273-80.

100. **Betz JM, Gay ML, Mossoba MM, et al.** Chiral gas chromatographic determination of ephedrine-type alkaloids in dietary supplements containing Ma Huang. J AOAC Int. 1997;80:303-15.

101. FDA proposes constraints on ephedrine dietary supplements. Am J Health Syst Pharm. 1997;54:1578.

101a. **Haller CA, Benowitz NL.** Adverse cardiovascular and central nervous system events associated with dietary supplements containing ephedar alkaloids. N Engl J Med. 2000;343:1833-8.

102. **Linde K, Ramirez G, Mulrow CD, et al.** St John's wort for depression: an overview and meta-analysis of randomised clinical trials. BMJ. 1996;313:253-8.

103. **Cott JM.** In vitro receptor binding and enzyme inhibition by *Hypericum perforatum* extract. Pharmacopsychiatry. 1997;30(Suppl 2):108-12.

104. **Bladt S, Wagner H.** Inhibition of MAO by fractions and constituents of *Hypericum* extract. J Geriatr Psychiatry Neurol. 1994;7(Suppl 1):S57-S59.

105. **Dulloo AG, Duret C, Rohrer D, et al.** Efficacy of a green tea extract rich in catechin polyphenols and caffeine in increasing 24-h energy expenditure and fat oxidation in humans. Am J Clin Nutr. 1999;70:1040-5.

105a. **Dulloo AG, Seydoux J, Girardier L, et al.** Green tea and thermogenesis: interactions between catechin-polyphenols, caffeine and sympathetic activity. Int J Obes. 2000;24:252-8.

106. **Kritetos AD, Thompson HR, Hill JO.** Hydroxycitric acid does not affect energy expenditure and substrate oxidation in adult males in a post-absorptive state. Int J Obes. 1999;23:867-73.

107. **Heymsfield SB, Allison DB, Vasseli JR, et al.** *Garcinia cambogia* (hydroxycitric acid) as a potential antiobesity agent: a randomized controlled trial. JAMA. 1998;280:1596-600.

108. **Guerciolini R, Radu-Radulescu L, Boldrin M, Moore R.** Fecal fat excretion induced by treatment with orlistat or chitosan: a 3-week randomized crossover design study. Obes Res. 2000;8:43S.

109. **Brenot F, Herve P, Petitpretz P, et al.** Primary pulmonary hypertension and fenfluramine use. Br Heart J. 1993;70:537-41.

110. **Thomas SH, Butt AY, Corris PA, et al.** Appetite suppressants and primary pulmonary hypertension in the United Kingdom. Br Heart J. 1995;74:660-3.

111. **Abenhaim L, Moride Y, Brenot F, et al.** Appetite-suppressant drugs and the risk of primary pulmonary hypertension. International Primary Pulmonary Hypertension Study Group. N Engl J Med. 1996;335:609-16.

112. **McCann UD, Seiden LS, Rubin IJ, Ricaurte GA.** Brain serotonin neurotoxicity and primary pulmonary hypertension from fenfluramine and dexfenfluramine: a systematic review of the evidence. JAMA. 1997;278:666-72.

113. **Chambers HF, Neu HC.** Penicillins. In: Principles and Practice of Infectious Diseases. Mandell GL, Bennett JE, Dolin R, eds. New York: Churchill Livingstone; 1995:233-46.

114. **Redfield MM, Nicholson WJ, Edwards WD, Tajik AJ.** Valve disease associated with ergot alkaloid use: echocardiographic and pathologic correlations. Ann Intern Med. 1992;117:50-2.

115. **Robiolio PA, Rigolin VH, Wilson JS, et al.** Carcinoid heart disease: correlation of high serotonin levels with valvular abnormalities detected by cardiac catheterization and echocardiography. Circulation. 1995;92:790-5.

115a. **Gardin JM, Schumacher D, Constantine G, et al.** Valvular abnormalities and cardiovascular status following exposure to dexfenfluramine or phentermine/fenfluramine. JAMA. 2000;283:1703-9.

116. **Weissman NJ, Tighe JFJ, Gottdiener JS, Gwynne JT.** An assessment of heart-valve abnormalities in obese patients taking dexfenfluramine, sustained-release dexfenfluramine, or placebo. Sustained-Release Dexfenfluramine Study Group. N Engl J Med. 1998;339:725-32.

117. **Choong CY, Abascal VM, Weyman J, et al.** Prevalence of valvular regurgitation by Doppler echocardiography in patients with structurally normal hearts by two-dimensional echocardiography. Am Heart J. 1989;117:636-42.

118. **Yoshida K, Yoshikawa J, Shakudo M, et al.** Color Doppler evaluation of valvular regurgitation in normal subjects. Circulation. 1988;78:840-7.

119. **Klein AL, Burstow DJ, Tajik AJ, et al.** Age-related prevalence of valvular regurgitation in normal subjects: a comprehensive color flow examination of 118 volunteers. J Am Soc Echocardiogr. 1990;3:54-63.

120. **Reid CL, Gardin JM, Yunis C, et al.** Prevalence and clinical correlates of aortic and mitral regurgitation in a young adult population: the CARDIA study [Abstract]. Circulation. 1994;90:I-282.

121. **Akasaka T, Yoshikawa J, Yoshida K, et al.** Age-related valvular regurgitation: a study by pulsed Doppler echocardiography. Circulation. 1987;76:262-5.

122. **Reginster F, Jadoul M, van Ypersele de Strihou C.** Chinese herbs: nephropathy, presentation, natural history and fate after transplantation. Nephrol Dial Transplant. 1997;12:81-6.

123. **Sporer KA.** The serotonin syndrome: implicated drugs, pathophysiology and management. Drug Saf. 1995;13:94-104.

124. **Brown TM, Skop BP, Mareth TR.** Pathophysiology and management of the serotonin syndrome. Ann Pharmacother. 1996;30:527-33.

125. **Gardner DM, Lynd LD.** Sumatriptan contraindications and the serotonin syndrome. Ann Pharmacother. 1998;32:33-8.

126. Executive Summary of the Clinical Guidelines on the Identification, Evaluation, and Treatment of Overweight and Obesity in Adults. Arch Intern Med. 1998;158:1855-67.

127. **Collins RW, Anderson JW.** Medication cost savings associated with weight loss for obese non-insulin-dependent diabetic men and women. Prev Med. 1995;24: 369-74.

128. **Greenway FL, Ryan DH, Bray GA, et al.** Pharmaceutical cost savings of treating obesity with weight loss medications. Obes Res. 1999;7:523-31.

129. Shrink your weight while keeping your wallet plump. Money. 1997;26:162-3.

130. **Martin LF, Tan TL, Horn JR, et al.** Comparison of the costs associated with medical and surgical treatment of obesity. Surgery. 1995;118:599-606.

10

■ ■ ■

Weight Loss Surgery

Lou-Ann Galibert, MD
John Kral, MD, PhD

Although surgical treatment of obesity can achieve significant sustained weight loss, it is just beginning to be widely accepted as a viable therapeutic option. This reluctance is due in part to the many complications of the early operations (intestinal bypass) and in part to the inherent invasiveness of surgery for a disease perceived often as a self-inflicted cosmetic condition rather than as a threat to health and longevity. Progress has been slow in not only educating the public but the medical community as well to accept obesity as a serious chronic disease, which in some cases requires surgery. Because there is no alternative method capable of sustaining medically meaningful weight reduction in the severely obese, and as minimally invasive techniques have become available, surgery is increasingly being considered as an option for treating obesity by the physician (to reduce comorbidities) and the patient (to improve quality of life).

Patient Selection

Case Study 1: Patient Selection for Weight Loss Surgery

Mrs Smith is 38 years old with a BMI of 38.2. She has mild hypertension controlled with a beta-blocker and was recently diag-

nosed with type 2 diabetes mellitus. She also is being treated with an SSRI for mild depression and has been on a stable dose and fully functional for 2 years. Her past attempts at weight loss have included participation in Weight Watchers on two occasions; she was able to maintain a BMI of 30 when an active participant and daily exerciser. After starting a family, however, it has been difficult for her to find time to maintain the program. Her use of an SSRI has precluded the use of centrally acting antiobesity agents, and a trial of orlistat under the supervision of her physician was not well tolerated. She is considering weight loss surgery.

Criteria

There are a number of accepted indications for surgical treatment of obesity, all based on weight. Historically, the primary criterion was a weight 100% in excess of life insurance standards for height. A slightly more liberal criterion is an excess weight of 45.5 kg (100 lb) above such standards. In an effort to standardize measurements, the 1991 National Institutes of Health Consensus Development Conference suggested use of a BMI > 40 kg/m² or a BMI > 35 kg/m² with comorbid conditions (Table 10.1) (1). The more comprehensive weight management report published by the NIH Obesity Education Initiative Expert Panel in 1998, which now supersedes the 1991 report in authoritativeness, includes guidelines for weight loss surgery supporting the earlier criteria (2). However, the 1998 report applies more stringent criteria to selecting patients for surgery. The Expert Panel recommends surgery be considered only "for carefully selected patients with clinically severe obesity (BMI > 40 kg/m² or BMI > 35 kg/m² with comorbid conditions) when less invasive methods of weight loss have failed and the patient is at high risk for obesity-associated morbidity or mortality". By inference, this recommendation proposes that at least 6 months of lifestyle intervention and, if unsuccessful, a trial of antiobesity medication (if not contraindicated) be tried before embarking on surgical intervention. Left unaddressed is whether patients with a BMI < 35 and comorbidities should be considered. This criterion has been recommended by some (3) and are an inclusion criterion for patients in the landmark Swedish Obesity Study (SOS) that is expected to study 10,000 patients assigned to either surgical intervention or control (lifestyle intervention) conditions (4). In fact, with the advent and anticipated approval of laparoscopic procedures that will minimize surgical risk, some have been so bold as to question whether a BMI > 30 might be a reasonable threshold for invasive intervention. The 1998 guidelines remain more cautious and conservative.

Because of its convenience as a unidimensional measure, BMI has become the accepted method for expressing relative weight. Although it is generally accurate for evaluating obesity, it has limited utility in assessing the

Table 10.1   Obesity-Related Conditions

Metabolic
  Diabetes
  Hypertension
  Dyslipidemia
  Infertility

Pulmonary
  Sleep apnea
  Obesity-related hypoventilation
  Pickwickian syndrome

Increased intraabdominal pressure
  Urinary incontinence
  Venous stasis disease
  Gastroesophageal reflux disease
  Pseudotumor cerebri

Osteoarthritis
  Spine
  Hips
  Knees

Cancer
  Colon
  Rectal
  Prostate
  Breast
  Uterine (cervical and endometrial)
  Ovarian
  Gallbladder
  Biliary tract

individual patient's risk for surgery. The goal of preoperative assessment is to identify pathologic conditions in order to optimize the patient's medical status. The Obesity Severity Index (Table 10.2) presents an attempt to stratify such risk and aid in selecting surgical candidates as well as allowing a more precise comparison of treatment results (5). However, the inherent risk from surgery using currently accepted procedures turns out to be quite low. Serious complications encountered in the postoperative period are rare (less than 10%) but include pulmonary embolism, wound infection, respiratory insufficiency, myocardial infarction, and death (less than 1%) (6).

Weight loss surgery has been shown to improve all comorbidities including, but not limited to, glucose intolerance, type 2 diabetes, dyslipidemia, hypertension, sleep apnea, and obesity-associated hypoventilation

Table 10.2   Obesity Severity Index

Male	1	Uncontrolled blood pressure	2
Age > 40 years	1	Cardiomegaly	2
Sleep apnea history	1	Smoker	2
Thromboembolism	1	Neck/thigh > 0.7	2
Diabetes	1	Hyperinsulinemia	2
Hemoglobin > 15 g/L	1	BMI: 28-31 = 1; 32-40 = 2; >40 = 3	
Pco_2 > 45 mm Hg	1		
		Maximum = 20 points	

(1, 2, 7). Moreover, preliminary data from the SOS study (4) have demonstrated a twofold to 32-fold decrease in the incidence of new-onset type 2 diabetes, hypertension, and hyperlipidemia 2 years into the study (8, 9); for diabetes, this continues to be true at 6 years (10). It is well recognized that the incidence, prevalence, and severity of these conditions increase with age and thus, given the outcomes of surgery, using age as a criterion is problematic. The increased mortality rate among the obese, which increases with duration of obesity and is more pronounced in those under 60 years of age, has been shown to revert toward normal levels with significant weight loss (11, 12). Whether individuals older than age 60 should be considered for surgery is questionable because there may not be an impact on prolonging long-term survival (3). However, age is not a criterion for most other surgeries and there is no question that weight loss surgery can be tolerated by older patients and result in improved quality of life (13). Setting a lower age limit for surgery is also a contentious issue; there is reluctance to use these procedures in children, adolescents, and, in some cases, young adults. Further research is needed to address this dilemma.

Screening and Risk Assessment

In general, screening and risk assessment procedures for weight loss surgery are similar to those conducted for any surgery requiring general anesthesia. However, there are certain facets of the assessment in the severely obese patient that may require special attention.

Secondary Causes
Under optimal circumstances the patient being evaluated for surgery has already had an evaluation by the nonsurgical physician (e.g., primary care physician, endocrinologist) for the rare reversible causes of obesity (e.g.,

Cushing disease). If not done previously, however, the surgeon should conduct the same type of evaluation as described in Chapter 5.

Psychological Assessment

In addition to being in optimal medical condition to undergo anesthesia, the consenting patient must be a fully informed, motivated adult with realistic expectations of projected weight loss as well as the ability to comply with the postoperative regimen. This regimen includes behavioral changes as well as lifelong monitoring and supplementation of certain vitamins and minerals, most notably vitamin B_{12}, folate, calcium, and iron (14). Unfortunately, research is inadequate to indicate how the general presurgical psychiatric and psychosocial profiles of a patient affect overall outcomes. The overwhelming majority of patients, of course, do quite well. Nevertheless, identifying psychologically appropriate patients for surgery is the most problematic component of the presurgical assessment process. What makes it difficult is the lack of good screening tools and predictors of who will adjust psychologically and do well long term. However, there are some "red flags" that warrant further evaluation.

Major Psychiatric Disorders

The prevalence of psychiatric disease, particularly depression, is no higher in moderately obese individuals than in the nonobese population; however, major depression is probably much higher in severely obese patients (15). Some serious psychiatric conditions, including major depression, active substance abuse, schizophrenia, and in some cases borderline personality disorder, can be serious and even life-threatening. In these situations, surgery is contraindicated unless the patient is well controlled, closely monitored, and has a postoperative treatment plan to continue managing the condition (3).

Ironically, the "Catch 22" with psychiatric illness is the propensity for weight gain caused by many psychotropic medications that make other noninvasive means of weight loss treatment ineffective and, in the case of some antiobesity medications, contraindicated due to potentially dangerous medication interactions. However, numerous studies indicate that well-controlled major depression has no effect on weight loss outcomes in the surgical patient (15). In contrast, new episodes of depression, including those leading to suicide, can occur postsurgically in any patient; unfortunately, there are no predictors to identify in whom this may occur (15).

Thus the overall approach to psychiatric illness is that if these individuals are stable and functional on medication, can give informed consent, and can carefully follow postoperative instructions, then psychiatric illness is not a basis for contraindication. Certainly input from a mental health professional is essential in making this decision. For those without a history of psychiatric illness, screening tools should be used (e.g., the Beck Depression Inventory (16)) along with general queries about the patient's psychological state as part of the comprehensive preoperative history and physical examination (as recommended in Chapter 5).

Binge-Eating Disorder

The prevalence of binge-eating disorder (BED) in obese patients is high (>30%) and is associated with a constellation of other psychological problems, including low self-esteem, anxiety, depression, and personality disorders (15). Some small studies suggest that this eating behavior persists after surgery and leads to poorer long-term outcomes (15). In the presurgical setting BED can be difficult to diagnose because some patients are so intent on having surgery that they are less than forthright about symptoms when queried. Some screening tools may be useful (e.g., the Eating Disorder Inventory (16)).

Psychopathology and Weight Loss

Although significant preoperative psychopathology predicts postoperative medical complications (17), the literature is divided over its effect on weight loss. The high prevalence of BED in obese persons and the poor outcomes associated with it, in conjunction with other common psychiatric problems that occur independently, argue in favor of every presurgical patient having a formal psychological evaluation. Because its cost-effectiveness is unknown, a formal psychiatric assessment is performed by many centers on an "as-needed" basis only.

Gastrointestinal Status

Gastrointestinal imaging should be considered in all symptomatic patients. Although a routine work-up is not mandatory, evaluation might prove helpful, especially in candidates for gastric bypass in which a portion of the GI tract will be excluded and virtually impossible to image after the procedure. Although formation of gallstones is a possible complication of any form of weight loss (18), routine removal of the gallbladder is not entirely without risk. The gallbladder should definitely be removed if the patient is symptomatic. In the era of open surgery, intraoperative evaluation and incidental cholecystectomy were easily performed. With the current trend towards minimally invasive surgery, unless intraoperative ultrasound is to be used, preoperative assessment of the biliary tract seems prudent.

Cardiac Status

The hyperdynamic circulation of obese patients as evidenced by cardiomegaly, increased cardiac output, and stroke volume increases their surgical risk (19, 20). An electrocardiogram should be performed on all patients preoperatively. A prolonged QT interval and evidence of left-ventricular hypertrophy are risk factors for sudden cardiac arrest (see discussion in Chapter 4 (20)). Further cardiac work-up (echocardiogram, perfusion scans, and/or stress testing) should be performed as indicated by physical examination, history, and plans for preoperative exercise. In all patients with a history of taking certain diet pills, an echocardiogram should be performed (see Chapter 9).

Pulmonary Status

A preoperative chest x-ray and arterial blood gas evaluation should be obtained for most patients consistent with the standards of practice for abdominal surgery of any kind. Pulmonary function testing and work-up for sleep apnea should be performed on high-risk patients (see Chapter 5).

Case Study 1: A Consideration

The patient in Case Study 1 appears to be an appropriate surgical candidate by the foregoing criteria. Mrs Smith has a BMI < 40 but has comorbidities. Although she suffers from depression, the condition is stable and most likely there has never been a major episode because such a severe condition would be difficult to control without the use of more powerful psychotropic agents. One essential element in her past treatment may be lacking, however—professional nutrition counseling. Weight Watchers is an effective program for many individuals that includes nutrition intervention and behavior therapy in the form of a support group. However, when individuals are not successful long-term, intervention with the help of a registered dietitian is indicated. This less-invasive therapy has yet to be tried in Mrs Smith's case and may be particularly useful in implementing orlistat therapy, a treatment whose effectiveness is tied to controlled fat intake. Moreover, although not necessarily credentialed as a behavior therapist, most dietitians use the basic components of behavior therapy that have proven to be useful for weight control. Although it is recognized that dietitian intervention is likely to fail long-term, it is important to indicate to Mrs Smith that the primary goal is to teach her more about meal planning and behavior skills that will be essential to a successful surgical outcome.

Recognized Procedures

Malabsorptive Procedures

Surgical therapy for obesity began in the 1950s with the introduction of jejunoileal bypass (21, 22). This procedure consisted of an anastomosis between the proximal jejunum and the distal ileum, bypassing virtually all of the approximately 650 cm of small intestine. In spite of many modifications of the exact lengths of intestine bypassed, this operation was abandoned due to its many complications including, but not limited to, cirrhosis, liver failure, arthritis, enteritis, anemia, interstitial nephritis, kidney stones, osteoporosis, diarrhea, vitamin and mineral deficiencies, and severe malnutrition (23). At present, the only intestinal bypass performed is for hyperlipidemia, in which only the last 200 to 250 cm of ileum is bypassed (24). This procedure should only be performed in specialized centers accustomed to dealing with specific postoperative care.

There are large numbers of patients who still have their jejunoileal bypass intact. As a general rule, they can be medically managed with close monitoring, dietary supplementation, antibiotics, and a low fat, high protein diet (18, 24). However, should surgical intervention be necessary for complications, another bariatric procedure should be performed to prevent the almost certain regain of weight. Other malabsorptive procedures include biliopancreatic diversion (BPD) and the duodenal switch modification, which is reputed to have fewer side effects than BPD with similar weight loss (25). Neither procedure is commonly practiced in the United States due to increased operative morbidity and mortality as well as a relatively high incidence of protein malnutrition.

Restrictive Procedures

In 1982 Mason described vertical banded gastroplasty (VBG), today the most commonly performed restrictive procedure (26). It consists of a vertically stapled pouch approximately 5 cm in length with the outlet restricted by a polypropylene band measuring 5 cm in circumference (Fig. 10.1, *A*).

In 1983 gastric banding for morbid obesity was introduced clinically by Bo and Modalsli (27), although it had been demonstrated to fail in animal experiments performed in 1974 (28). A silicone band is placed around the proximal stomach to create a small (15 to 30 cm^3) pouch with a restricted outlet. Like VBG, this is a purely restrictive procedure; however, it has the benefit of being completely reversible because neither stapling nor cutting of the stomach is performed. Initial results were poor, with a high incidence of late regain of weight and partial gastric outlet obstruction (6). In 1992 Kuzmak described an adjustable band connected to a subcutaneous injectable "well" similar to a chemoport (Fig. 10.1, *B*) (29). Saline may be injected or aspirated to decrease or increase the diameter of the new gastric outlet in accordance with the patient's food tolerance. The adjustable band has been placed laparoscopically in Europe and Australia since 1993 with promising results and is currently under FDA trial in the United States (30).

Combined Procedures

The gastric bypass was introduced in 1967 by Mason and Ito (31). Over the years it has undergone a number of modifications. A small gastric pouch (15

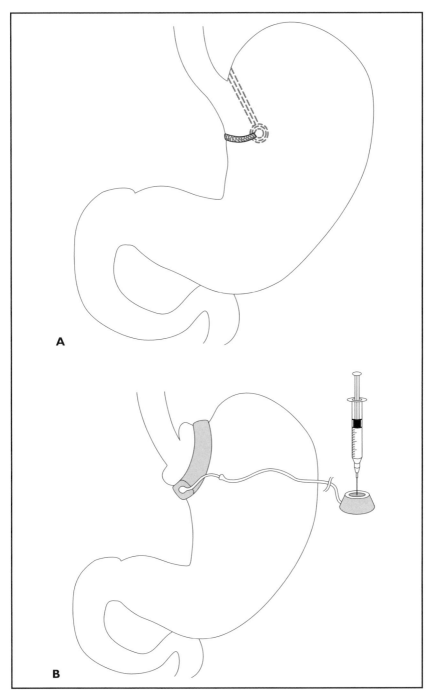

Figure 10.1   Gastric restrictive operations. *A,* Vertical banded gastroplasty. A 15 to 30 cm³ pouch is stapled off with the outlet restricted by a band 5 cm in circumference. *B,* Adjustable gastric banding. A 15 to 30 cm³ pouch is formed by placing a silicone band around the proximal stomach. The band is attached to a subcutaneous injectable port placed over the rectus muscle, through which the inner circumference may be adjusted.

to 30 cm³) is stapled off. A limb of small intestine 50 cm distal to the ligament of Treitz is brought up to maintain continuity of the gastrointestinal tract (Fig. 10.2, *A*). This operation functions by limiting the amount of food that may be ingested at one time as well as imposing a mild malabsorptive state. In the superobese patient (BMI > 50 kg/m²), a more malabsorptive procedure called a *distal gastric bypass* may be performed (Fig. 10.2, *B*).

Outcomes

Because the goals of therapy for severe obesity are significant weight loss maintained over time and the amelioration of comorbid conditions, these are the measures by which the various surgical procedures must be judged. A number of weight loss criteria have been proposed to standardize evaluation of surgical results (32). With all surgical procedures maximum weight loss occurs over the first 1 to 2 years, with gradual weight gain during the 2 to 5 years following surgery (1). Therefore it is important that patients be followed at least 5 years to properly evaluate the results of a procedure. Unfortunately not all authors are in agreement on the best method with which to evaluate outcomes, and the results are reported in the literature in a variety of ways. *Failure*, for example, has been defined as "regain to greater than preoperative weight" or, alternatively, "to 80% of preoperative weight".

Weight Loss

Vertical Banded Gastroplasty
An average loss of 50% of excess body weight is sustained at 5 years in patients undergoing VBG (18). Usually weight loss plateaus at about 12 months (33). However, 40% of patients will lose less than this amount or will start to regain weight. The main failure of this procedure is maladaptive eating behavior in which the patient ingests large quantities of liquid or "melting" high-calorie substances that pass directly through the restricted outlet. Other reasons for poor weight loss or weight regain include enlargement of the pouch and/or breakdown of the gastric staple line. Both complications are promoted by repeated ingestion of large amounts of insufficiently chewed solid food. Recent technical modifications have reduced the incidence of staple line disruption.

Gastric Bypass
Approximately 63% of excess body weight is lost in 90% of patients followed for greater than 5 years after gastric bypass (18). Weight loss plateaus between 12 to 18 months (33). This weight loss occurs through a number of mechanisms. The gastric restrictive portion limits the amount of solid food

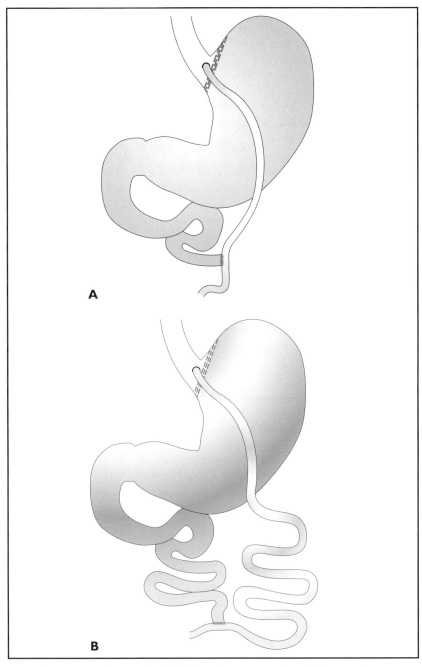

Figure 10.2 Gastric bypass. The shaded portion corresponds to the bypassed segment of the gastrointestinal tract. *A,* 15 to 30 cm³ blind pouch is stapled off. The jejunum is divided 50 cm distal to the ligament of Treitz. The distal limb is anastomosed to the gastric pouch, and the proximal limb is anastomosed 50 cm away. *B,* Distal gastric bypass. The jejunojejunostomy is performed 150 cm distal to the gastrojejunostomy, decreasing the length of the common channel.

that can be ingested at one time. There is mild-to-moderate malabsorption depending upon the amount of intestine that is bypassed. Food intake is also reduced by undigested food in the distal small intestine eliciting satiety and/or dumping through the release of gut neuropeptides (34-37).

Laparoscopic Procedures

There are few data on the 5-year follow-up results of laparoscopically placed adjustable gastric banding. A review of the literature reveals an approximate 60% reduction in excess weight at 2 years (38, 39). Some studies have shown a continuous (albeit slow) weight loss for up to 4 years (40). The laparoscopic procedure has been adapted to the Roux-en-Y gastric bypass as well, and short-term results are promising. A series of 275 patients followed for 1 to 31 months indicates that the subsets followed for 24 and 30 months have an excess weight loss of 83% and 77%, respectively (41).

Reduction in Comorbidities

Surgical therapy of severe obesity often has drastic effects on comorbid conditions. Some of the more commonly encountered comorbidities and their cure rates are discussed below.

Diabetes

Glucose and insulin levels can be normalized following both gastric bypass and restrictive procedures before any significant weight loss (7). It has been shown that following gastric bypass 83% of patients with type 2 diabetes mellitus will have normal blood glucose and glycosylated hemoglobin levels and 99% of patients with impaired glucose tolerance will be euglycemic (7).

Hypertension

From 66% to 75% of hypertensive patients become normotensive or display a significantly reduced need for antihypertensive medication following weight reduction surgery. This change does not require a large weight loss and occurs soon after surgery (42).

Sleep Apnea and Hypoventilation Syndrome

Five years postoperatively approximately 66% of patients with sleep apnea and 75% of those with hypoventilation syndrome will be asymptomatic (42). This effect is realized soon following surgery, but symptoms may return with relatively little regained weight after reaching a nadir.

Dyslipidemia

The major effect seen postoperatively on the lipid profile is a lowering of the triglycerides with a long-term increase in HDL.

Glucose Homeostasis

In a small study of morbidly obese women with preoperative normal glucose tolerance but low insulin sensitivity and compensatory hyperinsulinemia, postoperative weight loss to BMI < 25 normalized these parameters (compared with matched controls) (43).

Infertility

Weight loss may improve fertility but raises concerns of proper nutrition for the developing fetus. Large series of pregnancies following bariatric surgery have not demonstrated increases in neural tube defects; in fact, they have demonstrated improved safety for mother and child (44). There was, however, a higher miscarriage rate and incidence of premature delivery in pregnancies conceived during the rapid weight loss phase. Therefore reliable forms of birth control should be used during the first 1 to 2 years following surgery.

Psychological Outcome and Quality of Life

Overall, surgically induced weight loss substantially improves the patient's quality of life, particularly physical functioning, and is likely the most important factor motivating patients to seek surgical treatment of obesity. However, some studies now suggest that only short-term psychological gains are attained and that after 3 years much of the improvement dissipates (15). In fact, there is often an increase in interpersonal conflicts, particularly within a marital relationship, after surgery. If there are underlying psychosocial problems before surgery, the patient needs to understand that many of those issues will not be resolved by surgery because the overall environment in which the patient lives does not necessarily change simply because the patient had surgery. Thus it is important to reorient the patient's motivation to emphasize improved health and to encourage the patient to remain involved in support groups, and therapy if needed, to develop the social skills necessary for adjustment and lifelong success.

Complications

Case Study 2: Complications of Weight Loss Surgery

Mrs Smith (the patient discussed in Case Study 1) has surgery and an uneventful postoperative course. She is doing well until about 8 months postoperatively when, after having lost 50 lb, she begins to have frequent episodes of diarrhea associated with palpitations, diaphoresis, and nausea. Her weight has increased 10 lb in 2 weeks, and she returns to her physician for an evaluation.

Complications and Side Effects

A distinction must be made between complications and side effects of surgery. Side effects are expected, generally controllable (and sometimes helpful) results of surgery. Complications are neither expected nor desired. Mortality rates for the commonly performed surgical treatments of obesity are less than 0.5% in specialized centers (6, 45). Wound complications (incisional hernia, wound infection) can occur in approximately 20% of cases depending on the type of operation (24). Open gastric bypass, for example, has significantly more such complications than purely restrictive procedures. Wound complications are virtually eliminated by the laparoscopic approach. Peritonitis from gastrointestinal leak (anastomotic or iatrogenic perforation) occurs in 1% or 2% of cases (23). Symptomatic gallstones occur in approximately 10% of patients (6).

Vertical Banded Gastroplasty

The most commonly encountered side effect is vomiting, which is usually due to dietary indiscretion. If the patient is unable to identify the reason for vomiting (too high a volume or too rapid a rate) and is unable to tolerate liquids after 4 h of fasting, a mechanical complication should be considered. In addition, if vomiting begins occurring months after surgery, it should not be assumed the patient is overeating. Endoscopic evaluation may not only reveal the diagnosis but facilitate treatment (dilation of a stricture).

Failure of weight loss must be considered a complication, one that occurred in as many as 48% of patients in some series before introduction of certain technical modifications (6). Other than failure to lose weight, complications are low with this procedure (approximately 10%) and consist of band erosion, staple line disruption, gastroesophageal perforation (<0.5%), esophageal reflux, and rare nutritional deficiencies (18). Conversion to gastric bypass generally is successful in treating weight loss failure and reflux problems.

Gastric Bypass

The gastric bypass best illustrates the distinction between side effects and complications. If adjustments in eating habits are not adhered to, the side effect of overdistension of the gastric pouch will cause vomiting, which reduces oral intake. Ingestion of the wrong foods (i.e., high-calorie liquids or foods high in fat or carbohydrate) often causes dumping, considered a complication of Roux-en-Y gastrojejunostomy when performed for other indications, but a desired side effect after gastric bypass for obesity. This food intolerance generally consists of palpitations, diaphoresis, lightheadedness, and tachycardia. The most common complications are related to the incision (11% superficial infection, 4% deep infection, 7% to 20% hernia), the anastomosis (1% leak, 1% gastric staple line disruption, 13% marginal ulcer), or 2% deep vein thrombosis (6). Nutritional deficiencies (particularly calcium, vitamin B_{12} and iron) can become a problem if not properly monitored and prophylactically supplemented (14). Low levels of these micronutrients and minerals can be quite common, and clinical manifestations can occur in 12% to 25% of patients (33).

Laparoscopic Procedures

Although initial results of gastric banding were poor, the adjustable gastric band has shown good results. One European study found that most complications occurred within 11 months of surgery. There was a 13% reoperation rate, with most of the bands needing repositioning. Late complications included 5% pouch dilation and 8% stomach slippage. The complication rate dropped precipitously from 40% in the first 2 years to 4% subsequently (46). Another study showed a similar drop in complication rate (30% down to 2.5%) in the last 200 patients (40). This decrease corresponds to the learning curve as well as to improvements in the placement technique. Complications specific to this procedure include reservoir infection, band slippage, and leakage from the tubing (47). The experience with laparoscopic Roux-en-Y bypass is similar (41). Early major complications (within 30 days of the procedure) occurred in ~3% of patients, including peritonitis, abscess, small bowel obstruction, renal insufficiency, and pulmonary embolus (the latter resulting in death). Early minor complications (including atelectasis, gastrointestinal leak, wound infection, bleeding) occurred in 27% of patients. Late complications, such as prolonged nausea and vomiting and nutritional deficiencies, occurred in 47% of patients. Only three patients required a conversion to an open procedure. Within the series, as the procedure has been redefined, complication rates have fallen.

Preliminary Results from the Swedish Obesity Subjects Study

Because the SOS study is (and most likely will ever be) the largest single series on weight loss surgery, the preliminary results on complications warrant mention (9). The study uses a variety of procedures (gastric bypass, gastric banding, vertical banded gastroplasty) so the data reflect the combined complication/side effect rates. Postoperative mortality and complications are 0.12% and 13%, respectively. Two percent of patients suffering postoperative complications required re-operation during the initial hospitalization. Over the ensuing 4 years postoperatively, 22% required re-operation for repair or to convert to a more efficacious procedure to address weight loss failure.

Case Study 2: A Consideration

The patient in Case Study 2 requires a thorough evaluation. Mrs Smith's weight gain is a clear sign of a lapse. She also has symp-

toms consistent with the dumping-like syndrome that can occur with procedures that have a malabsorption component to their intended mechanism. Because these episodes of diarrhea have begun 8 months postoperatively, however, there is a high likelihood of dietary indiscretion that was not present earlier. High-calorie drinks, small chocolates, ice cream, and so on are foods typically eaten by patients that sabotage the effectiveness of these procedures. A more comprehensive examination and history are needed to ascertain 1) whether Mrs Smith truly has diarrhea and 2) whether there are other causes for her complaints. Nevertheless, it is highly likely that after a more thorough investigation it will be determined that she has lapsed and conceivably may be binging, a problem she carefully hid from those performing her original evaluation. It is imperative that both a dietitian and therapist be reintroduced into her care for further evaluation.

Conclusion

Surgery for the treatment of severe obesity and its attendant comorbidities is safe and effective. The increasing application of minimally invasive techniques and operations may modify the selection of both the patient and the procedure. The currently established indications may soon be expanded to include lower BMI levels, particularly in those patients with severe comorbid conditions. A multidisciplinary team is essential for preoperative assessment and long-term postoperative monitoring (1). A staged approach may be applied to surgical therapy. Most patients should initially be treated with the simplest, least invasive, and thus safest procedure. Those who fail to lose weight or who regain weight could be offered a more complex procedure.

In the final analysis, surgical therapy for severe obesity needs to be compared with medical treatment. To date, surgery is the only treatment that produces a significant sustained weight loss. In one study of costs in the United States, the cost/benefit ratio calculated as dollars per pound of weight lost favored surgery at five years (48). Especially in this current climate of fiscal restraint, surgery is likely to be considered more often in the treatment of severe obesity. Finally, given the employers' role in determining health care delivery and costs, it should be noted that recent evidence suggests that, after the year 1 postoperative disability cost increase expected with surgery, there is a significant reduction in sick days (up to 15%), which makes surgery an attractive benefit (49). Therefore there is substantial medical, economic, and social evidence that weight loss surgery is currently the most effective form of weight management and should be considered as a viable treatment for the severely obese patient.

◼ ◼ ◼

Key Points

- Weight loss surgery is the most effective form of weight management currently available, and the approved procedures are relatively safe in proper selected patients.

- The NIH has deemed that weight loss surgery is indicated in "carefully selected patients with clinically severe obesity (BMI > 40 kg/m^3 or BMI > 35 kg/m^3 with comorbid conditions) when less invasive methods of weight loss have failed and the patient is at high risk for obesity-associated morbidity or mortality".

- A multidisciplinary team approach is critical for appropriate patient selection, and lifelong medical monitoring, behavior support, meal planning, and exercise are essential for success.

- Vertical banded gastroplasty and gastric bypass are the only currently accepted procedures, but laparoscopic intervention will soon be feasible and widespread.

◼ ◼ ◼

REFERENCES

1. **NIH Consensus Development Conference.** Gastrointestinal surgery for severe obesity. Am J Clin Nutr. 1992;55(Suppl 2):487S-691S.
2. **NHLBI Obesity Education Expert Panel.** Clinical guidelines on the identification, evaluation, and treatment of overweight and obesity in adults: the evidence report. Bethesda, MD: National Institute of Health/National Heart, Lung, and Blood Institute. Report 98-4083. Sept. 1998; pp. 95-97.
3. **Balsiger BM, Murr MM, Poggio JL, Sarr MG.** Bariatric surgery: surgery for weight control in patients with morbid obesity. Med Clin North Am. 2000;84:477-89.
4. **Sjostrom L, Larsson B, Backman L, et al.** Swedish obese subjects (SOS): recruitment for an intervention study and a selected description of the obese state. Int J Obes. 1992;16:465-79.
5. **Kral JG.** Side-effects, complications and problems in antiobesity surgery: Introduction of the obesity severity index. In: Progress in Obesity Research. London: John Libbey;1996;7:655-61.
6. **Kellum JM, DeMaria EJ, Sugerman HJ.** The surgical treatment of morbid obesity. Curr Probl Surg. 1998;35:793-858.

7. **Pories WJ, Swanson MS, MacDonald KG, et al.** Who would have thought it? An operation proves to be the most effective therapy for adult-onset diabetes mellitus. Ann Surg. 1995;222:339-52.

8. **Sjostrom CD, Lissner L, Wedel H, Sjostrom L.** Reduction in incidence of diabetes, hypertension and lipid disturbances after intentional weight loss induced by bariatric surgery. The SOS Intervention Study. Obes Res. 1999;7:477-84.

9. **Ryan DH, Bray GA, Rossner S, Galasso GJ.** Conference Report - Obesity: New Directions, 27-29 June 1998, Charleston, South Carolina. Obes Res. 1999;7:303-8.

10. **Sjostrom CD, Lissner L, Sjostrom L.** Long-term effects of weight loss on hypertension and diabetes. SOS Intervention Study [Abstract]. Int J Obes. 1998;22:S78.

11. **Lew EA, Garfinkel L.** Variations in mortality by weight among 750,000 men and women. J Chronic Dis. 1979;32:563-76.

12. **Manson JE, Willett WC, Stampfer MJ, et al.** Body weight and mortality among women. N Engl J Med. 1995;333:678-85.

13. **Murr MM, Siadati MR, Sarr MG.** Results of bariatric surgery for morbid obesity in patients older than 50 years. Obes Surg. 1995;5:399-402.

14. **Kushner R.** Managing the obese patient after bariatric surgery: a case report of severe malnutrition and review of the literature. J Parenter Enteral Nutr. 2000;24:126-32.

15. **Hsu GLK, Benotti PN, Dwyer J, et al.** Nonsurgical factors that influence the outcome of bariatric surgery: a review. Psychosom Med. 1998;60:338-46.

16. **Food and Nutrition Board, National Institute of Medicine.** Assessment Instruments of Relevance to Obesity Treatment. Thomas PR, ed. Washington, DC: National Academy of Sciences; 1995;173-97.

17. **Valley V, Grace DM.** Psychosocial risk factors in gastric surgery for obesity: identifying guidelines for screening. Int J Obes. 1986;11:105-13.

18. **Kral JG.** Therapy of severe obesity. In: Gastroenterology. Philadelphia: WB Saunders; 1994:3231-9.

19. **Alexander JK.** The cardiomyopathy of obesity. Prog Cardiovasc Dis. 1995; 27:325-34.

20. **Kral JG.** Medical Management of the Surgical Patient. Philadelphia: JB Lippincott; 1995;415-23.

21. **Kremen AJ, Linner JH, Nelson CH.** An experimental evaluation of the nutritional importance of proximal and distal small intestine. Ann Surg. 1954;140:439-48.

22. **Payne JH, DeWind LT.** Surgical treatment of obesity. Am J Surg. 1969;118:141-7.

23. **Sugerman HJ, DeMaria EJ.** Mastery of Surgery. Boston: Little-Brown; 1997:982-91.

24. **Buchwald H.** Mastery of Surgery. Boston: Little-Brown; 1997:1358-65.

25. **Kral JG.** Surgical treatment of obesity. Clinical Obesity. 1998;545-63.

26. **Mason EE.** Vertical banded gastroplasty. Arch Surg. 1982;117:701-6.

27. **Bo O, Modalsli O.** Gastric banding, a surgical method of treating morbid obesity: preliminary report. Int J Obes. 1983;7:493-9.

28. **Wilkinson LH, Peloso OA.** Gastric (reservoir) reduction for morbid obesity. Arch Surg. 1981;116:602-5.

29. **Kuzmak LI.** Stoma adjustable silicone gastric banding. Probl Gen Surg. 1992;9:298-317.

30. **Belachew M, Legrand MJ, Defechereux TH, et al.** Laparoscopic adjustable silicone gastric banding in the treatment of morbid obesity: a preliminary report. Surg Endosc. 1994;8:1354-6.

31. **Mason EE, Ito C.** Gastric bypass in obesity. Surg Clin North Am. 1967;47:1345-51.

32. **Reinhold RB.** Late results of gastric bypass surgery for morbid obesity. J Am Coll Nutr. 1994;13:326-31.

33. **Benotti PN, Forse RA.** The role of gastric surgery in the multidisciplinary management of severe obesity. Am J Surg. 1995;169:361-7.

34. **Koopmans HS, Sclafani A.** Control of body weight by lower gut signals. Int J Obes. 1981;5:491-5.

35. **Naslund E, Gryback P, Backman L, et al.** Distal small bowel hormones: correlation to fasting antroduodenal motility and gastric emptying. Dig Dis Sci. 1998;43:945-52.

36. **Sirinek KR, O'Dorisio TM, Howe B, McFee AS.** Neurotensin, vasoactive intestinal peptide, and Roux-en-Y gastrojejunostomy. Arch Surg. 1985;120:605-9.

37. **Kellum JM, Kuemmerle JF, O'Dorisio TM, et al.** Gastrointestinal hormone responses to meals before and after gastric bypass and vertical banded gastroplasty. Ann Surg. 1990;211:763-71.

38. **Dargent J.** Laparoscopic adjustable gastric banding: lessons from the first 500 patients in a single institution. Obes Surg. 1999;9:446-52.

39. **Fielding GA, Rhodes M, Nathanson LK.** Laparoscopic gastric banding for morbid obesity. Surg Endosc. 1999;13:550-4.

40. **O'Brien PE, Brown WA, Smith A, et al.** Prospective study of a laparoscopically placed, adjustable gastric band in the treatment of morbid obesity. Brit J Surg. 1999;85:113-8.

41. **Schauer PR, Ikramuddin S, Gourash W.** Outcomes after laparoscopic Roux-en-Y gastric bypass for morbid obesity. Ann Surg. 2000;232:515-29.

42. **Kral JG.** Surgical treatment of obesity. In: Handbook of Obesity. Bray GA, Bouchard C, James WP, eds. New York: Marcel Dekker; 1997:977-93.

43. **Letiexhe MR, Scheen AJ, Gerard PL, et al.** Postgastroplasty recovery of ideal body weight normalizes glucose and insulin metabolism in obese women. J Clin Endocrinol Metab. 1995;80:364-9.

44. **Marceau P, Biron S, Hould FS, et al.** Outcomes of pregnancies after obesity surgery. In: Progress in Obesity Research. London: John Libbey; 1999:795-802.

45. **Yale CE.** Gastric surgery for morbid obesity: complications and long-term weight control. Arch Surg. 1989;124:941-6.

46. **Belachew M, LeGrand M, Vincent V, et al.** Laparoscopic adjustable gastric banding. World J Surg. 1998;22:955-63.

47. **Miller K, Hell E.** Laparoscopic adjustable gastric banding: a prospective 4-year follow-up study. Obes Surg. 1999;9:183-7.

48. **Martin LF, Tan TL, Horn JR, et al.** Comparison of the costs associated with medical and surgical treatment of obesity. Surgery. 1995;118:599-607.

49. **Narbo K, Agren G, Jonsson E, et al.** Sick leave and disability pension before after treatment for obesity: a report from the Swedish Obese Subjects (SOS) study. Int J Obes. 1999;23:619-24.

■   ■   ■

KEY REFERENCES

Hsu GLK, Benotti PN, Dwyer J, et al. Nonsurgical factors that influence the outcome of bariatric surgery: a review. Psychosom Med. 1998; 60:338-46.

Kellum JM, DeMaria EJ, Sugerman HJ. The surgical treatment of morbid obesity. Curr Probl Surg. 1998;35:793-858.

NIH Consensus Development Conference. Gastrointestinal surgery for severe obesity. Am J Clin Nutr. 1992;55(Suppl 2):487S-691S.

Pories WJ, Swanson MS, MacDonald KG, et al. Who would have thought it? An operation proves to be the most effective therapy for adult-onset diabete mellitus. Ann Surg. 1995;222:339-52.

11

■ ■ ■

Future Pharmacotherapy for Obesity: Integration of Metabolism and Body Weight Regulation

Jamie Dananberg, MD

History of Pharmacotherapy

For more than half a century, using pharmacotherapy in the treatment of obesity has met with varying degrees of success. The relative high failure rate was reflected in the historically very low proportion of health care dollars that were directed at pharmacotherapy relative to other treatment modalities. For example, in 1995 nearly $35 billion was spent in the United States on weight loss products and services such as diet foods and drinks (which accounted for ~$12 billion), exercise programs and equipment, and ancillary products. In the same year, roughly $500 million was spent on antiobesity pharmaceuticals. Although both perceived and real concerns over safety played an important role in limiting the use of pharmacotherapy, the mostly deserved reputation of limited overall efficacy has also greatly tempered enthusiasm for these agents.

There have been significant advances in the field of antiobesity pharmacotherapy since 1995. Both sibutramine and orlistat were approved for use in the treatment of obesity. Renewed interest in the sympathomimetic amine phentermine and other older agents such as mazindol, benzphetamine, and phendimetrazine surfaced just as fenfluramine and dexfenflu-ramine were withdrawn from the market over concerns of safety. None of these older agents, however, are FDA approved for use beyond the short term. Additionally, agents such as ephedrine, fluoxetine, and caffeine were studied for use in the treatment of obesity; none of these have been ap-proved for use by the FDA. Many of these compounds have only limited efficacy (1).

Research in the area of obesity treatment has clearly spotlighted the challenges facing the clinical development of new antiobesity drugs. First, all weight loss agents will be faced with the same apparent "counterregula-tory" mechanisms that impede weight loss by diet and exercise. In virtually all clinical trials, irrespective of treatment modality, weight loss reaches a plateau at 24 to 30 weeks. Perhaps owing to the power of counterregula-tion, weight invariably begins to rise from the plateau point through to the end of the study. Second, complicating all analyses of weight loss is the profound study effect on weight loss. Finally, dropout rates in clinical trials are exceedingly high, particularly in placebo arms. Given the true novelty of some of the targets chosen for drug development, there is growing ex-citement that new agents may overcome many of the shortcomings of their predecessors.

To appreciate the breadth of targets for which new pharmacotherapy is aimed is to understand the complexity of the physiologic regulation of weight and energy. Although our knowledge of discrete components of this regulation has exploded, our awareness of how these components piece together into an integrated regulatory system is still in its infancy. Presently, any number of efforts at drug discovery and development are aimed at the individual components of the weight homeostatic system. However, no single target is likely to be a panacea for obesity. More prob-able is that single or multiple agents affecting at two or more different but complimentary pieces of the regulatory machinary will have far greater im-pact on causing and maintaining real weight loss.

The different elements of the regulatory system controlling weight and energy homeostais can be subgrouped into signaling, integration, and ef-fector components. The signaling component involves sensory, somatic, and environmental messages that relay information regarding body compo-sition, energy balance, thermogenesis, and food availability. In addition, those signaling entities can be further grouped into lipostatic, glucostatic, and satiety signals (Fig. 11.1). Integration components are those peptides, receptors, and more generally, circuits within the central nervous system (CNS) that "interpret" the rich afferent source of signals. Finally, the CNS utilizes the effector components to elicit a response to protect or change weight and energy status. New pharmacologic targets to treat disorders of weight can be found in all three areas.

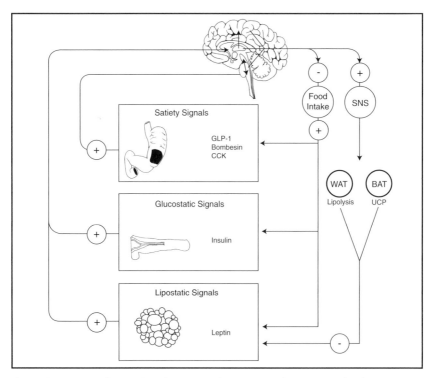

Figure 11.1   Signaling entities: lipostatic, glucostatic, and satiety signals. These signaling components, along with the integration and effector components, comprise the regulatory system controlling weight and energy homeostasis. (From Dananberg J, Caro J. Obesity. In: DeGroot LJ, Jamesone JL, eds. Endocrinology. Philadelphia: WB Saunders; 2001:615-30; with permission.)

Signaling Components

Lipostatic Signals

The regulation of body weight requires an integrated system of communication between the storage compartment and the regulatory compartment. White adipose tissue (WAT) comprises the major site for long-term energy storage in the form of triglycerides. Transmitting information regarding the relative amount of WAT was shown to be dependent on the hormone leptin (2). Leptin is the protein product of the *ob* gene, the deficiency of which was shown to be the etiology for obesity in the *ob/ob* mouse (2). The most important support for the role of leptin in regulating weight in man is the occurrence of genetic defects within the leptin-signaling pathway in two families (3, 4).

Leptin as a Therapeutic Target

The discovery of leptin held out great promise for a potential target at which to direct pharmacotherapy. However, the observation that leptin levels rise and fall with weight and reach very high levels in obese patients (5) led to the conclusion that most patients with obesity are resistant to the effects of leptin. There appears to be no major leptin receptor defect accounting for this level of resistance (6). Therefore resistance to leptin action appears related to 1) an inability of higher leptin concentrations to penetrate the blood-brain barrier to signal to a normally functioning receptor, or 2) a post-receptor signaling defect in patients with obesity, or 3) a combination of these. A trial of recombinant leptin at approximately 300 mg/day by subcutaneous injection in humans of up to 6 months achieved a significant decrease from initial weight of ~8 kg compared with the placebo effect of a decrease of ~2 kg (7). In a follow-up statement regarding this work, no significant effects on weight were achieved overall; however, a subset of patients did achieve a response that could be the subject of further investigation (8).

The leptin receptor is a member of the cytokine receptor superfamily. It has been speculated that other cytokines may alter feeding behavior and energy homeostasis through systems that may not be affected by those factors that induce leptin resistance. One such factor, ciliary neurotrophic factor (CNTF), which was effective in a leptin-resistant form of rodent obesity (9), is being explored as a treatment.

Fatty Acid Synthase

Fatty acid synthase (FAS) is an enzyme that facilitates the synthesis of long-chain fatty acids from acetyl-coenzyme A and malonyl-coenzyme A by adding the 2-carbon malonyl CoA fragments to the growing fatty acid chain. Recently, a compound (C75) was identified that could inhibit FAS and caused weight loss in mice without a reduction in metabolic rate (10). The studies also suggested that malonyl CoA may serve as an important signal generated in the periphery that suppresses appetite through suppression of NPY but through a mechanism independent of leptin. Further studies are needed to determine the efficacy and safety of this compound for treating obesity in humans.

Glucostatic Signals

Although insulin clearly plays a role in systemic fuel utilization, there are also data supporting its activity within the CNS to regulate energy homeostasis. There is evidence for insulin-regulated glucose metabolism within ventromedial hypothalamus neurons that may regulate autonomic outflow and, subsequently, metabolic rate in humans (11) and in animal models

(12, 13). Because insulin plays such a central role in glucose and lipid metabolism, target discovery in this area is difficult and may rely less on insulin than on the signaling pathways through which insulin acts.

Satiety Signals

Cholecystokinin

Among the earliest satiety factors identified was the gut peptide cholecystokinin (CCK) that dose-dependently regulated meal size in rats (14) and in baboons (15). The importance of CCK in the regulation of appetite and food intake was further established with the use of selective antagonists. Whereas CCK reduced meal intake by nearly half, a selective antagonist completely reversed this suppression. By itself, the CCK antagonist was able to increase food intake by approximately one-third (16).

Bombesin Family

Several factors have been identified that may play a role in meal size regulation, including the bombesin family of molecules. These molecules include bombesin, gastrin-releasing peptide, neuromedin C, and neuromedin B, all of which are able to suppress food intake. These molecules appear to act through a family of receptors, which have been initially grouped as neuromedin C preferring and gastrin-releasing peptide preferring (17-19).

Incretins

Another family of gastrointestinal peptides are the incretins. These peptides, secreted by enteroendocrine cells of the large and small intestine, were first identified as being responsible for the incremental release of insulin that occurs following oral administration of glucose relative to that following an equivalent amount of glucose administered intravenously (20, 21). The most studied of the family members are glucose-dependent insulinotropic peptide (GIP) (22) and glucagon-like peptide 1 (GLP-1). Intracerebroventricular administration of GLP-1 significantly decreased food and water intake (22). It was shown that many of these peripheral satiety factors signal the brain via afferent nerves or by acting as circulating factors that interact with specific receptors in the brain (15, 23-25). However, chronic administration was not shown to significantly affect body weight (26).

Glucocorticoids

Although glucocorticoids have long been acknowledged to have profound effects on fat and muscle mass, it has been difficult to isolate the role they play in signaling in the CNS from peripheral metabolic effects. Other parts of the hypothalamic-pituitary-adrenal axis that may be more amenable to pharmacologic manipulation are discussed below.

Satiety Signals as Therapeutic Targets

Several of these peripherally circulating peptides have also generated some interest as potential primary or adjunctive therapies for obesity including cholecystokinin (CCK) (24), glucagon-like peptide (GLP-1) (27), and bombesin (28). These molecules may be helpful by altering the meal termination signal. The key question is whether these agents, by themselves, can help regulate weight, or whether they will serve more importantly as adjunctive therapy or weight maintenance therapy following effective weight loss by other means.

Integration Components

A number of orexigenic and anorexigenic signals within the brain have been identified. Many of the inputs to the brain integrate within the hypothalamus. This is underscored by the observation that mRNA for the functional long form of the leptin receptor has been identified in numerous nuclei throughout the hypothalamus including the arcuate nucleus (ARC), dorsomedial hypothalamus (DMH), paraventricular nucleus (PVN), ventromedial hypothalamus (VMH), and lateral hypothalamus (LH), ventral premammillary and medial mammillary nuclei, and lateral olfactory nucleus (29). The cross-talk within and between these nuclei, and even within single neurons, is only now being understood and systematically explored.

Orexigenic Signals

Neuropeptide Y

A characteristic of post-leptin-receptor signaling is the inhibition of neuropeptide Y (NPY). NPY is a neurotransmitter widely expressed throughout the brain. However, NPY neurons within the hypothalamus were shown to be an important part of regulating energy consumption and feeding behavior following the discovery of leptin. NPY is overexpressed in the leptin-deficient *ob/ob* mouse and in the leptin-receptor deficient *db/db* mouse (30, 31). Furthermore, NPY overexpression can be reversed by leptin administration in the *ob/ob* mouse but not in the *db/db* mouse (32). In normal animals, leptin administration to animals that have been fasted prevents the increase in hypothalamic NPY normally seen with food restriction (33, 34). NPY injected directly into the PVN of the hypothalamus causes a marked increase in food intake, weight, and body fat within 10 days in female rats (35). The metabolic changes induced by centrally administered NPY mimic those changes seen in obesity (36). Furthermore, centrally administered NPY reduces sympathetic nervous system efferent activity to brown adipose tissue (BAT) with a subsequent decrease in energy expenditure (37, 38).

In that NPY is among the most potent orexigenic peptides identified, selective blockade of NPY at the "feeding" receptor may decrease appetite and food-seeking behavior. Because the NPY-1 and NPY-5 receptors appear to be the most important subtypes with respect to feeding and weight regulation, several development programs are underway for identification of selective antagonists at these receptors. However, NPY is a component of an important feedback loop and experiments in transgenic animals suggest that the role of NPY in weight regulation and feeding behavior is complex. Mice deficient in NPY have normal body weight, feeding behavior, and body composition (39, 40). Furthermore, NPY-5 receptor knockout mice gain more weight, not less, between 12 and 20 weeks of age compared with heterozygous knockout or wild-type mice. This weight gain is associated with increased amounts of food consumption and fat pad weight (41). In the NPY-1 receptor knockout mouse weight is increased as well but is associated with decreases in energy expenditure during the active period and with no change in food intake compared with heterozygous knockout or wild-type mice (42). Therefore the relative importance of the NPY and the various NPY receptor subtypes will require additional work with more selective antagonists and transgenic animals with combinations of gene disruptions.

Melanin Concentrating Hormone

Melanin concentrating hormone (MCH) is a circulating peptide first discovered in chub salmon that regulates fish scale color by aggregating melanonosomes (43). It was implicated in weight homeostasis when MCH was identified in the hypothalamus of the *ob/ob* mouse by differential display polymerase chain reaction. Injection of MCH into the lateral ventricles causes an increase in food intake (44). Recently it has been shown that transgenic mice produced with targeted deletions of the MCH gene had lower body weight, hypophagia, and increased metabolic rate despite lower levels of both leptin and POMC mRNA within the arcuate nucleus (45). Interestingly, these mice had a hyperphagic response to starvation (45) similar to that seen in mice lacking expression of NPY (40).

Galanin

Galanin, a hypothalamic peptide found in abundance in the PVN, is associated with preference for dietary fat (46). Galanin expression is significantly upregulated by increases in dietary fat, more so in obese-prone strains than in obese-resistant strains (47). However, chronic central administration of galanin does not result in hyperphagia or obesity (48).

Orexins

Two closely related hypothalamic neuropeptides have been identified that also may play a role in weight homeostasis. Orexin-A and orexin-B (hypocretin-1 and -2, respectively), derived from the same parent precursor molecule, are upregulated with fasting. Central administration of either protein stimulates food intake (49).

Opiods

The proopiomelanocortin (POMC) polypeptide is the parent molecule of several peptides with potential weight regulating properties. Among those with orexigenic properties are the endogenous opioid peptides. Opioids have been known for years to stimulate appetite, but it was the identification of the endogenous opioid peptides β-endorphin, dynorphin A, and enkephalins that led to increased interest in this system as it relates to energy balance. Long-acting enkephalin analogues (possibly via the δ-opiod receptor), β-endorphin (possibly via the μ-opiod receptor), and dynorphin A (possibly via the κ-opioid receptor) have all been shown to increase feeding behavior (50, 51).

Orexigenic Signals as Therapeutic Targets

The newly discovered neuropeptides MCH and orexins as well as CRH, galanin, and opiod antagonists are all considered potential targets in the race to develop effective antiobesity agents. In addition to these novel peptides, there is ongoing work in the area of selective agonists of the 5-HT$_{2c}$ receptor subtype that may have a significantly better therapeutic index than any of the predecessor compounds to date.

Anorexigenic Signals

Proopiomelanocortin System

In addition to the opiod molecules that stimulate feeding behavior, the POMC polypeptide yields a number of anorexigenic molecules as well. α-Melanocyte-stimulating hormone (α-MSH) elicits effects that are opposed to the effects of NPY and MCH. The action of α-MSH is mediated through the melanocortin family of receptors, of which five have been identified. α-MSH activation of the melanocortin-4 (MC-4) receptor and possibly the MC-3 receptor appears to inhibit feeding behavior and increase energy expenditure as deduced from antagonist and gene knockout experiments. Agouti protein, a naturally occurring antagonist to all melanocortin receptors and normally produced only in skin, causes obesity when ectopically overexpressed in the brain of the yellow agouti (A^y) mouse (52). Furthermore, transgenic mice deficient in MC-4 receptor have a hyperphagic and obese phenotype (53). Finally, agouti-related protein (AGRP), another endogenous protein that is an antagonist at the MC-3 and MC-4 receptors, when overexpressed in transgenic mice also produces an obese phenotype (54).

Serotonergic Systems
For a number of years, there has been speculation that serotonergic neurons had integrative and regulatory functions related to feeding behavior and weight homeostasis. Several studies have suggested a role specifically for the 5-HT$_{2c}$ receptor. Obesity develops in mice with mutations of the 5-HT$_{2c}$ receptor (55). The compound meta-chlorophenylpiperazine, an agent with agonist activity at the 5-HT$_{2c}$ receptor, has been reported to cause weight reduction but is associated with anxiety and nausea (56, 57).

Corticotropin Releasing Hormone
Corticotropin releasing hormone (CRH) (58) and the related urocortin reduce food intake and body weight when administered directly to the brain (59). Additionally, leptin administration increases the expression of CRH mRNA in the hypothalamus (33). Last, the increase in weight seen in glucocorticoid excess states may in part be due to the attendant suppression of CRH (60, 61).

Cocaine and Amphetamine Regulated Transcript
The neuropeptide cocaine and amphetamine regulated transcript (CART) was identified by differential display identifying those genes expressed following acute administration of cocaine and amphetamine to rats. The C-terminal 48-amino-acids of the prohormone predicted by the sequence of the gene appears to be the biologically active form and is a potent inhibitor of feeding (62). CART mRNA has been shown to be highly expressed in multiple nuclei of the hypothalamus, many of which are important in feeding behavior and appetite regulation. The potential role of CART in energy balance was suggested by showing that leptin coordinately regulated CART expression and furthermore that CART inhibited the feeding response induced by either fasting or by NPY (63).

Neurotensin
Neurotensin (NT), a 13-amino-acid peptide first discovered due to its vasodilatory activity and isolated and purified from bovine hypothalamus, is found throughout the brain and the gastrointestinal tract. In the brain, its highest concentrations are in the hypothalamus with a nuclei pattern consistent with its role as an anorexigenic peptide (50). NT decreases both spontaneous and norepinephrine-induced feeding. The regulation of NT is inverse to that of NPY in *ob/ob* mice and in Zucker obese (fa/fa) rats. However, the role of NT in the daily regulation of feeding behavior, caloric intake, and satiety has not yet been established.

Other Peptides

As discussed above, GLP-1 may be an important signaling peptide from the periphery. However, several lines of evidence also suggest that GLP-1 may be a central anorexigenic molecule as well. It is known that GLP-1 has potent central effects. Furthermore, concentrations of GLP-1 administered centrally have effects that are not reproduced when administered peripherally. Finally, GLP-1 has been found in several hypothalamic nuclei responsible for energy balance (50).

Other neuropeptides that have been identified as possibly affecting weight homeostasis include somatostatin, thyroid-stimulating hormone (independent of thyroid hormone), calcitonin-gene-related peptide, norepinephrine, and growth hormone-releasing hormone.

Anorexigenic Signals as Therapeutic Targets

To date, only poorly selective 5-HT_{2c} agonists have been studied in humans and the efficacy has not outweighed the side effect profile. However, it is possible that many of the side effects are related to other receptor pharmacologies, such as the 5-HT_{2a} receptor. Therefore, concerted efforts are underway to identify a selective 5-HT_{2c} agonist. Many of the other peptides discussed above are important potential targets for drug discovery. Considerable interest in drug development has been focused recently on the products of the POMC gene as well as on the melanocortin receptors through which they act in part due to the occurrence of mutations of POMC processing enzymes (64, 65) and of the MC-4 receptor (66) that appear to be responsible for rare cases of human obesity.

Effector Components

The peripheral systems involved in energy balance can be divided into efferent signals from the brain and their respective receptors and the effector molecules that translate these efferent signals into an increase or decrease in energy expenditure. The two most studied efferent signal systems are the adrenergic nervous system and the thyroid hormone axis.

Thyroid Hormone Axis

Although thyroid hormone clearly plays a role in the basal state of energy utilization, the long half-life of thyroxine as well as its long-term genomic effects suggest that this system is most important in affecting energy balance on a long-term basis. The discovery of several isoforms of the thyroid hormone receptor with differential tissue distributions opens the possibility of regulation of energy through specific receptor subtypes (67).

Adrenergic Nervous System

The daily variations in energy expenditure are more likely to occur via the adrenergic nervous system. The effector molecules that separate fuel oxidation from ATP synthesis (i.e., potential chemical energy) reside within a subset of the family of mitochondrial transport protein known as uncoupling proteins (UCPs). The adrenergic nervous system regulates energy expenditure at the cellular level by regulating the expression of uncoupling proteins and at the whole animal level by enhancing total and basal oxygen consumption (68), increasing thermogenic responses, and increasing BAT mass (69). The α- and β-adrenergic receptors mediate catecholamine responses.

β_3-Adrenergic Receptor

The β-adrenergic receptors were first subtyped by Lands et al into β_1- and β_2-adrenergic receptors (70). However, evidence grew that the pharmacology of known adrenergic agonists in adipose and gastrointestinal tissue was not explained by the known β-adrenergic receptors (71). In 1984, it was proposed that the atypical β-adrenergic receptor within adipose tissue be considered a third β-receptor subtype (72). Although all three receptor subtypes are found within adipocytes, the β_3-adrenergic receptor is most highly expressed in BAT, the tissue most likely responsible for the thermogenic effect of food (73) and acclimation to cold (74).

The β_3-adrenergic receptor is a member of the seven transmembrane G-protein coupled receptor family and is 95% homologous to the β_1- and β_2-adrenergic receptors. Despite having sequence information on the β_1- and β_2-adrenergic receptors for a number of years, the cloning of the human β_3-adrenergic receptor did not occur until 1989 (75). Additional work led to the discovery that the human isoform of β_3-receptor was unique to the rat receptor in that it had a second exon with an additional six amino acids on the C terminus (76). This change in protein structure was not expected to cause significant interspecies differences in pharmacology. However, many of the pharmacologic agonists synthesized and optimized for activity at the rat β_3-receptor were actually weak partial agonists at the human receptor. This was a possible explanation for the failure of β_3-receptor agonists to increase energy expenditure in humans (77). A unique aspect of the β_3-receptor, in contrast to the β_1-and β_2-adrenergic receptors, was the lack of acute homologous downregulation by serine kinases (78).

β_3-receptor pharmacology and/or receptor mRNA has also been identified in tissues other than fat with considerable variation existing between species: skeletal muscle (79), ileum-colon (80-82), gastric fundus (83), neural tissue (84), bronchial smooth muscle (85), vasculature (86), and heart tissue (87).

A polymorphism in the β_3-adrenergic receptor gene has been identified that leads to a single amino acid substitution within the molecule at position 64 replacing a tryptophan with an arginine (88). Many studies have examined whether the occurrence of this polymorphism links to any of a number of abnormalities including obesity, diabetes, insulin resistance, glucose intolerance, and the relative risk of each of these conditions. The evidence suggests that if this polymorphism has any effect on development of obesity or diabetes, it is relatively minor.

Human adipocytes express α-adrenergic receptors to a high level. The α_2-adrenergic receptors are the predominant subtype. The α-adrenergic receptor, under catecholamine stimulation, acts to suppress lipolysis. The differences in the relative expression of the α- and β-adrenergic receptors have been used to explain some of the uniqueness of human forms of obesity. Unlike lower mammals, human adipocytes tend to express relatively fewer β- and higher α-adrenergic receptors. Therefore, on balance, human adipose is relatively resistant to lipolytic effects of catecholamines and hence are more likely to store fat.

β_3-Adrenergic Receptor as a Therapeutic Target

The β_3-adrenergic receptor is highly expressed in human BAT and to a limited degree in human WAT (89). Several studies in animals have indicated that this receptor is a potential target for antiobesity therapy. Administration of a β_3-adrenergic receptor agonist has been shown to cause weight loss, an increase in energy expenditure, or both in several species (90-97). In addition, β_3-adrenergic receptor agonists have been shown to have antihyperglycemic effects that appear to be, at least in part, independent of their antiobesity effects (98, 99).

Dampening much of the initial enthusiasm for this class of agent is the fact that there has been little or no efficacy of β_3-adrenergic receptor agonists in humans, although one agent was able to induce a shift in the respiratory quotient, indicating an alteration in lipid oxidation (77). Furthermore, it is argued that the small amount of BAT in adult humans limits the maximal effect on energy expenditure. However, several factors have been identified that explain some of the shortfalls of the first-generation molecules. All of the compounds used in clinical trials before 1998 were optimized for activity at the rat β_3-adrenergic receptor. It was discovered only after these agents entered clinical development that the pharmacology of the rodent receptor is distinct from human and other species homologues. It is also argued that reduced amount of target BAT in humans will not impair the potential for efficacy. In animals treated with β_3-adrenergic receptor agonists, there is a significant expansion of the BAT compartment (100, 101). Humans have the potential for induction of BAT as demonstrated in patients with pheochromocytoma in whom brown fat is markedly increased (102). Lastly, β_3-adrenergic receptors do not appear to undergo acute, agonist-induced downregulation (78), which suggests that the weight loss effect may require activity over a period of time.

Significant optimism toward this class of agent was recently generated when it was demonstrated for the first time that a β_3-adrenergic receptor agonist could increase energy expenditure in humans (103). It is likely that additional information on the potential for β_3-adrenergic receptor agonists for use in the treatment of obesity will be forthcoming in the near future.

Uncoupling Proteins

The first uncoupling proteins (now called UCP-1) were identified in the mid-1970s (104, 105) as mitochondrial proteins that bound to purine nucleotides and fatty acids and were involved in energy dissipation. This protein family belongs to the mitochondrial anion carrier proteins that also include ADP/ATP-carrier, phosphate, and oxogluturate carriers. UCP-1 is primarily expressed in BAT (106). In mitochondria derived from other cell types, oxidation of fuels is tightly coupled to the generation of ATP. The mitochondrial respiratory chain produces a proton gradient across the inner mitochondrial membrane. ATP synthesis from ADP by the protein ATP synthase is driven by the coupled movement of protons down this electrochemical gradient. If ADP substrate is limited, proton flux through ATP synthase is inhibited and the gradient is maintained. In BAT mitochondria, protons may move down the gradient in a manner that is uncoupled from ATP synthesis (107). The uncoupling of the potential energy of the gradient from ATP generation provides a mechanism for both the dissipation of excess calories and for the production of heat.

The activity of UCPs is highly regulated within BAT. In addition to receptor-mediated changes in cAMP, free fatty acids are important intracellular activators of UCP-1 activity (108, 109). Cytosolic ATP inhibits UCP-1 activity, perhaps in a negative feedback loop. In addition to allosteric or transport-level regulation, it is likely that there is transcriptional regulation. The UCP-1 protein is acutely upregulated by catecholamines via the β_3 adrenergic receptor (79) as well as by the other β-receptor subtypes, particularly during development (110). The adrenergic-mediated upregulation of UCP-1 also accounts for increased expression with cold exposure and explains, to some extent, diet-induced thermogenesis (111, 112).

Two additional cloned uncoupling proteins, UCP-2 and UCP-3, have different tissue-specific expression and transcriptional regulation. At least one report has shown that the proton transport activity of UCP-1 is dependent on the presence of an intact histidine pair that is absent in both UCP-2 and UCP-3 (113). UCP-2 is expressed in BAT, but unlike UCP-1, is expressed in a broad range of tissues.

Uncoupling Proteins as Therapeutic Targets

There is difficulty in targeting uncoupling proteins because the need to deliver compounds to the intracellular, and possibly the intramitochondrial, compartments represents a true challenge. Furthermore, attempts to upregulate the expression or activity of UCPs in a tissue-specific manner may also be a difficult hurdle. UCP-2, for example, though highly expressed in BAT and skeletal muscle, is also in immune-response tissue, cardiocytes, and the brain. Uncoupling oxidative respiration in these tissues may lead to unfavorable toxicology. UCP-1, found only in BAT, may be expressed insufficiently to have an impact on human forms of obesity.

■　■　■

Key Points

- The potential for new therapeutic targets has increased with greater understanding of the regulation of weight and energy homeostasis.

- These targets can be classified into those that interact with three areas of energy regulation: signaling (including lipostatic, glucostatic, and satiety signals), integration, and effector systems.

- No single target can be expected to treat all forms of obesity, which is likely to be a polygenic and environmental disorder of complex etiology.

- β_3-adrenergic receptor agonists will be among the first group of novel receptor targets to be tested in humans for the treatment of obesity.

▓　▓　▓

REFERENCES

1. **Munro JF.** Clinical aspects of the treatment of obesity by drugs: a review. Int J Obes. 1979;3:171-80.

2. **Zhang Y, Proenca R, Maffei M, et al.** Positional cloning of the mouse obese gene and its human homologue. Nature. 1994;372:425-32.

3. **Montague CT, Farooqi IS, Whitehead JP, et al.** Congenital leptin deficiency is associated with severe early-onset obesity in humans. Nature. 1997;387:903-8.

4. **Clement K, Vaisse C, Lahlou N, et al.** A mutation in the human leptin receptor gene causes obesity and pituitary dysfunction. Nature. 1998;392:398-401.

5. **Sinha MK, Opentanova I, Ohannesian JP, et al.** Evidence of free and bound leptin in human circulation: studies in lean and obese subjects and during short-term fasting. J Clin Invest. 1996;98:1277-82.

6. **Considine RV, Considine EL, Williams CJ, et al.** The hypothalamic leptin receptor in humans: identification of incidental sequence polymorphisms and absence of the *db/db* mouse and *fa/fa* rat mutations. Diabetes. 1996;45:992-4.

7. **Greenberg AS, Heymsfield SB, Fujioka K, et al.** Preliminary safety and efficacy of recombinant methionyl human leptin administered by SC injection in lean and obese subjects. In: Eighth International Congress on Obesity. Vol. 22, Supplement 3. Despres J-P, Macdonald I, eds. Paris: Stockton Press; Supplemental Distribution; 1998.

8. Amgen reports solid third-quarter results and announces additional $1 billion stock repurchase plan. Amgen Press Release. Amgen, Thousand Oaks, CA; 1998.

9. **Gloaguen I, Costa P, Demartis A, et al.** Ciliary neurotrophic factor corrects obesity and diabetes associated with leptin deficiency and resistance. Proc Natl Acad Sci U S A. 1997;94:6456-61.

10. **Loftus TM, Jaworsky DE, Frehywot GL, et al.** Reduced food intake and body weight in mice treated with fatty acid synthase inhibitors. Science. 2000;288:2379-81.

11. **Rowe JW, Young JB, Minaker KL, et al.** Effect of insulin and glucose infusions on sympathetic nervous system activity in normal man. Diabetes. 1981;30:219-25.

12. **Sakaguchi T, Bray GA.** The effect of intrahypothalamic injections of glucose on sympathetic efferent firing rate. Brain Res Bull. 1987;18:591-5.

13. **Young JB, Landsberg L.** Impaired suppression of sympathetic activity during fasting in the gold thioglucose-treated mouse. J Clin Invest. 1980;65:1086-94.

14. **Gibbs J, Young RC, Smith GP.** Cholecystokinin decreases food intake in rats. J Comp Physiol Psych. 1973;84:488-95.

15. **Figlewicz DP, Sipols A, Porte D Jr, Woods SC.** Intraventricular bombesin can decrease single meal size in the baboon. Brain Res Bull. 1986;17:535-7.

16. **Reidelberger RD, O'Rourke MF.** Potent cholecystokinin antagonist L 364718 stimulates food intake in rats. Am J Physiol. 1989;257:R1512-8.

17. **Gibbs J, Fauser DJ, Rowe EA, et al.** Bombesin suppresses feeding in rats. Nature. 1979;282:208-10.

18. **Stein LJ, Woods SC.** Gastrin releasing peptide reduces meal size in rats. Peptides. 1982;3:833-5.

19. **Ladenheim EE, Wirth KE, Moran TH.** Receptor subtype mediation of feeding suppression by bombesin-like peptides. Pharmacol Biochem Behav. 1996;54:705-11.

20. **Perley MJ, Kipnis DM.** Plasma insulin responses to oral and intravenous glucose: studies in normal and diabetic subjects. J Clin Invest. 1967;46:1954-62.

21. **Elrick H, Stimmler L, Aria et al.** Plasma insulin response to oral intravenous glucose administration. J Clin Invest. 1964;24:1076-82.

22. **Drucker DJ.** Glucagon-like peptides. Diabetes. 1998;47:159-69.

23. **Figlewicz DP, Sipols AJ, Porte D Jr, et al.** Intraventricular CCK inhibits food intake and gastric emptying in baboons. Am J Physiol. 1989;256:R1313-7.

24. **Moran TH, Shnayder L, Hostetler AM, McHugh PR.** Pylorectomy reduces the satiety action of cholecystokinin. Am J Physiol. 1988;255:R1059-63.

25. **Smith GP, Jerome C, Norgren R.** Afferent axons in abdominal vagus mediate satiety effect of cholecystokinin in rats. Am J Physiol. 1985;249:R638-41.

26. **West DB, Fey D, Woods SC.** Cholecystokinin persistently suppresses meal size but not food intake in free-feeding rats. Am J Physiol. 1984;246:R776-87.

27. **Wang Z, Wang RM, Owji AA, et al.** Glucagon-like peptide-1 is a physiological incretin in rats. J Clin Invest. 1995;95:417-21.

28. **Ohki-Hamazaki H, Watase K, Yamamoto K, et al.** Mice lacking bombesin receptor subtype-3 develop metabolic defects and obesity. Nature. 1997;390:165-9.

29. **Elmquist JK, Bjorbaek C, Ahima RS, et al.** Distributions of leptin receptor mRNA isoforms in the rat brain. J Comp Neurol. 1998;395:535-47.

30. **Chua SC Jr, Brown AW, Kim J, et al.** Food deprivation and hypothalamic neuropeptide gene expression: effects of strain background and the diabetes mutation. Brain Res Mol Brain Res. 1991;11:291-9.

31. **Wilding JP, Gilbey SG, Bailey CJ, et al.** Increased neuropeptide-Y messenger ribonucleic acid (mRNA) and decreased neurotensin mRNA in the hypothalamus of the obese (*ob/ob*) mouse. Endocrinology. 1993;132:1939-44.

32. **Stephens TW, Basinski M, Bristow PK, et al.** The role of neuropeptide Y in the antiobesity action of the obese gene product. Nature. 1995;377:530-2.

33. **Schwartz MW, Seeley RJ, Campfield LA, et al.** Identification of targets of leptin action in rat hypothalamus. J Clin Invest. 1996;98:1101-6.

34. **Seeley RJ, van Dijk G, Campfield LA, et al.** Intraventricular leptin reduces food intake and body weight of lean rats but not obese Zucker rats. Horm Metab Res. 1996;28:664-8.

35. **Stanley BG, Kyrkouli SE, Lampert S, Leibowitz SF.** Neuropeptide Y chronically injected into the hypothalamus: a powerful neurochemical inducer of hyperphagia and obesity. Peptides. 1986;7:1189-92.

36. **Zarjevski N, Cusin I, Vettor R, et al.** Chronic intracerebroventricular neuropeptide-Y administration to normal rats mimics hormonal and metabolic changes of obesity. Endocrinology. 1993;133:1753-8.

37. **Billington CJ, Briggs JE, Grace M, Levine AS.** Effects of intracerebroventricular injection of neuropeptide Y on energy metabolism. Am J Physiol. 1991;260:R321-7.

38. **Bray GA.** Peptides affect the intake of specific nutrients and the sympathetic nervous system. Am J Clin Nutr. 1992;55:265S-271S.

39. **Erickson JC, Hollopeter G, Palmiter RD.** Attenuation of the obesity syndrome of *ob/ob* mice by the loss of neuropeptide Y. Science. 1996;274:1704-7.

40. **Erickson JC, Clegg KE, Palmiter RD.** Sensitivity to leptin and susceptibility to seizures of mice lacking neuropeptide Y. Nature. 1996;381:415-21.

41. **Marsh DJ, Hollopeter G, Kafer KE, Palmiter RD.** Role of the Y5 neuropeptide Y receptor in feeding and obesity. Nat Med. 1998;4:718-21.

42. **Pedrazzini T, Seydoux J, Kunstner P, et al.** Cardiovascular response, feeding behavior and locomotor activity in mice lacking the NPY Y1 receptor. Nat Med. 1998;4:722-6.

43. **Nahon JL.** The melanin-concentrating hormone: from the peptide to the gene. Crit Rev Neurobiol. 1994;8:221-62.

44. **Qu D, Ludwig DS, Gammeltoft S, et al.** A role for melanin-concentrating hormone in the central regulation of feeding behaviour. Nature. 1996;380:243-7.

45. **Shimada M, Tritos NA, Lowell BB, et al.** Mice lacking melanin-concentrating hormone are hypophagic and lean. Nature. 1998;396:670-4.

46. **Akabayashi A, Koenig JI, Watanabe Y, et al.** Galanin-containing neurons in the paraventricular nucleus: a neurochemical marker for fat ingestion and body weight gain. Proc Natl Acad Sci U S A. 1994;91:10375-9.

47. **Leibowitz SF, Akabayashi A, Wang J.** Obesity on a high-fat diet: role of hypothalamic galanin in neurons of the anterior paraventricular nucleus projecting to the median eminence. J Neurosci. 1998;18:2709-19.

48. **Smith BK, York DA, Bray GA.** Chronic cerebroventricular galanin does not induce sustained hyperphagia or obesity. Peptides. 1994;15:1267-72.

49. **Sakurai T, Amemiya A, Ishii M, et al.** Orexins and orexin receptors: a family of hypothalamic neuropeptides and G protein-coupled receptors that regulate feeding behavior. Cell. 1998;92:573-85.

50. **Kalra SP, Dube MG, Pu SY, et al.** Interacting appetite-regulating pathways in the hypothalamic regulation of body weight. Endocr Rev. 1999;20:68-100.

51. **Morley JE.** Neuropeptide regulation of appetite and weight. Endocr Rev. 1987;8:256-87.

52. **Cone RD, Lu D, Koppula S, et al.** The melanocortin receptors: agonists, antagonists, and the hormonal control of pigmentation. Recent Prog Horm Res. 1996;51:287-317; discussion 318.

53. **Huszar D, Lynch CA, Fairchild-Huntress V, et al.** Targeted disruption of the melanocortin-4 receptor results in obesity in mice. Cell. 1997;88:131-41.

54. **Ollmann MM, Wilson BD, Yang YK, et al.** Antagonism of central melanocortin receptors in vitro and in vivo by agouti-related protein. Science. 1997;278:135-8.

55. **Heisler LK, Chu HM, Tecott LH.** Epilepsy and obesity in serotonin 5-HT2C receptor mutant mice. Ann N Y Acad Sci. 1998;861:74-8.

56. **Dourish CT.** Multiple serotonin receptors: opportunities for new treatments for obesity? Obes Res. 1995;3(Suppl 4):449S-462S.

57. **Sargent PA, Sharpley AL, Williams C, et al.** 5-HT$_{2c}$ receptor activation decreases appetite and body weight in obese subjects. Psychopharmacology. 1997;133:309-12.

58. **Rothwell NJ.** Central effects of CRF on metabolism and energy balance. Neurosci Biobehav Rev. 1990;14:263-71.

59. **Spina M, Merlo-Pich E, Chan RK, et al.** Appetite-suppressing effects of urocortin, a CRF-related neuropeptide. Science. 1996;273:1561-4.

60. **Schwartz MW, Seeley RJ.** Seminars in medicine of the Beth Israel Deaconess Medical Center: neuroendocrine responses to starvation and weight loss. N Engl J Med. 1997;336:1802-11.

61. **Flier JS, Maratos-Flier E.** Obesity and the hypothalamus: novel peptides for new pathways. Cell. 1998;92:437-40.

62. **Kristensen P, Judge ME, Thim L, et al.** Hypothalamic CART is a new anorectic peptide regulated by leptin. Nature. 1998;393:72-6.

63. **Thim L, Kristensen P, Larsen PJ, Wulff BS.** CART, a new anorectic peptide. Int J Biochem Cell Biol. 1981;30:1281-4.

64. **Jackson RS, Creemers JW, Ohagi S, et al.** Obesity and impaired prohormone processing associated with mutations in the human prohormone convertase-1 gene. Nat Genet. 1997;16:303-6.

65. **O'Rahilly S, Gray H, Humphreys PJ, et al.** Brief report: impaired processing of prohormones associated with abnormalities of glucose homeostasis and adrenal function. N Engl J Med. 1995;333:1386-90.

66. **Yeo GS, Farooqi IS, Aminian S, et al.** A frameshift mutation in MC4R associated with dominantly inherited human obesity. Nat Genet. 1998;20:111-2.

67. **Murata Y.** Multiple isoforms of thyroid hormone receptor: an analysis of their relative contribution in mediating thyroid hormone action. Nagoya J Med Sci. 1998;61:103-15.

68. **Hauge A, Oye I.** Effect of adrenaline and adrenergic blocking agents on the basal oxygen consumption of the perfused rat heart. Nature. 1966;210:998-1000.

69. **Rothwell NJ, Saville ME, Stock MJ.** Sympathetic and thyroid influences on metabolic rate in fed, fasted, and refed rats. Am J Physiol. 1982;243:R339-46.

70. **Lands AM, Arnold A, McAuliff JP, et al.** Differentiation of receptor systems activated by sympathomimetic amines. Nature. 1967;214:597-8.

71. **Furchgott RF.** In: Catecholamines. Blaschko H, Muecholl E, eds. Berlin: Springer-Verlag; 1972;283-335.

72. **Tan S, Curtis-Prior PB.** Characterization of the beta-adrenoceptor of the adipose cell of the rat. Int J Obes. 1983;7:409-14.

73. **Rothwell NJ, Stock MJ.** A role for brown adipose tissue in diet-induced thermogenesis. Obes Res. 1997;5:650-6.

74. **Himms-Hagen J.** Brown adipose tissue thermogenesis and obesity. Prog Lipid Res. 1989;28:67-115.

75. **Emorine LJ, Marullo S, Briend-Sutren MM, et al.** Molecular characterization of the human beta 3-adrenergic receptor. Science. 1989;245:1118-21.

76. **Granneman JG, Lahners KN, Rao DD.** Rodent and human beta 3-adrenergic receptor genes contain an intron within the protein-coding block. Mol Pharmacol. 1992;42:964-70.

77. **Weyer C, Tataranni PA, Snitker S, et al.** Increase in insulin action and fat oxidation after treatment with CL 316,243, a highly selective beta 3-adrenoceptor agonist in humans. Diabetes. 1998;47:1555-61.

78. **Nantel F, Bonin H, Emorine LJ, et al.** The human beta 3-adrenergic receptor is resistant to short-term agonist-promoted desensitization. Mol Pharmacol. 1993;43:548-55.

79. **Nagase I, Yoshida T, Kumamoto K, et al.** Expression of uncoupling protein in skeletal-muscle and white fat of obese mice treated with thermogenic beta 3-adrenergic agonist. J Clin Invest. 1996;97:2898-2904.

80. **McLaughlin DP, MacDonald A.** Evidence for the existence of 'atypical' beta-adrenoceptors (beta 3-adrenoceptors) mediating relaxation in the rat distal colon in vitro. Br J Pharmacol. 1990;101:569-74.

81. **van der Vliet A, Rademaker B, Bast A.** A beta-adrenoceptor with atypical characteristics is involved in the relaxation of the rat small intestine. J Pharmacol Exp Ther. 1990;255:218-26.

82. **Taneja DT, Clarke DE.** Evidence for a noradrenergic innervation to "atypical" beta-adrenoceptors (or putative beta 3-adrenoceptors) in the ileum of guinea pig. J Pharmacol Exp Ther. 1992;260:192-200.

83. **McLaughlin DP, MacDonald A.** Characterization of catecholamine-mediated relaxations in rat isolated gastric fundus: evidence for an atypical beta-adrenoceptor. Br J Pharm. 1991;103:1351-6.

84. **Esbenshade TA, Han C, Theroux TL, et al.** Coexisting beta 1- and atypical beta-adrenergic receptors cause redundant increases in cyclic AMP in human neuroblastoma cells. Mol Pharmacol. 1992;42:753-9.

85. **Webber SE, Stock MJ.** Evidence for an atypical or beta 3-adrenoceptor in ferret tracheal epithelium. Br J Pharmacol. 1992;105:857-62.

86. **Oriowo MA.** Different atypical beta-adrenoceptors mediate isoprenaline-induced relaxation in vascular and non-vascular smooth muscles. Life Sci. 1995;56:L269-75.

87. **Kaumann AJ, Molenaar P.** Differences between the third cardiac beta-adrenoceptor and the colonic beta 3-adrenoceptor in the rat. Br J Pharmacol. 1996;118:2085-98.

88. **Shuldiner AR, Silver K, Roth J, Walston J.** Beta 3-adrenoceptor gene variant in obesity and insulin resistance. Lancet. 1996;348:1584-5.

89. **Krief S, Lonnqvist F, Raimbault S, et al.** Tissue distribution of beta 3-adrenergic receptor mRNA in man. J Clin Invest. 1993;91:344-9.

90. **Ghorbani M, Himmshagen J.** Appearance of brown adipocytes in white adipose tissue during CL316,243-induced reversal of obesity and diabetes in Zucker *fa/fa* rats. Int J Obes. 1997;21:465-75.

91. **Santti E, Huupponen R, Rouru J, et al.** Potentiation of the anti-obesity effect of the selective beta 3-adrenoceptor agonist BRL 35135 in obese Zucker rats by exercise. Br J Pharmacol. 1994;113:1231-6.

92. **Umekawa T, Yoshida T, Sakane N, et al.** Anti-obesity and anti-diabetic effects of CL316,243, a highly specific beta(3)-adrenoceptor agonist, in Otsuka Long-Evans Tokushima fatty rats: induction of uncoupling protein and activation of glucose transporter 4 in white fat. Eur J Endocrinol. 1997;136:429-37.

93. **Yoshida T, Sakane N, Wakabayashi Y.** Anti-obesity effect of CL 316,243, a highly specific beta 3-adrenoceptor agonist, in mice with monosodium-L-glutamate-induced obesity. Eur J Endocrinol. 1994;131:97-102.

94. **Yoshida T, Sakane N, Wakabayashi Y, et al.** Anti-obesity and anti-diabetic effects of CL 316,243, a highly specific beta 3-adrenoceptor agonist, in yellow KK mice. Life Sci. 1994;54:491-8.

95. **Yoshida T, Hiraoka N, Yoshioka K, et al.** Anti-obesity and anti-diabetic actions of a beta 3-adrenoceptor agonist, BRL 26830A, in yellow KK mice. Endocr J. 1991;38:397-403.

96. **Collins S, Daniel KW, Petro AE, Surwit RS.** Strain-specific response to beta(3)-adrenergic receptor agonist treatment of diet-induced obesity in mice. Endocrinology. 1997;138:405-13.

97. **Sasaki N, Uchida E, Niiyama M, et al.** Anti-obesity effects of selective agonists to the beta 3-adrenergic receptor in dogs. II. Recruitment of thermogenic brown adipocytes and reduction of adiposity after chronic treatment with a beta 3-adrenergic agonist. J Vet Med Sci. 1998;60:465-9.

98. **deSouza CJ, Hirshman MF, Horton ES, et al.** CL-316,243, a beta(3)-specific adrenoceptor agonist, enhances insulin-stimulated glucose disposal in nonobese rats. Diabetes. 1997;46:1257-63.

99. **Liu X, Perusse F, Bukowiecki LJ.** Mechanisms of the antidiabetic effects of the beta 3-adrenergic agonist CL-316243 in obese Zucker-ZDF rats. Am J Physiol. 1998;274:R1212-9.

100. **Champigny O, Ricquier D.** Evidence from in vitro differentiating cells that adrenoceptor agonists can increase uncoupling protein mRNA level in adipocytes of adult humans: an RT-PCR study. J Lipid Res. 1996;37:1907-14.

101. **Champigny O, Ricquier D, Blondel O, et al.** Beta 3-adrenergic receptor stimulation restores message and expression of brown-fat mitochondrial uncoupling protein in adult dogs. Proc Natl Acad Sci U S A. 1991;88:10774-7.

102. **Ricquier D, Nechad M, Mory G.** Ultrastructural and biochemical characterization of human brown adipose tissue in pheochromocytoma. J Clin Endocrinol Metab. 1982;54:803-7.

103. **Miller JW, Farid NA, Johnson RD, et al.** Stimulation of energy expenditure by LY377604, a beta 3-adrenergic receptor agonist with beta1/2-antagonist properties, in healthy male subjects. Obes Res. 1999;7:121S.

104. **Ricquier D, Kader JC.** Mitochondrial protein alteration in active brown fat: a sodium dodecyl sulfate-polyacrylamide gel electrophoretic study. Biochem Biophys Res Commun. 1976;73:577-83.

105. **Heaton GM, Wagenvoord RJ, Kemp A Jr, Nicholls DG.** Brown-adipose-tissue mitochondria: photoaffinity labelling of the regulatory site of energy dissipation. Eur J Biochem. 1978;82:515-21.

106. **Gura T.** Uncoupling proteins provide new clue to obesity's causes. Science. 1998;280:1369-70.

107. **Lowell BB, Flier JS.** Brown adipose tissue, beta 3-adrenergic receptors, and obesity. Ann Rev Med. 1997;48:307-16.

108. **Strieleman PJ, Schalinske KL, Shrago E.** Fatty acid activation of the reconstituted brown adipose tissue mitochondria uncoupling protein. J Biol Chem. 1985;260:13402-5.

109. **Bukowiecki LJ.** Regulation of energy expenditure in brown adipose tissue. Int J Obes. 1985;9:31-41.

110. **Silva JE, Rabelo R.** Regulation of the uncoupling protein gene expression. Eur J Endocrinol. 1997;136:251-64.

111. **Carmona MC, Valmaseda A, Brun S, et al.** Differential regulation of uncoupling protein-2 and uncoupling protein-3 gene expression in brown adipose tissue during development and cold exposure. Biochem Biophys Res Commun. 1998;243:224-8.

112. **Florez-Duquet M, Horwitz BA, McDonald RB.** Cellular proliferation and UCP content in brown adipose tissue of cold-exposed aging Fischer 344 rats. Am J Physiol. 1998;274:R196-203.

113. **Bienengraeber M, Echtay KS, Klingenberg M.** H+ transport by uncoupling protein (UCP-1) is dependent on a histidine pair, absent in UCP-2 and UCP-3. Biochemistry. 1998;37:3-8.

12

■ ■ ■

Weight Loss Recidivism and Relapse Prevention

John C. Guare, PhD

Angela Schulze, BS

Long-term management of obesity is a major clinical challenge. Although significant progress has been made in helping people lose weight, efforts to prevent recidivism (weight regain) have been less successful. However, recent research addressing weight maintenance/relapse prevention is providing guidance in assisting patients with long-term weight management efforts.

Behavioral Interventions

The goal of behavior therapy is to facilitate changes in lifestyle habits pivotal to regulating energy intake and expenditure. Strategies typically used in behavioral therapy include self-monitoring, goal setting, stimulus control (e.g., minimizing exposure to food cues), cognitive restructuring (e.g., changing thought processes, particularly irrational and negative "self-talk"), social support mechanisms, stress management, and problem-solving skills (1). Note that behavior modification is only one component of behavior therapy and that this type of therapy is skills oriented rather than insight oriented. The psychological paradigm is a pragmatic one that focuses on goals, process, and small changes (2). This approach stresses changing behaviors (changes that all of us are capable of making) rather than a psychotherapeutic or analytical approach. This does not mean that psychotherapy is unnecessary for some patients. In some cases, there are obstacles to success that require more attention. However, all obese individuals need to focus on developing skills that translate into behavior change.

Behavioral weight loss interventions have steadily improved since their introduction in the 1960s. Wadden's review (3) notes average weight losses for behavioral studies in 1974, 1984, and 1988-90 of 3.8 kg, 6.9 kg, and 8.5 kg, respectively. One of the most striking changes is the duration of treatment, increasing from an average of 2 months in 1974 to a typical 5 to 6 month intervention at present. (Note that the standards of practice established by the 1998 NIH report states at least 6 months of lifestyle intervention is indicated (1).) The rate of weight loss has not changed over time, remaining at 0.4 to 0.5 kg/wk.

Interventions of 6 months are helpful because they provide participants time to begin to develop and practice new habits and skills while actively working with professional clinicians. Longer programs (e.g., 48 wk) have produced greater losses of 13.5 to 17.3 kg (4), which suggests the possible superiority of programs extending beyond 6 months. In contrast, other research has shown that the "window of opportunity" for effective weight loss seems to be the first 6 months; an additional 16 to 26 weeks yields a much slower rate of weight loss (5). Nonetheless, some studies suggest one of the best predictors of long-term weight loss is length of treatment (3, 6).

Long-Term Results

Preventing recidivism is the major challenge in the treatment of the obese patient. When health care professionals began addressing weight management in a systematic fashion, it was not unusual for patients to regain one-third to one-half of their weight loss during the first year following active intervention and to return to pretreatment weight within 3 to 5 years (3, 7). However, recent studies suggest progress in achieving more favorable long-term outcomes. In a general random phone survey, ~10% of individuals who had a history of overweight/obesity had lost and maintained at least 10% weight loss for at least 5 years (8). In a larger, hospital clinic based research study, 19% of participants maintained weight loss within 5 lb annually over a period of 5 years of follow-up (9). Approximately 30% of individuals participating in a nationwide, proprietary, comprehensive weight management program have been able to achieve the NIH goal of 10% sustained weight loss (10). Weight Watchers also has demonstrated long-term efficacy among Lifetime Members who had previously reached their goal weight (11). At 5 years, ~19% of participants remained within 5 lb of goal weight and ~43% had maintained at least 5% weight loss. These improved outcomes are thought to be due to the longer initial intervention period, a multidisciplinary team approach to treatment, better patient education, and implementation of relapse prevention strategies after completing the intensive treatment period.

Thus a significant number of patients are able to maintain weight loss. Regrettably, however, the vast majority of patients are still failing to sustain weight loss long-term that meets the NIH goal. Such results have led experts in the field to view obesity as a chronic health problem that requires lifelong treatment (12).

Weight Maintenance and Relapse Prevention

Extended Treatment

The 1998 NIH report made an uncompromising statement regarding relapse: "Lost weight usually will be regained unless a weight maintenance program consisting of dietary therapy, physical activity, and behavior therapy is continued indefinitely" (13). To that end, Perri (6) reviewed a series of studies investigating the impact of extending treatment. Several studies provided subjects with a weekly behavior therapy program for 5 to 6 months followed by a second phase of continued contact (i.e., biweekly sessions for another 6 months). Other investigations compared two groups: subjects who were randomly assigned to either 1) a standard (20 to 26 wk) behavioral program, or 2) the standard program plus extended treatment (an additional 20 to 52 wk). Results indicated that subjects who received extended treatment did not achieve additional weight loss beyond that obtained at 5 to 6 months, but did maintain all of their initial 5 to 6 month loss. Subjects who did not receive extended treatment regained one-third of their weight loss during the extended treatment period. In addition, during a (no treatment) follow-up period, extended treatment subjects regained weight. Overall, the findings from this body of research demonstrate that 1) lengthening treatment beyond 5 or 6 months does not produce greater weight loss but does promote weight loss maintenance, and 2) when treatment and contact with the patient is discontinued, weight regain occurs.

Recent research (14) demonstrates the danger of waiting too long to re-enter a weight loss program. All subjects participated in a follow-up weight loss program after participating in an initial program. Subjects who waited longer than 6 months to return to a weight loss program gained significantly more weight during their hiatus than those who re-entered treatment within 6 months of their initial program. Interestingly, even in those subjects who regain weight, the psychological impact may not be significant. To the contrary, many subjects report improved mood and reduced binging despite lack of follow-up, which suggests that patients benefit from participating in a program even if their weight does not reflect this (15). Nevertheless, the evidence strongly suggests the need for a treatment and management model that promotes long-term, ongoing care in order for patients to fully benefit from weight loss.

Maintenance of Key Behaviors

Why does lengthening treatment help? One explanation is that continued care promotes continued adherence to important lifestyle behavior changes. Subjects who received extended treatment reported better maintenance of key weight control behaviors compared with those who did not receive extended treatment (6). The need to place greater emphasis on maintenance of weight control behaviors is also demonstrated by French and colleagues (16). Subjects participating in a weight gain prevention program were followed over a 4-year period. The duration of using key behaviors (e.g., exercise, lower fat intake) was correlated with long-term weight outcome. Two key findings emerged: 1) the duration of performing specific behaviors was brief, and 2) there was a dose-response relationship between duration of key behaviors and long-term weight control. Therefore helping patients persist in developing and maintaining proper health behavior habits is essential.

Although a number of behaviors enhance long-term weight control (e.g., eat low-fat foods, refuse food offers), two key behaviors are self-monitoring of food intake and exercise.

Self-Monitoring

Keeping a food log is one of the best predictors of weight loss maintenance. Subjects who consistently write down their food intake have better long-term weight loss than those who do not (17-19). Convincing subjects to continue their efforts is difficult, but when self-monitoring is performed on a long-term basis it becomes streamlined and more efficient as patients find what method works best for them (i.e., which method is the least time-consuming yet most effective) and creates feedback that is positive reinforcement for maintaining weight (20).

Unfortunately, few individuals record their food intake consistently (21). Simplifying food logs, re-emphasizing the value of self-monitoring, and helping patients avoid the negative "self-talk" when they overeat (which can lead to disengagement of self-monitoring) may help encourage record keeping. Research needs to move beyond demonstrating the importance of self-monitoring to identifying strategies that assist patients in this skill.

Exercise

Exercise is also extremely important in preventing weight regain. Most studies comparing diet with diet + exercise demonstrate the superiority of diet + exercise for weight loss at end of treatment (22). It is extremely diffi-cult to maintain weight loss without maintaining exercise (23, 24). For ex-ample, subjects reporting >200 min versus <150 min of exercise/week lost 13.1 kg versus 3.5 kg, respectively, at 18 months (25). It is important to note that the former group maintained their 6-month loss at 18 months, whereas the latter group regained weight during months 6 to 18. The same pattern of results has been observed by other investigators: Subjects who exercise the most maintain (not enhance) their 6-month loss, whereas the least-active participants show weight regain (26).

The type of exercise that best promotes long-term weight control has also been investigated. Overweight women were placed on a 1200 kcal/day diet and randomly assigned to either a structured aerobic exercise program (aerobic classes 3×/week) or a moderate lifestyle activity program (short bouts of walking, use of stairs, etc.) (26). Each group lost approxi-mately 8 kg at the end of the 16-week program. At 1-year follow-up, the aerobic group regained 1.6 kg versus 0.08 kg for the lifestyle group. Given the challenges of attending structured exercise classes on a lifelong basis, emphasizing small but sustainable changes in lifestyle exercise appears promising.

Relapse Prevention Training

Individuals who have successfully lost weight are all faced with the chal-lenges of lapses and relapse. A *lapse* is a short term "slip" that results in some weight regain, whereas *relapse* refers to a situation in which all weight loss is regained. The ongoing challenge the patient faces in pre-venting recidivism is not whether overeating will occur but how one reacts to overeating episodes. Relapse prevention training (RPT) can be used to teach individuals how to 1) avoid lapses in eating and exercise behavior, and 2) respond effectively when a lapse occurs so that a relapse does not occur. Avoiding lapses requires identifying and avoiding high-risk situa-tions, planning ahead for unavoidable high-risk scenarios, and so on.. Re-sponding appropriately utilizes cognitive restructuring to help patients identify their automatic (and often irrational) thoughts in response to a lapse, understand the lapse accurately, and use healthy "self-talk" to get back on track. Weight maintenance programs utilizing RPT and other weight control strategies have been shown to prevent recidivism (6). RPT is a set of learned skills and requires consistent practice. Otherwise, individu-als may "throw the baby out with the bathwater" in response to a lapse, give up completely, fall into a pattern of learned helplessness, and return to old habits. Professionally supervised programs, often in groups, are very useful in helping assist patients with this process. In addition, some low-cost/no-cost programs are effective for some individuals in providing this type of help (e.g., Overeaters Anonymous, Weight Watchers, TOPS).

One way to demonstrate the need for effective coping is to show patients the following steps:

(a) Healthy Eating/Activity → (b) Slip/Lapse → (c) Relapse → (d) Collapse

The goal is for individuals to engage in healthy eating and activity behaviors most of the time. When a lapse occurs, how one responds dictates if the person cycles back to step (a) or moves to step (c) or even (d). From a process management perspective, the key is to avoid steps (c) and (d) and cycle through steps (a) and (b) as appropriate.

Successful Losers: The National Weight Control Registry

The National Weight Control Registry (NWCR) was established in 1994. Its purpose is to register individuals who are successful at long-term weight loss and to study the behaviors and habits related to weight loss maintenance (27). To be eligible for NWCR, a person must have lost >30 lb and kept it off for >1 year. NWCR currently has data on over 2500 individuals who, on average, have lost 66 lb and maintained at least a 30 lb loss for 5.5 years. Participants provide assessment (questionnaire) data on an ongoing basis.

Data from the NWCR for individuals who have met the aforementioned criteria include 1) an average caloric intake of 1380 kcal/day, 2) ~24% of daily calories from fat, and 3) >1 h of moderate activity per day (27-32). Exercise data indicate that participants expend 2800 cal/wk in physical activity, a figure much higher than that of the general public (27). In sum, those individuals who are highly successful at long-term weight control eat a low-calorie/low-fat diet and have incorporated consistent and substantial physical activity into their daily routine.

Many people who have lost weight and try to sustain their lower weight have a difficult time exercising at a comparable level. More research is needed to determine if strategies can be developed to help the majority of people achieve a sustained level of high physical activity. Conversely, given the challenges of a lifelong high level of exercise and the health benefits of maintaining a moderate 5% to 10% weight loss, the goal of decreasing body weight by only 5% to 10% has received recent support (6, 22).

Other Key Strategies for Weight Loss Maintenance

In addition to the strategies already mentioned, other strategies helpful for weight loss maintenance include (17, 33, 34)

- Refuse food offers
- Set specific and realistic goals
- Be mindful when eating/Do nothing else when eating
- Do not use food as a source of comfort or escape; instead, develop other coping methods
- Do not reward self with food
- Seek support when appropriate
- Assume personal responsibility for weight control
- Weigh self regularly (get feedback)
- Tailor maintenance strategies to self

The NWCR results indicate that successful weight losers long-term emphasize multiple strategies to maintain weight loss but, ultimately, these strategies lead to the common characteristics of ongoing low-calorie, low-fat consumption and high levels of physical activity (35, 36).

Pharmacotherapy

It is becoming increasingly evident that pharmacotherapy will become a key component in long-term weight control. Although development of these medications focuses on weight loss, their long-term use indicates that the major role will be to sustain weight loss. This has been implicitly incorporated in FDA regulations for extended clinical trials of new agents (currently a one-year double-blind phase and a second-year open-label phase). Furthermore, a critical characteristic of an effective antiobesity agent is that a weight loss plateau occurs but there is a lack of tachyphylaxis. Patients reach and sustain a nadir in weight (which often is still in the overweight or obese BMI range) but, if the agent is discontinued, recidivism is inevitable unless major lifestyle changes have been successfully implemented. Thus antiobesity agents should be strongly considered when a patient is lapsing.

Recent research has investigated the use of sibutramine for weight maintenance (37). Following a 6-month weight loss trial (using sibutramine 10 mg/d), subjects were randomly assigned to sibutramine or placebo for an additional 18 months. Nutritional and exercise advice was provided throughout the extended study period. At the end of 2 years, sibutramine subjects lost 7.2 kg more than placebo subjects; 58% and 49% of subjects in each group, respectively, completed the trial.

A more intriguing trial was the introduction of sibutramine after a 4-week run-in with a very-low-calorie diet in patients who had lost at least 6 kg (38). As expected, sustained weight loss after 1 year was better in the sibutramine group than in the placebo group. However, what was particularly interesting was the additional 5.2 kg weight loss that occurred (compared with an average regain of 0.5 kg in the control group). Moreover, 75% of the sibutramine-treated group sustained their weight loss compared with 42% of controls.

Another agent demonstrating sustained weight is orlistat (39, 40). Data pooled from the major clinical trials of orlistat indicate that significantly greater weight loss was observed at 2 years for orlistat subjects (8.7 kg) versus placebo subjects (6.5 kg) and sustained 10% weight loss was 43% higher in the orlistat-treated subjects compared with controls. Although these data are promising, it is always important to consider that 1) such weight maintenance pharmacotherapy trials usually only select subjects who respond positively to the initial trial of medication after a run-in phase; and 2) potential trade-offs exist between the benefits of the greater weight loss induced by medication (beyond placebo) and the associated side effects. Nevertheless, pharmacotherapy will be playing an increasingly significant role in long-term weight management and RPT.

As reviewed above, behavior therapy is the cornerstone to RPT and the multidisplinary approach critical to long-term outcomes (41). This is true even when using pharmacotherapy to address lapses and prevent recidivism. Wadden and colleagues (42) observed that subjects receiving 15 mg/d of sibutramine + group behavior modification + a 1000 kcal/d portion-controlled diet (combined treatment) lost 17.1% of body weight at 6 months. Subjects receiving the first two components lost 11.5%, and those receiving just medication lost 5.2%. These results confirm the superiority of the combined treatment. Continued use of sibutramine is being assessed in this study to determine if it promotes maintenance of weight loss.

Public Health Model for Promoting Long-Term Weight Control

Weight maintenance data from the National Weight Control Registry (27, 31) and commercial weight loss programs (11) indicate that many individuals can lose weight and keep it off. However, it is clear that the prevalence of overweight and obese persons is increasing dramatically in the United States. The recent rise in weight gain is due primarily to environmental/cultural factors such as technology/machines reducing the need to expend calories in our daily routine (thus promoting a sedentary lifestyle), an increase in the number of fast-food restaurants, the relatively inexpensive cost of restaurant food, the enormous portion sizes at fast-food and other restaurants, reliance on automobiles to move even short distances, and the lack of easy access to sidewalks and bicycle/walking trails. In other words, our environment supports obesity, not a healthy weight. Preventing recidivism is therefore a formidable task. Weight loss interventions (behavioral and/or pharmacotherapy) are helpful, but more is needed for long-term weight control.

Viewing obesity as a public concern and the need to intervene at a societal level is gaining momentum. Obesity experts are calling for a greater recognition of the overweight epidemic in the United States and the development of interventions at the environmental, cultural, and public health levels (43-45). This would require health care professionals, public health professionals and educators, leaders of local health care organizations, community and business leaders, and state and federal legislators, among others, to work together to generate a public health policy and an environmental milieu that promotes weight control and physical activity. The United States is currently applying this approach in an effort to control the use of tobacco. By adopting a similar comprehensive approach for the management of obesity, overweight individuals trying to lose weight and maintain their weight loss would benefit.

■   ■   ■

Recommendations

1. Health care professionals and overweight individuals need to view obesity as a chronic problem that can be managed but not cured.

2. Effective long-term management of obesity may require a continuous care model for many overweight persons, much like that used in the management of diabetes.

3. Behavioral and/or pharmacotherapy interventions can help patients maintain weight loss long-term.

4. Because the problem of maintaining weight loss is exacerbated by our current environment and cultural milieu that supports a sedentary lifestyle and easy access to an abundance of (high-fat) food, a comprehensive public health model should be developed to promote healthy eating and activity. A more supportive environment is necessary to prevent obesity and enhance weight loss maintenance. Examples of possible changes include *a*) public health educational initiatives to promote the health risks of obesity and what individuals can do to lose weight, *b*) easy access to sidewalks in local communities, *c*) the development of bicycle trails to promote recreational activity and provide an alternative method of workplace transportation, *d*) large work sites that actively recruit and support on-site healthy food vendors, and *e*) employers that reward overweight employees for losing weight and maintaining weight loss.

■ ■ ■

Key Points

- Although recidivism (weight regain after weight loss) rates are still quite high, recent data indicate that a significant number of patients are able to sustain 10% weight loss long-term.

- Behavior strategies that maintain low calorie intake and high levels of physical activity are essential to weight maintenance.

- Recent studies suggest that pharmacotherapy is effective in maintaining weight loss and preventing regain.

- Most data indicate that, with exception of weight loss surgery, long-term success for most patients results in a nadir weight being achieved at ~6 months without additional weight loss but weight maintenance with adequate intervention to prevent recidivism.

■ ■ ■

REFERENCES

1. **NHLBI Obesity Education Expert Panel.** Clinical guidelines on the identification, evaluation, and treatment of overweight and obesity in adults: the evidence report. Bethesda, MD: National Institutes of Health/National Heart, Lung, and Blood Institute; Report 98-4083; Sept. 1998; pp. 81-82.

2. **Wadden TA, Foster GD.** Behavioral treatment of obesity. Med Clin North Am. 2000;84:441-61.

3. **Wadden TA.** Treatment of obesity by moderate and severe caloric restriction: results of clinical research trials. Ann Intern Med..1993;119(7 pt 2):688-93.

4. **Wadden TA, Vogt RA, Foster GD, Anderson DA.** Exercise and the maintenance of weight loss: 1-year follow-up of a controlled clinical trial. J Consult Clin Psychol. 1998;66:429-33.

5. **Nonas CA, Funkhouser ABS, Pi-Sunyer FX.** Window of opportunity in 6 months for successful weight loss [Abstract]. Obes Res. 1999;7(Suppl 1):99S.

6. **Perri MG.** The maintenance of treatment effects in the long-term management of obesity [Review]. Clinical Psychology Science and Practice. 1998;5:526-41.

7. **Miller WC.** How effective are traditional dietary and exercise interventions for weight loss? Med Sci Sports Exerc. 1999;31:1129-34.

8. **McGuire MT, Wing RR, Hill JO.** The prevalence of weight loss maintenance among American adults. Int J Obes. 1999;23:1314-9.

9. **St. Jeor ST, Brunner RL, Harrington ME, et al.** Who are the weight maintainers? Obes Res. 1995;3:249s-259s.

10. **Wadden TA, Frey DL.** A multicenter evaluation of a proprietary weight loss program for the treatment of marked obesity: a five-year follow-up. Int J Eat Disord. 1997;22:203-12.

11. **Lowe MR, Miller-Kovach K, Phelan S.** Weight-loss maintenance one to five years following successful completion of a commercial weight loss program [Abstract]. Obes Res. 1999;7(Suppl 1):43S.

12. **Perri MG, Sears SB, Clark JE.** Strategies for improving the maintenance of weight loss: towards a continuous care model of obesity management. Diabetes Care. 1993;16:200-9.

13. **NHLBI Obesity Education Expert Panel.** Clinical guidelines on the identification, evaluation, and treatment of overweight and obesity in adults: the evidence report. Bethesda, MD: National Institutes of Health/National Heart, Lung, and Blood Institute. Report 98-4083. Sept. 1998, p. 73.

14. **Funkhauser ABS, Thorton JC, Nonas CA, Pi-Sunyer FX.** Length of time away from a weight loss program affects re-entry outcomes [Abstract]. Obes Res. 1999;7(Suppl 1):43S.

15. **Foster GD, Wadden TA, Kendall PC, et al.** Psychological effects of weight loss and regain: a prospective study. J Consult Clin Psychol. 1996;64:752-7.

16. **French SA, Jeffery RW, Murray D.** Is dieting good for you? Prevalence, duration and associated weight and behaviour changes for specific weight loss strategies over four years in US adults. Int J Obes. 1999;23:320-7.

17. **Guare JC, Wing RR, Marcus MD, et al.** Analysis of changes in eating behavior and weight loss in Type II diabetic patients: which behaviors to change. Diabetes Care. 1989;12:500-3.

18. **Head S, Brookhart A.** Lifestyle modification and relapse-prevention training during treatment for weight loss. Behav Ther. 1997;28:307-21.

19. **Boutelle KN, Kirschenbaum DS.** Further support for consistent self-monitoring as a vital component of successful weight control. Obes Res. 1998;6:219-25.

20. **Klem ML, Wing RR, Lang W, et al.** Does weight loss maintenance become easier over time? Obes Res. 2000;8:438-44.

21. **Brownell KD, Jeffrey RW.** Improving long-term weight loss: pushing the limits of treatment. Behav Ther. 1987;18:353-74.

22. **Wadden TA, Sarwer DB.** Behavioral treatment of obesity: new approaches to an old disorder. In: The Management of Eating Disorders and Obesity. Goldstein DJ, ed. Totowa, NJ: Humana Press; 1999:173-99.

23. **McGuire MT, Wing RR, Klem ML, Lang W.** What predicts weight regain in a group of successful weight losers? JCCP.1999;67:177-85.

24. **Mannix ET, Dempsey JM, Engel RJ, et al.** The role of physical activity, exercise, and nutrition in the treatment of obesity. In: The Management of Eating Disorders and Obesity. Goldstein DJ, ed. Totowa, NJ: Humana Press; 1999:155-72.

25. **Jakicic JM, Winters C, Lang W, Wing RR.** Effects of intermittent exercise and use of home exercise equipment on adherence, weight loss, and fitness in overweight women: a randomized trial. JAMA. 1999;282:1554-60.

26. **Anderson RE, Wadden TA, Bartlett SJ, et al.** Effects of lifestyle activity versus structured aerobic exercise in obese women. JAMA. 1999;281:335-40.

27. **Klem ML, Wing RR, McGuire MT, et al.** A descriptive study of individuals successful at long-term maintenance of substantial weight loss. Am J Clin Nutr. 1997;66:239-46.

28. **McGuire MT, Wing RR, Klem ML, Hill JO.** Long-term maintenance of weight loss: do people who lose weight through various weight loss methods use different behaviors to maintain their weight? Int J Obes. 1998;22:572-7.

29. **McGuire MT, Wing RR, Klem ML, Hill JO.** Behavioral strategies of individuals who have maintained long-term weight losses. Obes Res. 1999;7:334-41.

30. **Shick SM, Wing RR, Klem ML, et al.** Persons successful at long-term weight loss and maintenance continue to consume a low-energy low-fat diet. J Am Diet Assoc. 1998;98:408-13.

31. **Leermakers EA.** Strategies for successful weight loss and maintenance. Weight Control Digest. 2000;10:875, 881-83.

32. **Schoeller DA, Shay K, Kushner RF.** How much physical activity is needed to minimize weight gain in previously obese women? Am J Clin Nutr. 1997;66:551-6.

33. **Fletcher AM.** Thin for Life: 10 Keys to Success from People Who Have Lost Weight & Kept It Off. Shelburne, VT: Chapters Publishing; 1994.

34. **Clark MM, Szymanski LA, King TK.** Maintenance strategies: an individualized approach. Weight Control Digest. 1997;7:585,592-4.

35. **McGuire MT, Wing RR, Klem ML, Hill JO.** Long-term maintenance of weight loss: do people who lose weight through various weight loss methods use different behaviors to maintain their weight? Int J Obes. 1998;22:572-7.

36. **McGuire MT, Wing RR, Klem ML, Hill JO.** Behavioral strategies of individuals who have maintained long-term weight losses. Obes Res. 1999; 7:334-41.

37. **James P, Astrup A, Finer N, et al.** Sibutramine trial in obesity reduction and maintenance (STORM) [Abstract]. Obes Res. 1999;7(Suppl 1):50S.

38. **Apfelbaum M, Vague P, Ziegler O, et al.** Long-term maintenance of weight loss after very-low-calorie diet: a randomized blinded trial of the efficacy and tolerability of sibutramine. Am J Med. 1999;106:179-84.

39. **Hauptman J, Lucas C, Boldrin M, Segal KR,** Long term weight loss with orlistat: impact of selection algorithm on outcomes [Abstract]. Obes Res. 1999;7(Suppl 1):50S.

40. **McNeely W, Benfield P.** Orlistat. Drugs. 1998;56:241-9.

41. **Brownell KD.** The central role of lifestyle change in long-term weight management. Clin Corner. 1999;2:43-51.

42. **Wadden TA, Berkowitz RI, Sarwer DB, et al.** Behavior therapy improves the pharmacologic treatment of obesity [Abstract]. Obes Res. 1999;7(Suppl 1):51S.

43. **Koplan JP, Deitz WH.** Caloric imbalance and public health policy. JAMA. 1999;282:1579-81.

44. **Mokdad AH, Serdula MK, Dietz WH, et al.** The spread of the obesity epidemic in the United States, 1991-1998. JAMA. 1999;282:1519-22.

45. **Hill JO.** Obesity: a call for action [Editorial]. Weight Control Digest. 1999;9:796.

Clinical

Vignettes

Assessment and Management of Obesity in an Overweight Patient Who Does Not Present for Weight Loss Therapy

SD is a 47-year-old African American male presenting for the pre-employment physical required for a new job. He last visited a physician 10 years ago.

Problem List	SD indicates no current or past significant medical problems, but by visual inspection it is clearly evident that he is overweight.
Medications	None.
Obesity History	SD has not been concerned with his weight. Upon raising *your* concern, he acknowledges a slow weight gain since graduating college, at which time he entered the work force and gradually reduced his activity. He has never taken any medication chronically, has never received nutrition instruction, and has not attempted to lose weight. His lowest adult weight was in college (175 lb) and his highest is his current weight (stated weight is 210 lb).
Family History	Mother was overweight/obese but lost and maintained weight loss for 30 years; hypertension.
Social History	SD is a lawyer who has accepted a new position with a private law firm after previously working as a public defender; rare alcohol use; does not smoke or use street drugs.
Review of Systems	DOE, which he attributes to deconditioning and weight.
Nutrition	A brief assessment by the physician indicates frequent snacking by the patient, often fatty foods. He drinks approximately 2 cups of coffee and 6 colas daily. He skips meals, particularly breakfast. He walks to and from the subway (one-half mile round trip) but has no programmed activity.
Psychological Screening	Beck Depression Inventory (BDI) = 3; no acute psychopathology or unusual eating behaviors.

Physical Examination

- *Vital Signs:* Weight, 225.1 lb; height, 73 in.; BP, 160/90; HR, 80
- *General:* Well-developed, well-nourished individual
- *Eyes:* EOMs intact; PERRLA without gross retinopathy
- *Neck:* Without thyromegaly or carotid bruits
- *Chest:* Clear to auscultation
- *Heart:* Regular without murmur, S3, S4
- *Abdomen:* Soft, nontender without organomegaly
- *Extremities:* 2+ pulses without edema
- *Labs* (obtained through new employer as part of pre-employment exam): Total cholesterol, 232; other chemistries and CBC normal

■ **QUESTIONS**

1. What is SD's BMI? In which obesity category would you place him?
2. What are the obesity-related illnesses in this patient's history? In his family history?
3. What other anthropometric data should be obtained to help determine this patient's obesity-related health risk?
4. What additional medical history and diagnostic tests are needed to evaluate this patient's obesity-related health risk?
5. Are there any general risks to treating this patient? Any risks from specific treatment modalities or contraindications?
6. Define treatment goals and outline a treatment plan.

■ **ANSWERS**

1. BMI = 29.7 with a measured weight significantly higher than the weight he reported; overweight category (BMI = 25-29.9).
2.   a) *Personal History:* possible hypertension (need to confirm with repeat BP measurement at a follow-up visit); borderline hypercholesterolemia (based on current National Cholesterol Education Program categorization)
   b) *Family History:* obesity; hypertension
3. Waist circumference.
4. A complete fasting lipid panel; fasting plasma glucose if pre-employment tests were nonfasting; TSH screening (per American Thyroid Association recommendation as well as the remote possibility that SD's borderline hypercholesterolemia is due to hypothyroidism). Although SD has a history of DOE, there are no other signs or symptoms that indicate an exercise tolerance test should be performed.

5. Overall, the risk of treatment by any modality is low; unless a comorbidity is present (hypertensive or hypercholesterolemic), antiobesity agents are not approved for use in patients with BMI < 30. Weight loss surgery is contraindicated in SD's BMI category.
6. A more thorough assessment of motivation and readiness is needed before determining the treatment goal. Based on the above, it is not clear that this patient has an understanding of the health implications of his weight. If the patient is not ready for weight loss, counseling to prevent weight gain with general advice on portion control, diversity of food intake, and increasing physical activity is indicated.

■ DISCUSSION

If SD demonstrates readiness, weight loss is indicated. The weight loss also can be first-line therapy for potential cardiovascular risk factors uncovered during his evaluation (that remain to be confirmed with further testing). The approach to treatment is more comprehensive than simple weight gain prevention. Each component of lifestyle intervention needs to be addressed systematically, and regular follow-up with members of the health care team is imperative. However, there is no urgency; thus the treatment regimen should be implemented at a pace that will not overwhelm him.

- *Nutrition*—SD has a number of modifiable habits that can be initially addressed in the primary care clinic by taking pragmatic steps such as

  - ◆ Increase fruit and vegetable intake.

  - ◆ Initiate regular consumption of breakfast or, if not feasible or he is resistant, consider a daily liquid nutritional supplement.

  - ◆ Eliminate high-caloric consumption of colas that account for up to 900 cal/d. (Weaning schedule should be instituted to avoid caffeine withdrawal syndrome.)

  - ◆ Increase water intake to maintain hydration.

  - ◆ Eat healthier snacks and, if meals are skipped during the day, eat the snacks at regular intervals.

  It is often more effective to implement these changes stepwise (e.g., patient should choose one or two). Additional queries about eating habits (e.g., fish consumption) can be made as SD successfully implements these steps.

- *Behavior*—Keeping a food and activity log is the most fundamental behavioral intervention for weight loss. However, it is only of value if at least one member of the health care team reviews it on a regular basis to provide feedback and positive reinforcement. This can be done through a variety of mechanisms, but the periodic visits to the office/clinic to monitor weight, vital signs, and general well-being (as outlined in Chapter 5) should also include reviewing the log. Involvement in a support group should be strongly recommended, and SD should find one with which he is comfortable (e.g., Weight Watchers, Overeaters Anonymous, TOPS).

- *Physical Activity*—Both spontaneous and programmed activity should be discussed. Pragmatic approaches (e.g., choosing an earlier subway stop to increase walking) should be considered. Together, SD and the physician should determine a programmed activity that can be implemented as well. Identifying exercise that SD will find appealing and likely to continue long-term is essential. Having him start the exercise program slowly and only a few times weekly to avoid injury and frustration is also important. To avoid overwhelming the patient, it may be best to allow him to adjust to changes in nutrition and lose some weight before addressing exercise.

■ COMMENTS

After a period of weeks or months, if progress is inadequate, referrals for SD to appropriate allied health professionals should be considered: registered dietitian, exercise physiologist, and/or therapist. It might be more effective to refer SD to a comprehensive weight management program rather than use individual referrals to address his needs. If after 6 months SD has not reached the 10% weight loss goal, then, assuming his hypertension and/or hypercholesterolemia is confirmed during the initial assessment, antiobesity agents may be considered.

Management of Obesity in a Patient with Type 2 Diabetes Mellitus and a History of Depression

RT is a 30-year-old white female requesting antiobesity medication.

Problem List
1. Obesity
2. Type 2 diabetes mellitus (1998)
3. Depression (various pharmacotherapies, 1995-98)

Medications
1. Metformin 1000 mg bid
2. Rosiglitazone 4 mg qd

Obesity History

RT dates the onset of obesity to approximately age 12 (during late puberty) when progressive weight gain occurred. Her maximum adult weight is her current reported weight of 184 lb. Her adult minimum was 154 lb. She identifies at least five episodes of weight cycling (±20 lb). The longest duration of weight loss maintenance was 6 months. She has participated in Weight Watchers and NutriSystem. She reports that NutriSystem was particularly good because it provided structure through the purchase of their products. She states that she "hates counting calories" and this may have interfered with her progress during Weight Watchers. She has never been treated with antiobesity medication or had weight loss surgery. She is concerned about her weight because of her recent diagnosis of diabetes.

Family History

Mother and grandmother obese; diabetes mellitus.

Social History

She is an accountant for a private business firm and works long hours; no tobacco, alcohol, or drug use.

Review of Systems

Normal, regular menses; decreased libido; high anxiety, including hyperventilation, in social situations; sinus headaches; occasional severe headaches that are enhanced by light and are global in nature with no relief from Tylenol but improvement with Excedrin to a certain degree; low-back pain and tenderness (negative CT scan) history.

Nutrition (Report by Registered Dietitian)   RT dines out frequently, choosing high-fat foods and often overeating until uncomfortably full at dinner. She often chooses convenience-type foods and lacks eating awareness because of her busy work/home life. Her diet rarely includes fruit, and vegetable intake is inadequate. She does not report eating in response to emotions but will overeat pleasurable foods. From a dietary perspective her excess calories are mainly a result of poor meal planning and structure. She has been very active in the past. She reports enjoying physical activity, but time and current weight are significant barriers.

Psychological Screening   BDI = 23 (score in moderate depression range); no evidence of acute psychopathology; no history of eating disorder, including no binging or purging.

Physical Examination
- *Vital Signs:* Weight, 184 lb; height, 64.5 in.; BMI, 31.1; waist, 36 in.; blood pressure, 138/92; heart rate, 84; obese female in no acute distress
- *Eyes:* EOMs intact; PERRLA without retinopathy
- *Neck:* Without thyromegaly or bruits
- *Chest:* Clear to auscultation
- *Heart:* Regular without murmur, S_3, S_4
- *Abdomen:* Soft, nontender without organomegaly
- *Extremities:* Unable to palpate femoral pulses; without edema
- *Neurological Signs:* Cranial nerves are grossly intact; DTRs 2+, symmetric; intact to vibration sensation
- *Labs:* HbA_{1c}, 9.2%; CBC, chemistry, ALT within normal limits

■ **QUESTIONS**

1. What are the unique obesity-related highlights (medical, psychological, nutritional, exercise) of RT's situation?
2. What additional medical history and diagnostic tests are needed to evaluate this patient's obesity-related health risk?
3. Is antiobesity medication warranted? If so, which medications are indicated?

■ ANSWERS

1. *Highlights*
   - RT is suffering from a significant obesity-related illness, type 2 diabetes mellitus. Some of her weight gain may be related to use of rosiglitazone; this needs to be considered in designing her treatment plan but is only a contributing factor because her weight problem predates use of this agent. Her glycemic control is poor and should improve with weight loss. Thus, discontinuing her thiazoladinedione would be a good strategy, and during the active phase of weight loss, intensive home glucose monitoring is warranted to avoid hypoglycemia (although as monotherapy, metformin should not induce such a problem).
   - The history of weight cycling ("yo-yo" dieting) indicates this will be a challenging case. RT's past experiences should be used to help design a treatment plan. Because she has had interventions that included reputable resources, it would not be wise to allow her to undergo treatment too long without progress because frustration will be a major obstacle to long-term improvement. Therefore medication intervention is warranted sooner rather than later.
   - RT may have a social phobia that if not addressed could place limits on her ability to lose weight. In particular, she would benefit from participating in a support group, but this may not feasible if it creates too much anxiety for her.
   - This case is an example of the value of a thorough evaluation by an experienced registered dietitian. RT exhibits a number of behaviors that make weight management difficult for her. Yet many of these behaviors are not intractable, suggesting that in the appropriate treatment environment positive outcomes from lifestyle intervention could occur. The modifiable behaviors include excessive eating out (which makes control of meal portions and composition challenging), a paucity of fruit and vegetable intake, and time rather than attitude being the obstacle to increasing physical activity. With a systematic problem-solving approach, these are behaviors that can be modified with the help of the health care team members.

2. *Additional History and Diagnostic Testing*
   - There are no obvious signs of secondary causes of obesity that warrant further evaluation. TSH screening is worthwhile (see Chapter 5), but it is important the patient understand that thyroid disease would not explain this degree of obesity.
   - RT has a history of sinus headaches but may also have headaches in the migraine class. Further evaluation is warranted.
   - As noted above, RT seems to have a social phobia. Although she

would benefit from a group support system, she may find it overwhelming at this time. She also has a BDI score in the depression range and has not received pharmacotherapy for at least 2 years. Thus she would benefit from a more complete evaluation with appropriate intervention. Because some of the antidepressant medications cause weight gain, close consultation with her psychiatrist is important in devising an integrated treatment plan.

- Standard diabetic surveillance should be conducted, including urinalysis for microalbuminuria, a fasting lipid panel, and an ophthalmologic exam. Unless additional history warrants, there is no indication for formal exercise testing in patients with type 2 diabetes under age 35.

3. *Antiobesity Medication*
- Medication is an option that should be considered sooner rather than later. It is important to discuss this option at the initial meeting with RT to set parameters for when and how this will be used. Because this is a patient with past experience in weight management in part derived from reputable sources, waiting 6 months through another cycle of lifestyle intervention is not justified if the patient's weight loss plateaus quickly. However, implementing pharmacotherapy immediately is not wise; a period of lifestyle monitoring to verify that the patient is making attempts at re-establishing the foundation for long-term success is important. Unless the patient is placed on an antidepressant, all medication options are available and, based on her history, an appetite suppressant may be very useful. However, a lipase inhibitor is a reasonable choice as well, particularly because there is indirect evidence to suggest a disproportionate decline in cholesterol with such an agent, an important feature for any patient with diabetes.

Management of Obesity in a Patient with a Complex History of Health Problems

AB is a 49-year-old white female who is referred for the treatment of obesity and obesity-related illnesses.

Problem List
1. CVA with R hemiparesis; 2° major trauma from a motor vehicle accident (1991)
2. R mastectomy (breast cancer, 1993)
3. Chronic headaches
4. Costochondritis
5. TMJ
6. Chronic peripheral edema
7. Degenerative disk disease
8. Depression

Medications
1. Fluoxetine 40 mg qd
2. Relafen 1000 mg qd
3. Dolobid 500 mg pm
4. KCl
5. HCTZ 50 mg qd
6. "Vitamins, antioxidants, garlic"

Obesity History   Adult onset of obesity with two periods of major weight gain: postpartum (age 28) and in conjunction with her post-trauma/CVA recovery. Her highest weight was 250 lb; the lowest sustained weight as an adult (for 1 year) was 130 lb. Several attempts at weight loss with periodic success have occurred in conjunction with active interventions including Weight Watchers, anorexiants, and hypnosis. The most recent attempt at weight loss occurred 2 years ago. AB notes that physical activity is difficult, which she attributes to her weight rather than to neurologic deficit. She has significant concerns about her overall health and how her weight is affecting other medical problems.

Family History	Hypertension
	Diabetes
	Obesity
	Lung cancer
	Prostate cancer
Social History	Previous smoker (D/C, 1994); no alcohol or drug use; currently unemployed and on permanent disability.
Review of Symptoms	AB has multiple somatic complaints due to the afore-mentioned problems. She also has occasional palpitations, which she describes as "pounding", and shortness of breath while sleeping.

Physical Examination

- *Visual Signs:* Weight, 108.8 kg; height, 161 cm; BP, 118/76; HR, 84
- *Eyes:* PERRLA; EOMs intact; no retinopathy
- *Neck:* Without thyromegaly
- *Chest:* Surgical scar, R breast; no breast masses; lungs clear to auscultation
- *Heart:* RRR without S_3, S_4, or murmur
- *Abdomen:* Midline scar without organomegaly
- *Neurological Signs (Screening Exam Only):* Mild R arm and leg weakness

Labs

Sodium 135	Protein (total) 7.7
Potassium. 4.3	Albumin 4.2
Chloride 99	Uric Acid . . . . . . 6.9 *H
CO_2 (total) 27	Cholesterol . . . . 248 *H
BUN 14	AST 31
Creatinine. 1.0	HGB 13.7
Glucose 78	HCT 39.1
Calcium 9.4	WBC. 5.5
Phosphorus 3.0	RBC . . . . 4.09 *L
Bilirubin (total) . . . 0.6	

■ **QUESTIONS**

1. What is AB's BMI? How would you categorize her?
2. What are the obesity-related illnesses in this patient's history? In her family history?
3. What other anthropometric data should be obtained to help determine this patient's obesity-related health risk?
4. What additional medical history and diagnostic tests are needed to evaluate this patient's obesity-related health risk?

5. Are there any general risks to treating this patient? Any risks from specific treatment modalities?

6. Outline a treatment plan.

■ ANSWERS

1. 42.0 kg/m^2; >40 is extreme (morbid) obesity

2.   a) *Personal History:* breast cancer; degenerative disk disease; chronic peripheral edema (possibly obesity-related)
   b) *Family History:* HTN; diabetes if type 2; prostate for males only; *not* lung cancer

3. *Waist Circumference:* Although not useful for defining risk when BMI > 35, waist circumference is a parameter that can be followed for positive reinforcement as the patient loses weight.

4. *History and Tests to Consider*
   - Query patient on sleep apnea (e.g., snoring and witnessed apnea, excessive daytime drowsiness) and consider sleep study.
   - Query cardiac status due to shortness of breath and "palpitations". AB needs a more thorough pulmonary and cardiac evaluation for heart failure (left- and/or right-sided) that may warrant a referral to a specialist.
   - Details on OTC medicines (e.g., antiobesity agents such as herbal phen-fen or stimulants, diuretics, laxatives).
   - Echocardiogram due to anorexiant history (per recommendations of FDA).
   - Fasting lipid panel essential to evaluate risk.
   - TSH because hypothyroidism is common. (However, the latter only contributes to obesity; it does not cause the degree of obesity from which this patient suffers.)
   - More information is needed about AB's depression and adequacy of treatment.

5. *Treatment Risks*
   - Due to AB's history of stroke, avoid hypovolemia, which is more likely to occur in initial stages of dieting; VLCD is not recommended due to greater diuresis; may need to discontinue diuretic.
   - Slight elevation in uric acid may require monitoring, but with no history of gout allopurinol is generally not recommended.
   - If pharmacologic therapy is to be considered, the centrally acting agents are contraindicated due to the current use of fluoxetine and potential drug interactions that have never been rigorously evaluated in clinical trials (see Chapters 5 and 9); orlistat can be considered.
   - There are no absolute risks to weight loss surgery, but there certainly is a higher risk to surgical intervention in AB that must be considered

when determining the risk:benefit ratio.

- A comprehensive discussion about past nontraditional interventions is needed so that open communication can be established about future interventions that AB may use. This ensures that these interventions will be brought to the attention of the health care team and can be factored into ongoing monitoring for risk (and discouraged when unsafe or ineffective).

6. *Treatment Plan:* Based on NIH criteria, intervention is indicated. However, this is a highly complex case that needs extensive pretreatment diagnostic evaluation and a treatment plan with close monitoring. It is the type of case that may be best handled in a specialty weight management clinic. There will be limitations to implementing therapy due to AB's serious medical risks. Multiple attainable goals should be established and implemented in a progressive, stepwise plan (e.g., 4 lb in 1 month, then reevaluate). Improvement should be judged by how well the patient feels and risk factor reduction, rather than by the achievement of a predetermined weight.

Because AB has previously used reputable interventional resources (e.g., Weight Watchers), she has already had some or all of the NIH recommended 6 months of lifestyle intervention. Therefore, after a period of intervention, further options can be considered if there is a lack of progress.

- *Nutrition*—A more thorough evaluation, a reasonable meal plan, and follow-up by an RD is advisable. It is unlikely that nutrition intervention will have a major impact, but before considering more aggressive therapies, a foundation to optimize other therapeutic interventions, as well as to facilitate changing to healthier eating, needs to be established.

- *Behavior/Psychiatric State*—A more detailed history of depression should be sought to determine if her depression is well-controlled. If not, a re-evaluation of antidepression pharmacotherapy by a psychiatrist is warranted because this problem is an obstacle to effective intervention. Unfortunately, some medications chosen to treat her depression may impair weight loss or even promote weight gain. Thus an integrated plan that sets realistic goals must be established in consultation with the psychiatrist. Finally, more information is needed about AB's social support system, home environment, and what she views as obstacles to success.

- *Exercise*—Although AB states that weight is the factor that limits her physical activity, to optimize physical activity an evaluation by a physical therapist rather than by an exercise physiologist should be considered to determine limitations due to neurologic deficits, balance, and subtle physical constraints. (This is in addition to the cardiovascular/pulmonary evaluations noted above.)

Index

■ ■ ■